Sat
Paper matts for thansgiving
Group thank U card

Sun
Decorations fn party
　　　paper chains

Puzzles - making from scratch

1976002 — Shipped Wed. Nov. I.
confirmation #

- Contact charge nurse
- Call Sharon
- AP at 8578
        8590
        8591

Activity-Based Intervention Guide

With More Than
250 Multisensory Play Ideas

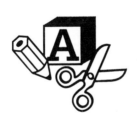

Marcia Cain Coling, M.A.

Judith Nealer Garrett, Ph.D., CCC-SLP

Therapy Skill Builders ✱®

a division of
The Psychological Corporation

3830 E. Bellevue / P.O. Box 42050
Tucson, Arizona 85733
1-800-763-2306

Dedication

To the families, children, and early interventionists who strive together to bring out the best in each other.

About the Authors

Marcia Cain Coling received the master of arts degree in special education from the University of Maryland, College Park, Maryland, and is pursuing her doctoral degree in education at The George Washington University, Washington, D.C. Ms. Coling is the Program Director of the Child Development Center of Northern Virginia where she is responsible for early intervention services through the Infant, Preschool, and At-Risk Programs. She is also an adjunct professor at George Mason University, Fairfax, Virginia, in the areas of early education and special education. Ms. Coling is the author of *Developing Integrated Programs*, published by Therapy Skill Builders.

Judith Nealer Garrett received the master of arts degree in speech-language pathology from the University of Tennessee, Knoxville, and the doctor of philosophy degree in early intervention/early childhood special education from George Mason University, Fairfax, Virginia. She holds the certificate of clinical competence in speech-language pathology. Dr. Garrett is an Assistant Professor in the Graduate School of Education at George Mason University where she teaches courses in early intervention and early childhood special education.

Contents

Acknowledgments

Several people contributed a substantial amount of time and expertise in reviewing various portions of this manuscript and making suggestions for improvements. They include Angela Dusenbury, M.A., P.T.; Philippa Hindman, M.A.; Patricia Hine, M.A., CCC-SLP; and Jane Stuart, M.A., O.T. This group deserves a large and public thank you for their efforts, interest, and support. Julia Glenn contributed to Appendix A: Program Planning Resources. Julia has done considerable work toward advancing literacy in both children and adults. She deserves more than a thank you for her generous contribution of time and expertise. Nancy Newman assisted with some of the research for Appendix A. Once again, the Technical Assistance Center #3 at George Mason University provided an excellent library of resources from which to base our research efforts.

We also want to acknowledge the intervention team members who helped to develop many of the activities described and who lived through the evolution from therapist-based to activity-based intervention firsthand: Kathy Ferrigno, Michelle Malanoski, Kerryn McMeans, Cindy Meranda, Denise O'Neil, Janet Thomas, and Karren Woods. Other co-workers too numerous to mention have also lent their ideas and support and provided the learning experiences that served as the foundation for this book.

Finally, we would like to thank our friends and families for their support throughout this project, even when we didn't have time to cook dinners.

▬▬ 1 An Introduction to Activity-Based Intervention

Why Did We Write This Book?

Each intervention session is a learning experience for the interventionist as well as for those receiving services. The young children and families with whom we have worked have taught us many things. One of the most important lessons was to appreciate the complex, and sometimes delicate, interactions that occur among children, adults, and the environment during intervention. We discovered that the most effective, enjoyable, and productive sessions were characterized by a relaxed and mutually supportive atmosphere. We also began to realize that the desired atmosphere usually developed when the sessions centered on situations such as bath time, baking cookies, or going to the playground. This realization marked the start of our commitment to activity-based intervention.

Our transition from a more traditional therapeutic approach to activity-based intervention has been gradual. We had to develop and refine our ability to read and respond to the cues of children, their families, and the environment. We also had to learn to relinquish control during intervention sessions. At times these changes were unsettling for us and we suspect that they may be troubling for others as well.

We hope that *Activity-Based Intervention Guide* will offer support to practitioners who are implementing activity-based intervention. This book:

- provides guidance on how to incorporate activity-based intervention into an existing practice

- discusses factors involved in planning and delivering activity-based intervention
- offers examples of activity-based units

This book does not discuss specific therapeutic techniques since we assume that readers are already skilled in their particular professional areas. Our aim is to help therapists and educators use their abilities in an activity-based setting.

What Is Activity-Based Intervention?

Activity-based intervention is a strategy for working with infants and young children that helps them develop functional abilities by embedding goals and objectives into routine, planned, and spontaneous activities (Bricker and Cripe 1992). It capitalizes on children's daily interactions with their social and physical environments to facilitate skill development. Activity-based intervention, which is based on an ecological approach to child development, emphasizes natural, functional, and meaningful interactions with the environment. This type of intervention is founded on the belief that real-life activities consist of sensory, motor, cognitive, communicative, and social components that should not be isolated from one another. Real-life activities, therefore, are the most appropriate milieu for conducting intervention and they can be structured to meet a child's developmental and therapeutic needs (Bricker and Cripe 1992).

What Types of Activities Are Included in Activity-Based Intervention?

Bricker and Cripe (1992) describe three different types of activities: routine, child-initiated, and planned. Routine activities are events that occur in the day-to-day life of the child. They include mealtimes, bathing, dressing, and other caregiving situations. Child-initiated activities occur spontaneously when an object or event catches and maintains a child's attention. Planned activities require adult organization. During planned activities, an adult sets the stage for a child's exploration and learning by providing selected toys, materials, and situations. One example of a planned activity is making cookies.

Although routine and child-initiated activities are briefly discussed, this book focuses on planned activities. Please refer to a resource such as Bricker and Cripe (1992) for a more thorough discussion of routine and child-initiated activities.

What Are the Characteristics of Activity-Based Intervention?

Activity-based intervention is distinguished by several important characteristics. It is engaging and integrated; it acknowledges the importance of play; and it emphasizes functional skill development and generalization (Bricker and Cripe 1992).

It is engaging. In order for learning to take place, a child must be attentively engaged in an activity. This engagement is more likely to happen when objects and events are chosen by the child rather than by an adult (Jones and Warren 1991). As a result, an important part of activity-based intervention involves creating a stimulating, responsive atmosphere and then following the child's lead as the child interacts with that environment.

It is integrated. Child development occurs in multiple domains that are intricately interrelated to one another. Development in one domain directly affects development in other domains. One example of this

relationship may be observed during the period that Piaget (1962) calls secondary circular reactions. As infants develop and refine motor abilities, they may unintentionally hit a mobile hanging over the crib. If this action results in a pleasing movement or sound, they will try to repeat the action that led to the interesting effect. In this example, motor exploration facilitated development of cognitive abilities. Our interventions must reflect developmental interrelatedness. Activity-based intervention provides an opportunity for children to practice a number of skills in different developmental domains during a single activity.

It recognizes the importance of play. The importance of play in the developmental process is documented in the literature (Fromberg 1987; Garvey 1977; Piaget 1962). Play is the strategy that children use to develop sensory, motor, cognitive, communicative, and social competence (Fromberg 1987; Garvey 1977; Piaget 1962). Unfortunately, intervention is sometimes far removed from a pleasurable, engaging, intrinsically motivating, child-directed activity. An activity-based approach is designed to capitalize on children's interests so that they are active explorers, rather than passive recipients, in the learning process.

It emphasizes functional skill development and generalization. Interventionists have become increasingly aware that abilities acquired in isolation often fail to generalize to real-life situations (Miller 1989). Research indicates, however, that skills can be gained very effectively in naturalistic environments and that these skills tend to be generalized across settings and times (Warren and Kaiser 1986). When goals are embedded in functional daily activities, maintenance and generalization are enhanced.

What Is the Role of the Interventionist in Activity-Based Intervention?

In this type of intervention, the adult has two basic responsibilities. The first is to construct a challenging and responsive environment in which learning can take place. The second is to facilitate, enhance, and expand the child's interaction with the environment.

What Is the Difference between Activity-Based Intervention and Play-Based Intervention?

Some people use these terms interchangeably. We believe that all intervention should be pleasurable for the participants but choose to use the term *activity-based intervention* because it encompasses a wider variety of activities than those typically considered play. For example, mealtimes provide excellent opportunities for children to acquire and refine skills. Mealtime, however, is not play in the traditional sense. In addition, some of the planned activities in this book require a degree of structure not usually associated with play.

What Are Some Advantages of Activity-Based Intervention?

Many advantages result from the use of activity-based intervention. It is easily used with groups of children but is also applicable for individual intervention sessions. It is appropriate for use in home-based, center-based, and integrated settings. This approach is particularly effective for accommodating groups of children with and without special needs. Activity-based intervention provides a natural way of including parents as active participants in intervention. It is also very compatible with the transdisciplinary approach to intervention that is frequently used by early intervention professionals.

What Is Contained in the Rest of this Book?

The remainder of this book includes information on how to put activity-based intervention into practice. We have found that a plan-implement-monitor-modify system of service delivery is efficient and successful. This book explains how to incorporate an activity-based approach at each stage of the service delivery sequence. Chapter 2 lays the foundation for activity-based intervention by describing how to choose activities, expand children's play schemes, and facilitate communication development. Other chapters present information on team building and working with families. Various ways to plan and conduct activity-based intervention in different settings, such as center-based programs, home programs, and integrated environments, are presented. *Activity-Based Intervention Guide* includes chapters on adapting activities and incorporating assistive technology into sessions. Chapter 10 contains a full year of activity-based lesson plans suitable for early intervention programs. Finally, we have included a list of resources that we have found helpful for implementing activity-based intervention with young children and their families.

≡ 2 Models for Activity-Based Intervention

Activity-based intervention can be implemented in almost any setting. It is really more of a mindset than a curriculum or theoretical approach, although it is well supported in current research (Bricker and Cripe 1992; Linder 1990, 1993). A wide variety of curricular themes can be introduced and taught using an activity-based approach. The purpose of this chapter is to introduce and establish the activity-based way of thinking so that the interventionist will be able to approach almost any content from an activity-based point of view. It contains a discussion of factors to consider when choosing activities and offers tips on transitioning from one activity to another. This chapter also provides guidelines for expanding children's play and discusses how to incorporate language into activities.

Activity-Based Intervention

Let's look for a moment at a traditional intervention program session and compare it with an activity-based session. Six children and their caregivers are participating in an intervention program. The children and their caregivers arrive at the session and sit in the circle space. As the children attempt to explore the room, their caregivers try to restrain them, offering the familiar toys they have brought from home in their diaper bags. The interventionists enter the room and begin the opening circle time with some announcements, followed by singing. Then they break into individual sessions or small group sessions with therapists who present the children with planned activities designed to move them toward achieving their IFSP goals. The parents or other caregivers observe these sessions but usually do not have the opportunity to participate directly in them.

Let's now assume that the same group of children and their caregivers are attending an activity-based intervention session. As the children and their caregivers enter the room, they find an activity already set up that relates to the session's theme. The children begin to explore the activity or perhaps find their favorite familiar activity in the room. The interventionists and caregivers play together with the children. The interventionists point out features of the activity that the children have not discovered or facilitate the child's motor skills to better enable the child to participate in the activity. As the children settle into the session, an interventionist brings out a related activity. The children drift over to explore it and it becomes the circle time activity. Other transitions between activities are managed similarly.

For more insight into this distinction, Toni Linder (1993) provides a wonderful description of traditional versus play-based intervention in *Transdisciplinary Play-Based Intervention* (pages 17-21).

The difference between activity-based intervention and traditional (adult-directed) intervention concerns whether the learner or the teacher drives the interactions. In traditional intervention, the teacher chooses the activities and sets the goals for the students. The learner is expected to conform to the teacher's agenda. In activity-based intervention, the learner chooses the activities and together the teacher and learner determine the goals to be accomplished. In this type of interaction, the teacher serves as a facilitator for the student's learning. As a facilitator, the teacher may present the learner with a variety of activities designed to help the learner accomplish the goals that have been set.

How can the learner help to determine goals when the learner is only an infant? By "reading" and interpreting the child's cues, a skilled facilitator can usually determine the child's goals in a particular interaction. For example, suppose an infant is lying on her back on a blanket. Two feet away is a musical toy. The baby keeps her gaze fixed on the toy as she stretches her arms in the direction of the toy. She kicks her feet at the same time. The facilitator deduces that the baby wants to reach the toy. Rolling, a skill not quite developed, would help the baby achieve that goal. The facilitator helps the baby roll over so that she can reach the toy. In this interaction, the baby is setting her own goal (reaching the toy) while at the same time learning the gross motor skills that her parents and therapists have been concerned that she achieve. The teacher and learner have worked together to establish the goals for this activity.

An activity-based intervention program allows children to make choices about the activities in which they will participate and about the way in which they will participate. Sometimes several activities may be available at the same time, as in the opening activity of the activity-based infant group session described above. An activity may include several stations for children to choose among. The Red Toys activity suggested for the first week in February (see chapter 10) is an example of this type of planning. Sometimes the children will select a component of an activity on which to focus or will vary the activity to better suit their needs and interests. For example, if the planned activity involves making snowpeople out of a soap flake paste, some children may focus on the sensorimotor aspects of manipulating their hands in the paste and making large movements on the smooth table, which are facilitated by the slippery soap.

The belief that learners know what they need and will act in such a way as to meet their needs is one of the cornerstones of the activity-based mindset. Learners are encouraged to choose activities and their choices are respected. Inappropriate behavior is interpreted as an ineffective attempt to address one's needs. The facilitator attempts to understand what needs the learner is trying to meet and then redirects the learner's behavior so that those needs can be met more effectively and appropriately. For example, the child who repeatedly runs into walls despite the ability to see the wall and stop in time may be seeking more proprioceptive input. Interventionists can redirect his behavior by providing other activities, such as wrapping up in a sleeping bag, jumping into a pile of mats, or exchanging bear hugs, that provide this kind of stimulation in a safer and more acceptable way.

Another important component of the activity-based mindset is the ability to see and facilitate the breadth of developmental goals inherent in a given activity. An activity-based intervention program can incorporate therapeutic goals from all disciplines into the planned activities. Pullout for individual therapy is kept to a minimum. Instead, therapists work with individual children as they are engaged in activities with their peers. In addition, all interventionists incorporate a transdisciplinary approach* so that goals from several developmental areas are built into a single activity and are addressed by whomever is interacting with the child at that time. For example, suppose an activity involves dress-up. The physical therapist might work directly with one child on improving balance skills. As they work together, the therapist and child talk about the actions involved, such as putting on, taking off, arm in, arm out, and over the head. This method incorporates some of the child's language goals in the physical therapy session. At the same time, the speech-language pathologist might be working with another child on expanding the length and variety of her sentences. They may have begun this work together with a preparatory activity as the therapist bounced the child gently on her knee to enhance the child's muscle tone and produce a more upright posture, thus facilitating some of her gross motor goals in addition to the language goals. As they try on different clothes and talk about their activities, the speech-language pathologist also helps the child plan how she will get the blouse over her head and how she will carry two clothing items back to the rack, for instance, again facilitating motor goals during the speech therapy session.

Any intervention program includes routine and child-initiated activities as well as planned activities. Planned activities, the focus of this book, provide the context for intervention. Choosing appropriate activities is both an art and a science—many times what ought to work does not and activities that may seem questionable to the interventionists are often big hits with the children. Nevertheless, the following section addresses some issues that may increase the chances that the activities you plan will be successful.

---

* The term *transdisciplinary approach* refers to a model in which all team members are aware of and support goals from all disciplines in their interactions with the child. We do not intend this term to imply a model of direct intervention with a single provider, although an activity-based approach can be appropriately used with such a model as well.

Choosing Activities

Many factors need to be considered when choosing activities for a group of children. Some of these factors are related to the children, whereas others concern the staff, the facility, and the larger community.

Factors Related to Children

Ability Level/Developmental Level

Two important factors to consider when choosing activities are the ability level and developmental level of the children in the group. First and foremost, the interventionist should plan activities that are developmentally appropriate for the group. The National Association for the Education of Young Children (NAEYC) has published excellent guidelines on developmentally appropriate practices for the care of young children (Bredekamp 1986). Several other sources are available as well (for example, Destefano, Howe, and Horn 1991; Elkind 1986; Widerstrom 1991).

Within the framework of developmentally appropriate activities, it is important to plan activities that match the children's ability level. In our experience working with infants and young preschoolers, we have found that it is easier to underestimate children's interests and abilities than to overestimate, especially when the children have special needs. Activities may often be planned to simply introduce young children to concepts without expecting the more detailed learning that would occur with older preschoolers. For example, the fishing activities described for the third week in June (see chapter 10) were developed for and implemented with toddlers in the 14- to 24-month age range, although the interventionist's 5- and 9-year-old sons also enjoyed the activities as did the older siblings of several of the children in the intervention group.

It is also important to note that children's abilities may differ markedly from one developmental domain to another. For example, a child may be very severely delayed in motor skills, yet have age-appropriate cognitive skills and interests. Keeping this in mind, consider the various components of activities as they are planned. What motor skills are involved? What language skills are required? What

are the sensory components of the activity? Each child should have appropriate challenges in each developmental area, but not necessarily in all areas at the same time.

Traditionally, interventionists have learned to teach for achievement and not necessarily for mastery. When an individual begins to demonstrate a desired behavior consistently, we say that he has achieved that goal. However, it may take a long while before the individual feels comfortable and at ease with the new skill, even though the skill may be used often by the individual. When the individual reaches that point of ease and comfort with the skill, we call it *mastering* the skill.

Think, for example, about learning to drive. When you first passed your driver's test, you had achieved the goal of learning to drive. Yet it took much longer, perhaps several months or years, before driving was a comfortable enough task that you could say you had mastered it. Even after years of mastery you may revert again to the achievement level; for example, when confronted with an unfamiliar freeway configuration while vacationing in another city. In our schools and early intervention programs we rarely give children the opportunity to work toward mastery of skills. As soon as they have achieved a goal, we move ahead to the next one. While it is appropriate to continue to work toward achieving new goals, it is also important to plan activities that allow children to continue to work for mastery of the skills they have already achieved.

On the other hand, it is also possible to bore even infants into a state of complete nonmotivation by continuing to present the same activity over and over again when they are not demonstrating the desired behavior, perhaps because they are not appropriately challenged by the activity in the first place. During assessment, we have probably all experienced initially estimating a child's ability too low and having the child fail to respond to item after item. When we tried something that we thought was too difficult as an experiment to see what would happen, we were surprised by a child who brightened, became motivated and interested, and who began performing appropriately.

These examples are a reminder to carefully consider all aspects of a child's ability level when planning activities. If the child does not respond to an activity as hoped, the activity may be too challenging or may not be challenging enough. It is also possible that the activity is too challenging in one developmental area but appropriate or not challenging enough in another.

Interest/Motivation

A child's interest and motivation are sometimes more closely related to ability level than we might think. An individual who is interested in something expresses curiosity about it. The person is motivated to explore it, to learn about it, and to master skills related to it. Interest is intrinsic, whereas individuals can be motivated through external rewards to explore, learn about, and master skills related to something in which they have little intrinsic interest. For example, children may work long division problems to avoid adult wrath and possibly to go out to recess sooner if they get the work done faster.

One way to select activities, especially for preschool-age and older children, is to take note of their spontaneous interests. What are they naturally drawn to? What toys or activities do they consistently choose during free play? What interests do they have at home? All of these ideas can be developed into activity-based units.

It is unusual for an entire class or group to show a similar level of interest in the same types of activities, but it can happen, especially with older children or groups that have been together for a significant period of time. Such interests may be sparked by a field trip, outing, or planned activity that the group indicates a wish to repeat or continue. Take advantage of these interests because motivation is highest when the whole group is intrinsically interested in exploring a particular theme.

More common is the situation in which a small group within the class is particularly interested in exploring a specific theme. Two or more such sub-groups often exist in a class. Activities could be planned for the small groups or for the whole class, with each small group having an opportunity to share its particular interest with the rest of the class.

Sometimes a single child's interests can suggest a theme for activities that the entire group can enjoy. One two-year-old in a preschool class was obsessed with cars. All he wanted to play with or talk about was toy cars. A week's worth of activities was planned around that theme, including a car wash and a gas station. The entire class participated with

enthusiasm, incorporating the one child more firmly into the group and greatly expanding his language and play behaviors at the same time.

Activities can also be planned with the intention of motivating children. For instance, activities that are particularly rewarding for a child can be planned after a less preferred activity, which provides motivation for the child to participate in the less preferred activity in order to get to the more preferred one. Activities with a preferred theme can provide the motivation to encourage children to attempt more challenging tasks. A child who loves balloons but is wary of the platform swing may be persuaded to swing on the swing while catching or holding onto a bunch of balloons. Finally, the participation of other children can, in itself, be a great motivator. Many children who would never go through an obstacle course alone, or with the physical therapist, have been motivated to follow other children through it.

Factors Related to Staff

While factors relating to the needs and interests of the children are usually considered first when planning activities, the needs and interests of the staff must also be taken into account. The main consideration is to ensure that enough adults will be available to assist with the activities planned. Some activities require more adult assistance than others; for example, one adult can probably manage a group of six children while they are coloring during a table-top activity, yet at least two might be needed to assist the same group during a finger-painting activity. If the team wants to plan activities that require more adults than are usually available, they may also want to recruit parents, community volunteers, or high school or college students to assist the group.

Not only is it important for enough adults to assist with the planned activities but the adults must also have the appropriate skills to help the children achieve their goals. If the team plans an obstacle course to facilitate Jermaine's gross motor skills, the physical therapist needs to assist Jermaine during the activity or be sure that another adult is trained in how to facilitate Jermaine's movements appropriately.

The selected activities should be of interest to the adults as well as the children. The adults' interests may be used as ideas for developing an interesting unit. One teacher's interest in quilt making provided the inspiration for a class quilt project. If the adults are bored, they will convey that attitude to the children, even if they try to conceal it. The real goal of many of the art activities planned for very young children is to provide sensory and fine motor experiences—touching different textures; squeezing; manipulating the hands and fingers to pick up objects of different sizes, shapes, and weights; and coordinating eye and hand movements. Planning these activities around themes gives them more meaning and interest. If a staff member has a real objection to a particular activity, it may be best to find an alternative activity or plan that activity for a time when that adult will not need to participate. For example, the team would not want to bring in a dog during pet week when the occupational therapist is scheduled to be working with the group if the occupational therapist is afraid of dogs. The dog could easily visit on another day.

When taking staff needs and interests into account, the team members must have enough trust in one another to be able to share concerns, such as a fear of dogs, when they are relevant to planning. The members of the team should respect one another enough to take such concerns seriously when they are voiced and take the time to address whatever issues arise. Chapter 3 discusses such teamwork issues in more detail.

Factors Related to the Environment

The physical environment and the resources available to your program will have an impact on what activities can be planned. For example, if your space lacks ready access to the outdoors, outdoor activities would have to be modified for indoor spaces. However, the program staff should take advantage of all available resources. If your facility has access to a heated indoor pool, for instance, you may be able to plan water-based activities throughout the year.

A word of caution about letting the present resources dictate planning is in order. It is important to be realistic and plan activities based on what is available. Nevertheless, if there are activities that the team would like to incorporate but cannot right now, that very fact provides guidance on future planning for the organization. Make those needs the target of fund-raising efforts or budget allocations.

Factors Related to the Community

Each community has its own unique ethnic, socio-economic, political, geographical, historical, and religious make-up. Interventionists will want to plan activities with the local community make-up in mind. When planning activities, try to incorporate themes that are relevant to your community as much as you can.

You will also want to consider the geographical region. Since we are from the mid-Atlantic region of the United States, we tend to plan activities based on four seasons—autumn, winter, spring, and summer. The winter/snow themes suggested for January (see chapter 10) may not be the most appropriate for intervention programs in the South, where it rarely, if ever, snows. Substitute activities that are more suitable for your region. For instance, themes featuring walks in the woods may not be appropriate activities for an intervention group based in a desert region. Walks through a dry riverbed or through a canyon might be more appropriate.

Also, try to include themes that are relevant to all of the ethnic and religious backgrounds represented in your intervention group. You may want to ask families to share the winter and spring holidays they celebrate. Many cultures have special celebrations during these seasons other than Christmas, Hanukkah, Easter, and Passover. These holidays may also be celebrated differently by various ethnic groups. Try to take into account the diversity represented in your group as you choose activities. Let your families guide you in how they would like to share their traditions. Respect their wishes if they prefer not to share information about their culture.

Know and be sensitive to different groups' taboos as well. Some religious groups forbid their members to participate in parties of any kind. Others may refuse to allow their photographs to be taken. Honor these differences and seek to incorporate members of these groups in other ways—perhaps by having them share some of their ideas, beliefs, stories, and special foods.

Whenever possible, incorporate ethnic and regional foods into planned activities. Find out whether there are special foods associated with certain celebrations or seasons. If feasible, plan to make those foods or to serve them during snack time. Incorporate any special stories that are associated with these foods.

If special costumes or other items are associated with a particular celebration or custom, have them available for the children to explore. If books, stories, or pictures are associated with regional, religious, or cultural celebrations, include these in the activities you plan. The more multisensory an activity can be, the more children are likely to learn from it.

On the other hand, try to avoid activities that might be offensive to the community or some segment of it. For example, some communities might find it offensive if a planned activity calls for children to dance to rock music. Activities that incorporate stereotyped ideas of any group should be avoided. In the Grandma's House activity (see November, Week 2, Activity 4) we specifically ask that you avoid portraying grandmothers as little old grey-haired ladies with rocking chairs and knitting needles. Very few grandmothers fit this stereotype. Accept the guidance that your community offers on what activities are appropriate.

This section has identified many factors to consider when planning activities for an intervention group. Some of these factors include the age and ability level of the children, the interests of the children and the staff, the number of staff and their skill level, the physical environment and available resources, and the make-up of the community. In general, planned activities need to be age-appropriate, challenging, and sensitive to the make-up of the community. Multisensory activities—those that incorporate elements of touch, taste, smell, movement, sight, and sound—are likely to be most effective. Activities in which children can participate on a variety of levels, depending on their needs, interests, and abilities, are easier to carry out with groups, especially when a range of abilities exists within the group.

Transitioning between Activities

Transitions are not typically among the things that infants and young children do well. Careful planning and attention to detail can often make transitions much easier to accomplish. While the focus of this section is on transitions between activities within an intervention session, many of the ideas presented here can be applied to other transitions as well.

The timing of transitions is critical. You will want to move from one activity to the next when the children have learned as much as they can from the first activity but have not yet become bored or restless. Moving them too quickly, while they are still engaged in the first activity, can be frustrating for them and can produce less than desirable behaviors. On the other hand, waiting until they are thoroughly bored and are searching the environment for something else that stimulates them is also frustrating and can produce another set of less than optimal behaviors.

How can you tell when it is time to move from one activity to the next? Usually, the group will provide signals. Children whose attention is waning will increasingly look away from the activity, move away from the activity, focus their attention elsewhere, and become more easily distracted by other sights or sounds in the environment. Older children may engage in distracting verbal behavior, such as asking the same questions over and over or making comments unrelated to the activity. Of course, these behaviors may be symptoms of a child's dysfunction. It is important to know the children well so that you can tell when these behaviors indicate a need to change activities and when they need to be addressed as targets for intervention. Usually, a balance between the two approaches is indicated.

When more than half of the group is starting to give "finished" signals, it is time to move to another activity. Sometimes these signals occur sooner than planned, especially if the activity is too challenging or not challenging enough. Follow the group's signals, though, even if you planned for the activity to take 20 minutes and the group is letting you know after 8 minutes that it is time to move on.

If the transition involves moving children to another place in the room or washing hands, for instance, begin the transition with those children who are the most "finished," that is, those who are giving the strongest "finished" signals. Allow those who still seem interested in the first activity to transition last. This procedure will give them added time to finish the activity and they will have the advantage of observing the other children transition, which will help them prepare for the change in activity.

If the children can stay in the same location, begin to introduce elements of the new activity while at the same time removing portions of the previous activity. For example, the first suggested activity for Week 1 in March (see chapter 10) involves popping paper bags. The second suggested activity involves balloons. As the children begin to lose interest in the paper bags, begin to gather them up in a trash can. At the same time, another adult can begin to introduce the balloons to the group. Children can be encouraged to trade—when a child gives you the paper bag, give the child a balloon.

Another technique is to begin to demonstrate the new activity while the children are finishing the previous one. For example, Week 4 in May (see chapter 10) has the theme of Water Carnival. The first suggested activity involves "painting" walls, fences, or each other with various-sized paintbrushes. The second suggested activity is a water slide. When the children begin to indicate that they are tired of the painting activity, an adult can turn on the hose to the water slide and begin testing the water and checking the angle of the hose. The adult's actions will probably begin to attract the children, who will gravitate naturally to the new activity.

Incorporating elements of later activities into earlier ones can also make transitions easier for some children. For example, suggested activities for the first week in February feature the color red. The first suggested activity is an obstacle course in which the children collect red beanbags. The beanbags are then used during the next activity, a beanbag toss game. Similarly, during the second week in February, the first suggested activity involves pulling the children on a large blanket or sheet. In the second activity, the same blanket or sheet is used to bounce balloons placed on top of it.

Building transitions into the activities themselves is another effective way to ensure that the group moves smoothly from one activity to the next. In May, the suggested activities for the third week involve a grocery store theme. The first activity involves gathering the items needed to go shopping and pretending to drive to the store. The group is then automatically moved to the next activity. Likewise, after they have completed the shopping, they get in their pretend vehicles and go "home," again automatically moving to the next activity area. This technique is, of course, more effective with children who are developmentally mature enough to understand the sequence of events and to pretend aspects of the activity.

Planning activities to follow a natural sequence or theme is also helpful. Again, this approach is most effective with children who are developmentally mature enough to understand the sequence. For example, a day's activities could be built around taking a "baby" to the doctor. The children could get the baby up, feed and dress her, take her in the car to the doctor's office, take her out for ice cream, and bring her home for a nap. By following the natural sequence of the events, the children will automatically move from one activity to the next.

Younger children, especially, can be helped with transition by using transition objects. In some cases, the object may be the familiar blanket brought from home to help the child transition from a familiar environment (home) to a less familiar one (intervention center). The blanket can also help the child move from one place in the center to another. Objects from the different activities can sometimes be used in the same way. For example, if the class goes on a leaf-collecting walk, carrying the leaves to the next activity can help a child transition to that activity more easily. This use of transition objects can be incorporated even if the objects are not going to be used in the next activity, as long as the use of these objects does not disrupt the activity or distract the children from the main activity.

Expanding Children's Play

The phrase "play is the natural work of children" has become a cliché. Play is a learning mechanism whereby children process their observations of the world around them, put these observations into terms and actions they can understand, and practice a variety of behaviors they are not yet ready to enact for real. Throughout this process they incorporate a great deal of knowledge about the physical properties of the world, such as ideas about how objects fit together with other objects, size and shape relationships, and the effects of different physical characteristics. They also practice both motor and social skills as they play.

While this theory holds true even for children with severe delays, it does not mean that children with special needs are always able to use play as effectively as their typically developing peers. An adult facilitator can often help children play in ways that expand their knowledge and improve their cognitive, motor, and social skills. Even children who are developing typically often benefit from such facilitation. Facilitating and expanding children's play is one of the primary roles for nursery and preschool teachers, as well as for parents, relatives, older siblings, and friends.

We begin expanding an infant's play by demonstrating how we use toys and other objects or by modeling interesting activities that can be repeated as a social game. When we shake a rattle or show the baby how to squeeze a squeaky toy, we are attempting to expand that baby's play skills. We also do so when we demonstrate peek-a-boo or pat-a-cake. This same technique can be used with older children by demonstrating how a toy train moves on train tracks, how to turn the key in the wind-up toy, or how to stack blocks to build a tall tower, for instance.

As children become more developmentally advanced, our demonstrations become more complex and more subtle. Making cookies with a group of children becomes a way to demonstrate a complex sequence that they can later reenact in play. In the same respect, a trip to the grocery store or to the beach also provides material for later play activities. Exposing children to many real-life events and activities gives them much material to use in their pretend play sequences. Children who have never been to a grocery store will be unable to effectively pretend to shop for groceries. Although unusual, some children may not have had these opportunities. Check with each child's family to see what kinds of experiences the child has had upon which to base complex play activities. Supplement these experiences with field trips or group activities. When the whole group participates in an activity together, they have a common base from which to develop play sequences.

Besides modeling activities, several other techniques are effective for expanding children's play. Adding new objects to the ones that children are already using is one simple approach. For example, let's say a group of children are building towers and other structures with blocks. Introducing some toy cars into the play scheme can encourage the children to "drive" the cars along roads or under bridges made from blocks. Giving small rolling pins and cookie cutters to children who are playing with play dough can turn what began as manipulative play into pretend play. If simply introducing the new materials into the play scheme doesn't have the desired effect, an adult can then model ideas for incorporating the new materials into the ongoing activities.

It is often useful to incorporate verbal approaches into adult attempts to expand play schemes. This is a good idea even when you think the children are not able to comprehend much language, as long as you also provide demonstrations or use nonverbal approaches along with the language cues. One way to do so is by asking questions. If children are giving a doll a bottle, an adult might ask if the baby wants some cereal or if the baby is waking up or going to bed. The first question is more concrete and more likely to be effective with developmentally younger children. The second question leads to many more play possibilities but might be too abstract for a younger group to appreciate.

Another way of asking questions is to pose to the group, "What might happen if . . ." This technique is rather sophisticated and is effective with developmentally more mature children. Suppose the group is making breakfast for the baby. The adult might ask, "What would happen if you ran out of cereal?" or "What would happen if Grandma came by for a visit right now?"

A variation on this theme involves the phrase, "I wonder . . ." It can be used to recall a past activity or event or to point out a relationship that the children may have missed. "I wonder what the lion would do about this," "I wonder what the mother would do," or "I wonder what the baby thinks," can encourage the children to expand their thinking in another direction.

As we think about expanding children's play, it is important to keep several guidelines in mind. The first guideline is that play belongs to the children, not to the adults. It is easy for adults to become so directive that they take over the play scenario. This may be great fun for the adults but it prevents the children from exploring and developing the themes that are of interest to them. Stick to themes that the children are already exploring. If they resist an idea, drop it for the time being. You can come back to it later, when they may be better prepared to incorporate it into their play. By making only one or two suggestions per session you can ensure that you won't dominate the activity.

Expand play only when expansion is needed. Children need time for mastery as well as achievement. They may enjoy repeating a particular activity that they can successfully perform. Sometimes, however, children seem to get stuck repeating a familiar activity over and over because it is familiar and may provide some security. This sort of repetition may interfere with the learning process because it prevents further exploration, achievement, and mastery. Adult facilitation is generally called for when children seem to be getting stuck in play that involves a familiar idea or activity.

Children may also need adult facilitation when they are developing play schemes around new concepts or experiences. Reminding them of aspects they may have forgotten or relationships they may not have fully understood can help them process the activity more fully. On the other hand, it is important to allow the play to develop and unfold at the children's pace. Initially, they may be able to incorporate or process only part of a new experience. As those portions of the experience are processed, the children are then ready to accept more input. For example, children playing "store" for the first time may just want to pick out their purchases and put them in the cart. Checking out and paying the cashier may be too much for them to process at first. These elements can be incorporated the next time the group plays "store."

Using Lots of Language

Children learn by doing. This means that they learn to communicate by communicating. Communication is a special kind of skill because learning to communicate always requires two agents: a sender of information and a receiver of information. A child's communication partner can exert great influence on the development of communication and language abilities. In recognition of this fact, we often advise parents and beginning interventionists to remember to "use lots of language." This section of the chapter discusses that advice and offers suggestions for implementing it.

Effective communication, whether it occurs in a company board room or a baby's nursery, involves give and take. You talk (or sign or use a communication board) and I listen. Then I talk and you listen. Unless an interaction involves some type of turn taking, efforts at effective communication have limited chance for success. Recognition of this exchange has two important implications for facilitating children's communication development:

- We must be listeners as well as speakers.
- We must help children develop the concept of reciprocity.

Adults as Receivers of Children's Communication

Adults must not become so busy using lots of language that they dominate the communicative interaction. They also need to wait, watch, and listen. To be a good communicative partner for children, adults need to attend to and respond to children's attempts at communication. Even children who do not talk are able to communicate in other ways. They use facial expressions, body movements, gestures, or vocalizations. The infant who averts her gaze from a toy being dangled in front of her face is telling us something. The toddler who gives us one of the rings he has been stacking on a cone is also communicating. In order for children to feel the empowerment that results from becoming a communicator, these initial attempts must be successful. In other words, the adult partner needs to carefully observe children for these cues and respond to them. The adult's actions help to establish the give-and-take nature of communication.

Developing Patterns of Reciprocity

Adults must help children develop the idea of reciprocity. Reciprocity develops early and can be established in nonverbal ways. Let's consider the toddler stacking rings. As you play with him, he puts a ring on his wrist. You then put a ring on your wrist. He puts a ring on his head and you put your ring on your head. You then hold the ring up to your eye and look through it. The toddler, having now figured out the game, imitates your action. What if he doesn't imitate you? The first thing to do is wait and remain holding the ring in front of your eye. In all communicative interactions, whether verbal or nonverbal, children require time to respond. Allow enough time for the child to receive the information, process it, and develop a response. If, after waiting a while, the toddler still doesn't imitate you, return to matching his actions. Common baby games such as peek-a-boo can also be used to establish this give-and-take pattern. These types of pleasant interaction reinforce the sender/receiver aspects of communication, sometimes without your ever saying a word.

Facilitation Techniques

Talking is a good way to help children learn about their world and attach meaning to their experiences. This means talking about people, objects, events, and emotions. It involves attributing meaning to actions and talking about sizes, shapes, colors, smells, tastes, textures, and temperatures. Words, language structures, and pace that are appropriate to the age and ability of the child should be used. Young children most easily process concrete words and short, simple sentence structures. One- and two-word utterances and exclamations carry a great deal of meaning. An adult who says "Whee" when swinging with a child or "Uh oh" as a block tower falls helps that child make an association between the world and the words we use to describe it. We should remember that meaning is carried not only by words but also by facial expressions and intonation patterns. Effective use of these nonverbal aspects of communication can make simple utterances even more valuable. No one who has ever heard a toddler precisely mimic a profanity will doubt that intonation can increase the impact that our words have on children. As children develop more sophisticated language and cognitive abilities, decontextualized language (talking about things that aren't physically present), abstract language (such as concepts and categories), and more complex syntax (longer, more complicated sentence structure) can be introduced into conversations.

Adults sometimes confuse using a lot of language with giving the child a lot of direction. Although directions are an important communicative function, we can include language in our activities in many other ways. One way that adults can help children attach meaning to the world is to describe their own actions as they interact with children. Statements such as, "I'm eating my cracker," or "I'm putting on my coat," help children make the association between actions and the linguistic symbols that represent them. Children's actions can also be described; for example, "You kicked the ball," "You took the red block," or "You finished your juice." These statements help children make the connection between words and their own behaviors. Adults can also use words to interpret a child's nonverbal communication. When a child pushes the ball away, an appropriate adult response could be, "You don't want to play ball." Describing and commenting on objects, events, and special aspects of the environment using phrases such as, "That's called a football," "Here comes Daddy," "I see the airplane," or "It's a big dog," also help establish the word/world connection. Adults who talk about their feelings, "I'm excited about seeing Uncle Kimoni," or "I'm sad because it's raining and I wanted to go outside," teach children the words that represent emotions. By contrast, giving lots of directions models only one pragmatic function and does not encourage children to explore the various forms and functions of language.

Adult responses to children's speech can also facilitate language development. One effective technique is to model a more grammatically sophisticated form of a sentence for the child, putting special emphasis on the correct form. For example, if a child says, "I falled down," an adult can reply, "Yes, you *fell* down." Another strategy involves expanding the child's utterance. This occurs when a child says, "big ball," and the adult responds, "a big, *blue* ball." A third way to increase expressive language is to extend the communication pattern into a simple conversation. This method is illustrated in the following exchange.

Child: "My car."

Adult: "We can go for a ride."

Communication and communicative exchanges should be infused throughout all of our interactions with children. Although adults sometimes feel self-conscious initially, especially when describing their own actions, talking with children is just like any other skill. We get better with practice.

Literacy

No discussion regarding the construction of a language-rich environment would be complete without at least a brief reference to literacy. Spoken language conveys meaning through oral symbols. Reading and writing convey meaning through visual symbols. As with oral language, literacy experiences are included in the lives of young children. Through these experiences, children learn that reading and writing can serve different functions. They realize that they can be entertained by a story, share and obtain information through letter writing, and be warned of danger by reading a sign. They also begin to recognize that written materials come in different forms, such as newspapers, books, magazines, and correspondence, as well as grocery lists, traffic signs, and billboard advertisements. Although children learn much of this information by observing adults, observation alone is not enough. Children must be actively involved in literacy activities from an early age. Many successful strategies exist for incorporating literacy into activities for young children.

Books, Storytelling, Scribbles, and Artwork

Just as children learn to talk by talking, they learn to read by reading. Children develop their attitudes about reading from the adults around them. If adults treat reading as important, then children will consider reading important, too. Even very young children can participate in reading activities. Little ones enjoy simple books with single pictures on a page. They "read" by patting the pictures or naming them. For slightly older children, very simple stories are appropriate. It's not always necessary to read stories to children word for word. Often it's more appropriate to tell or paraphrase a story based on pictures. Questions such as, "What do you think happened next?" or "How do you think she felt?" can allow the child to "read" the story with you. Children frequently like to hear familiar stories over and over and may be able to start "reading" the stories to an adult based on the pictures. Books can also be used to generate and support themes in an activity-based curriculum, as discussed in chapter 5. Books are valuable tools for creating learning environments.

Children are wonderful storytellers. Literacy is promoted when children are encouraged to dictate their stories to adults who record them in pictures and words. Stories can also be grouped together into books for which children provide the illustrations and covers. These child-inspired books can become valuable additions to the classroom or home library and are a source of great pride for the children.

In addition to the experience provided through books and storytelling, children must learn to ascribe meaning to the written symbols that they produce. Scribbling and artwork are excellent vehicles for this. Adults must help very young children attach meaning to their written productions. For example, an adult can sit down next to a toddler who is making random marks on a paper and say, "Oh, you're writing a story. Is it about the house you made in the block center?" Adults can facilitate the symbol/meaning connection for older children by asking them to

"read" the scribbles they've made on paper. Children can also be encouraged to create stories using pictures rather than words. Children can then "read" their stories to adults and other children.

Integrating Literacy into Play

An activity-based model provides many opportunities to unite literacy experiences and play. Reading and writing can become an important part of spontaneous, planned, and routine activities. By incorporating reading and writing materials into the environment, literacy can be promoted during child-initiated play. Integrating literacy goes beyond simply setting up a book corner. Toys and centers can be labeled with pictures and words. A housekeeping center might include a pad and crayon for making grocery lists for pretend shopping expeditions. An old telephone book and message pad can be kept with a toy telephone. Play medical kits can include paper for writing "prescriptions."

Planned activities also offer excellent opportunities for children to practice pre-reading and writing skills. During a cooking activity, adults may provide a recipe that uses pictures and words for the children to follow. A post office activity would provide an occasion for children to write, mail, deliver, and read letters.

Literacy can also be included in daily routines. Children can help take and record class attendance and contribute to notes sent home to families. At home, children can help plan menus, write shopping lists, and sort mail.

Children become functional communicators (listeners, speakers, readers, and writers) by having many opportunities to practice communication skills. An activity-based approach to intervention can create an environment in which communication abilities are developed in a functional, enjoyable manner.

About Snacks

There is one naturally occurring multisensory activity, appropriate for children and adults of all ages and functional levels, that is usually planned several times a day. It incorporates goals from all developmental areas and, in many cases, is intrinsically rewarding. It is called *mealtime*. Adults in America usually plan three meals a day. Young children typically have five or six each day, although some are much smaller than others. The extra little meals are called *snacks* and are critical to getting the young child successfully through the day. An early intervention program incorporates snacks into its planning for a variety of reasons, not the least of which is the fact that young children really do need to eat every couple of hours to maintain energy. Aside from this very practical consideration, snack addresses many other objectives. Snack is multisensory, incorporating smell, taste, and temperature, as well as texture and visual appearance. It sometimes incorporates sound, such as when celery crunches or popcorn pops. Children need to use motor schemes to consume snacks. They need to be positioned functionally for eating and they need to use gross and fine motor control to pick up the food or utensil, bring it to their mouths, bite, chew, and swallow. Children need to employ problem-solving skills, such as how to get the cereal out of the box, how to eat just the chocolate chips out of the cookie, and how to get the applesauce to stay on the spoon long enough to eat it. They need to develop communication skills to indicate that they want more, are finished, like or dislike certain foods, or want what the child across the table has. They learn the names for foods, actions, colors, textures, and relationships. Mealtime is also a tremendous opportunity for social interaction.

Even the most mundane snacks incorporate most, if not all, of the elements mentioned above. With careful planning, snack can be used to summarize the intervention session for the child. It can highlight the main cognitive concepts of the day and promote generalization and recall skills. In addition, snack time can reinforce language and social skills while addressing motor needs. When planning snacks to summarize the session, the team can start in one of two places—with the theme of the lesson or with the oral-motor and self-feeding needs of the group. Both areas must be considered. Let's say that the theme of the session is red. The intervention team could plan a snack that would reinforce the idea of red. Any red food would do, but to emphasize the color red and to promote generalization skills, the team chooses to include a variety of red foods. They know that the group includes Amy, who eats only puréed foods, and Nakeem, who is learning to bite and chew. Strawberry yogurt meets Amy's need for purée and can be modified by adding additional texture as she can accept it. The team includes cherry fruit leather for Nakeem.

Working from the opposite approach, the team recognizes that it needs to include foods with a crunchy texture for Eric and Nicole and finger foods for Starr, Glen, and Howard. The theme of the session is bubbles and balls. Snack possibilities include mini rice cakes, peanut butter balls rolled in crushed nuts or granola, crunchy cereal nuggets, or pretzel rounds, all of which are round, crunchy, finger foods.

Once you have planned the menu, it is time to consider what the rest of snack time will include. Eating is a wonderful time for socialization and language. Sharing naturally occurs as food and utensils are passed. Children who are ready can learn counting and one-to-one correspondence by passing out a spoon and napkin to each child. Turn taking, one of the foundations of language, is built into a group snack situation. Children must exchange turns with both adults and peers during snack. They learn about new foods and learn the words for these new items. Snack is a powerful, naturally occurring situation in which effective communication is necessary for children to meet their needs. The motivation to communicate is therefore strong. Snack is also a time when a group naturally comes together and can share how their day is going. Properly facilitated, such sharing can promote generalization and recall skills as children talk about the elements of the snack that relate to their previous activities.

For many children, snack is also a time to address oral-motor and self-help issues. It is important that mealtime be a pleasant experience for all participants. Peer modeling can often be one of the most powerful motivators in getting children to try new foods or to incorporate a spoon into the mealtime repertoire. The routine associated with mealtime can also support a child's oral-motor program. For instance, if the group routinely brushes teeth after snack, Chang, who has hypersensitivity to touch in and around his mouth, will be more likely to accept tooth brushing when the rest of the class brushes their teeth.

Cooking is a natural way to incorporate students at a variety of developmental levels and work on many different developmental goals. It is also a great motivator to encourage children to try new foods or other new feeding experiences. Children can help prepare their own snack and then eat it. Often if they've made something themselves, they will be more willing to try it, even new foods. When the theme of the session's activities is incorporated into a snack that the children have helped prepare, when their sensory and motor needs are addressed, and when snack becomes a time for social sharing and communication, it can be the culminating experience of the intervention session. As such, it can reinforce the session's objectives for each child and promote recall and carryover into other environments. Appendix C provides a list of resources for cooking and snack ideas. New Visions publishes a "Mealtimes" catalogue that offers a variety of adaptive feeding devices as well as materials related to oral-motor and feeding issues. You will find their address in Appendix C.

Summary

This chapter provided an orientation to activity-based intervention. It discussed strategies for choosing activities and transitioning between activities. It presented ideas for interacting with children, expanding their play, and facilitating communication and literacy. It also provided information on how to make snack a multi-domain learning activity. The following chapter discusses the people who work together to implement intervention programs and suggests strategies for team building and maintenance.

≡3 Team Building

Early intervention and special education are people-intensive fields of work. Although the traditional focus has been on the children, we have also begun to consider the important role that families and professional staff play in the process. Children are best served when everyone involved in their care works collaboratively. One of the foundations of activity-based intervention is that children's development is made up of many interrelated components. Each developmental domain influences and is influenced by the others. Intervention teams work much the same way in that each member of the team affects the other members and is affected by them.

Intervention Teams

A team, whether it's a baseball team, management team, or intervention team, is a group of people who work together for a common purpose. In the case of an intervention team, their shared purpose is the planning and provision of developmental and therapeutic services for young children with special needs. A child's intervention team must always include that child's parents or primary caregivers. Additional team members might include early childhood special educators, physical therapists, occupational therapists, speech-language pathologists, social workers, counselors, psychologists, educational or therapy assistants, nurses, and other medical personnel. Intervention teams may be of various sizes, compositions, and configurations. A team may be small, consisting of a parent and one interventionist, or it may have multiple members. For some teams, membership is defined by administrators and supervisors. This might occur in a center- or classroom-based program in which educators and related support staff are assigned to particular rooms or groups of children. In this instance, the staff remains fairly constant and team composition varies only slightly with the inclusion of different families. Other teams are formed to meet the needs of a particular child and family and team members may even come from different programs and agencies. No matter what the composition or configuration, each team must figure out how to work together to achieve its goals. This chapter explores team development and functioning and presents strategies for team building and maintenance.

Team Development and Functioning

No matter why they were formed, teams and work groups tend to follow a predictable pattern as they develop (Corey 1990; Swan and Morgan 1993). The first step in the sequence is an exploration of the group's purpose. Members ask themselves and each other, "Why are we here? What are we supposed to do? What is our mission?" As they answer these questions, the group moves on to another developmental phase. In the second phase, members clarify their roles and identify areas in which they find consensus. They also begin to recognize areas in which they possess different values, preferences, and opinions. The team must resolve these differences before it can progress to the next stage of development. Trust, mutual respect, and cohesion are hallmarks of the third, and final, phase of development. At this stage, team members have established effective communication systems and working relationships. They share responsibility for team outcomes. The most productive and efficient teams are the ones that reach this final stage of development.

Even teams that reach this final stage are not totally self-sustaining. Once they are formed, they must be tended, managed, and nurtured if they are to continue to be efficient and functional. This management is accomplished by the performance of task-related and maintenance-related functions (Daniels 1986). Task-related functions are activities that are directly related to the team's goals. Examples of task-related behaviors include introducing ideas and topics for discussion, providing information, and suggesting a course of action. Maintenance-related functions are activities that regulate and promote productive group interactions. These functions include supporting and encouraging group members, ensuring that all members have an opportunity to participate in group discussions, and facilitating harmony within the group. Effective team functioning is characterized by a balance of task-related and maintenance-related behaviors. If a team engages in too few task-related activities, they will not achieve their goals. If too few maintenance-related activities are performed, group process and interaction will suffer.

Team Building and Maintenance

Effective team building results in groups that not only achieve their goals, but do so in an atmosphere of mutual support and respect in which members can speak honestly without fear of being judged. No one enjoys working in strained, suspicious, or chaotic circumstances. Team-building efforts should attend to developing a work group that is comfortable as well as efficient. This is especially important if we want families to enjoy their team membership. It means making adjustments in recognition of cultural, ethnic, and language differences, including arrangements for interpreters and translations, so that all members can fully participate in the team.

Individuals who want to build a team need to accomplish at least two things:

- determine team structure and operating procedures
- develop a shared vision and philosophy

These steps may be conducted either formally or informally. For some groups the process will be relatively quick, but for others it may be rather time-consuming. Although a shared vision and philosophy is the foundation from which the team functions, the development of the philosophy may require multiple team meetings with time between meetings for members to digest and process information. Most teams don't have the luxury of unlimited time. They need to get to their task-related activities as soon as possible. As a result, teams typically begin by creating their operating procedures and then use these procedures to assist in developing their philosophy. In this way, the team can begin to engage in some task-related functions as their philosophy evolves.

As tempting as it may be to take short cuts, it is important for the potential team to engage in both steps of the process. Individuals who, on the surface, appear to be in agreement, may find that even small differences in values, perceptions, and expectations can influence team effectiveness. This is not to suggest that all differences are to be avoided, quickly smoothed over, or ignored; rather, the process of identifying differences, discussing their importance, and coming to some type of resolution about them builds a stronger and more cohesive team. The process often results in creative approaches that are more appropriate than the original ideas. It also helps to promote a sense that responsibility for decisions and responsibility for outcomes are shared by all team members.

Throughout the team-building process, members increasingly recognize the skills and abilities that others bring to the team. It is also important that team members begin to appreciate each other as individuals, which includes their likes and dislikes, learning styles, and coping strategies. Effective teams support their members and take care to ensure that the "human connection" is maintained. Some teams maintain this connection by creating opportunities for interaction in non-task-oriented situations. One of the authors served on an intervention team that met for lunch on a monthly basis. The purpose of the lunch was not to discuss business but to make sure that the team was interacting with one another as people, not simply as titles on an organizational chart. Other teams have developed similar strategies to help members establish and maintain an appropriate level of comfort and trust.

Let's take a look at the elements of the team-building process in more detail. This section presents strategies for building and maintaining effective teams and discusses some characteristics that facilitate team collaboration.

Team Structure and Operating Procedures

Team operating procedures determine how the team will conduct its business. They provide the ground rules for team operation. As an organizational framework, operating procedures need to be specific enough to provide support but not so rigid that team interactions become mechanized. Some teams like to document their procedures in writing; other teams are comfortable with a verbal agreement. At a minimum, operating procedures need to answer these questions:

- Who will be on the team?
- How will information be disseminated and communicated?
- How will the team make decisions?
- How will the team handle disagreements and conflicts?

Team ground rules may also contain elements such as frequency and length of meetings and other items that are important to the team.

Parents are always part of their child's intervention team. Other team members may include educators, therapists, and medical personnel. Some team members' participation is continuous while other individuals, such as a medical specialist or consultant, may participate on an intermittent basis. The members of the team and their roles must be established for effective functioning. Team members work well together when all members are considered to have equal status; however, members who participate on an intermittent basis may not engage in all discussions or participate in all team decisions. For example, a child's pediatrician can be a major, contributing team member, but the pediatrician's participation in decisions about whether home visits are scheduled at 2:30 or 3:00 is unnecessary. Families are special members of the team. Their importance and roles are discussed in more detail in chapter 4.

A team needs to decide how information will be disseminated. What are the lines of communication? Is any member serving as a liaison between the team and others? Will communication occur formally or informally? Lack of communication can be the source of significant problems for a team. Team members who see each other on a daily basis, such as a group assigned to a particular classroom, often develop informal mechanisms for communicating and conducting team business. Although this informal method can be an efficient way of managing certain responsibilities, care must be taken to ensure that family members, who may not be in constant contact with other team members, are not inadvertently excluded from the communication.

Teams must also determine how they will make decisions. Decisions can be made in several ways. One way is to designate one person as a leader to make final decisions for the team. Although this method results in quick decisions, it is the least preferred method because it does little to foster shared responsibility for outcomes. Voting is another decision-making strategy. An advantage of voting is that it promotes equality among members since each person casts one vote. Decisions are based upon the number of votes that each alternative receives and no one vote is more important than any other. Voting, however, can turn decision making into a win/lose proposition. Once again, this does not promote a sense of collaboration or shared responsibility for outcomes. Voting can polarize members of the group and, in the case of small teams, can put one member in the awkward position of casting the deciding vote. A third decision-making strategy is reaching consensus. Through discussion, the team develops a strategy or approach that all members agree to try. It does not necessarily mean that the option chosen is considered best by all members. It does mean, however, that every member will support the implementation of the team decision. Although reaching consensus may take more time than either authority decisions or voting, it is the preferred decision-making strategy for most teams because it facilitates the sense of shared responsibility needed for effective collaboration.

It is extremely difficult for teams to decide how to handle conflict when they are in the midst of one. Therefore, it is important for teams to develop a rational strategy for conflict resolution early in the team-building process. Differences of opinion are inevitable in even the most harmonious groups. These discrepancies are not necessarily bad. Creative tension that comes from diversity is often the driving force of innovation. Teams need to devise ways to manage conflict that are constructive rather than destructive. One way is for teams to address disagreements overtly. This means dealing with conflict within team meetings rather than in the hallway or over the telephone, which can lead to misunderstandings and bruised feelings. Some teams find it beneficial to devise a conflict resolution plan. The elements of this type of plan include:

1. *Identifying the critical issues.* In this step, the team examines the area of conflict and determines how the conflict is affecting team goals and team functioning.

2. *Identifying the source of the conflict.* Conflict can arise from a variety of sources, including insufficient communication, differing expectations, opposing values, or varied perspectives. Some conflicts, such as those resulting from poor communication, can be resolved relatively simply by addressing the source of the problem.

3. *Developing strategies and alternatives.* Teams problem solve to generate options for addressing the conflict area or resolving differences. This may involve a change in communication patterns or modification of another current practice.

4. *Choosing and implementing a plan.* This step involves selecting one of the alternatives that was generated by the group and trying it out.

5. *Evaluating the effect of the implemented option.* Although it is nice when a proposed solution works on the first try, that doesn't always happen. The team should check after a specified time period to make sure that the conflict has truly been resolved. If not, it may be necessary to generate and implement additional options.

6. *Securing additional help, if needed.* Teams are usually able to resolve conflicts using their team resources. Sometimes, though, attempts at conflict resolution become so burdensome to the team that they significantly hamper goal attainment and group functioning. In these instances, teams may find it useful to ask for help from someone who is not on the team. Often, a neutral facilitator can assist the team with identifying issues and generating solutions.

No matter what strategy a team develops for resolving conflict, it is important that the dignity and worth of all team members be acknowledged, supported, and preserved.

Shared Vision and Philosophy

The second aspect of team building involves the development of a shared vision and philosophy. For a group to fit even the loosest definition of a team, the members must be working toward collective goals. Unless they have a common purpose, each potential member may as well function as an independent agent. In addition to shared goals, the team will function more smoothly if it agrees on methods for reaching those goals. Members' attitudes and perceptions about various aspects of intervention should be explored. For instance, topics such as the role of the family; the role of the interventionist; natural environments and inclusive settings; and multi-, inter-, and transdisciplinary functioning might be discussed. Members need to recognize their own values and biases and be willing to share their opinions with other team members. Of course, it is much easier to engage in this type of dialogue when trust exists among members. It may take some time for this level of trust to develop. As a result, teams often agree on some basic guiding principles before beginning to work together on task-related functions.

The team's philosophy may be formally written or simply mutually agreed upon by its members. Although the specific content varies, the following are some examples of statements typically contained in an intervention team philosophy.

We believe that:

- our goal is to help (child's name) develop abilities and skills that are useful in all aspects of life.
- all team members have equal status, but the family is the primary decision maker for the child.
- services for (child's name) should be provided in environments in which other children of a similar age typically spend their time.
- intervention should be conducted as part of functional daily activities and play.

Team Maintenance

As mentioned earlier, even established teams need to be nurtured if they are to remain viable and useful. Teams will find it helpful to occasionally review their philosophies and operating strategies to ensure that they continue to remain appropriate and functional. As time passes and conditions change, teams may need to make adjustments in the way they do things. We are familiar with the "plan, implement, monitor, modify" sequence that we use to provide services. This same type of cycle in also important for building and maintaining intervention teams.

Personal Characteristics

The diversity of individuals makes teams strong. Through the unique contributions of each member, teams become richer in talent and resources. Our experience with teams, however, also indicates that certain personal characteristics enhance team building and operation. We have found that we are most beneficial to our teams when we:

- recognize and acknowledge our own values and biases
- take time to listen to what others are saying
- remain flexible and open to new ideas
- demonstrate respect and a positive regard for others
- are honest and candid
- display trust in other team members
- demonstrate patience with ourselves, our team members, and the team process
- maintain a sense of humor
- remember how much we enjoy working with children, families, and other professionals

4 Family-Centered Services

Family-centered services are a "hot" topic for those of us who work with infants and young children. We see this term frequently in journal articles, program brochures, and conference advertisements. When interventionists discuss their approach to services, they often describe it as family-centered. What do we mean by this term? Do we all mean the same thing? This chapter describes why families are important to infants and young children and how children with special needs can affect the family. Two major principles that guide family-centered services will be reviewed. Also included is an example of how a family and early intervention team work together to develop and implement an intervention program that "fits" the family.

The Importance of Families

At birth, human infants, as wonderful and amazing as they are, depend completely on others for survival. If someone does not provide food, shelter, and protection for them, neonates soon die. Even as children grow and learn to do more things for themselves, they remain highly dependent upon their caregivers. This essential caregiving function inextricably links children and their families from infancy through adolescence. Infants and young children depend on others not only for their physical survival but also for developmental and emotional growth. Individuals do not develop in isolation. Development occurs through the interaction of the individual and the environment (Bronfenbrenner 1979; Sameroff and Chandler 1975). Research indicates that isolated environments have a negative impact on the physical, cognitive, and social-emotional development of young children (Shonkoff and Meisels 1990). This impact occurs because the central nervous system contains synapses that, although genetically programmed before birth, must be stimulated by experiences in order to fully function (Anastasiow 1990). These experiences, such as hearing someone talk or seeing someone smile, are essential for brain development and maturation to occur. As a result, even though it is less formal than a classroom, a therapy session, or an intervention program, a child's initial learning environment is the home and families are the child's first teachers.

Home is where a child typically begins to move and explore the environment. Most children learn to communicate and care for themselves at home. Children learn many of the manners and customs of society from their families so that they can eventually assume roles as functioning members of society. Let's consider a typical home routine: mealtime. Jarvis, who is 18 months old, is eating a snack with his mother and sister, Mia, age 3. Jarvis is doing much more than enjoying his cheese and crackers. He is developing and refining his abilities in a variety of developmental areas. For example, he is practicing motor skills as he reaches for and grasps food and utensils. He communicates choices and learns the names of food items. He experiences the sensation of different tastes, smells, textures, and temperatures. Jarvis's conversation and interaction with Mia and his mother help him develop social skills. He becomes increasingly independent as he improves his ability to feed himself. In addition, Jarvis is using his cognitive abilities and problem-solving skills as he tries to figure out how to keep the cheese from slipping off his crackers. Throughout this learning process, Jarvis's mother and sister are acting as teachers as they model, guide, and expand his experiences with his environment.

The importance of the environment is supported by research conducted in the areas of vulnerability and resilience. Genetic patterns and biologic insult are not completely accurate predictors of child outcomes (Shonkoff and Marshall 1990). Often children with comparable genetic anomalies or organic insults display very different developmental outcomes. This variability of outcome is due to individual resilience, which is the result of the interaction of constitutional and environmental factors (Werner 1990). Both Jessica and Sarah have Down syndrome and were born only a month apart. Jessica is now able to walk independently. Sarah, who is a month older, is just beginning to take some steps while holding onto furniture or someone's hand. Although they are of a comparable age and have the same genetic anomaly, they are able to do different things. These differences occur because the girls are affected by different constitutional factors such as muscle tone, cardio-respiratory status, or general state of health. The girls' development is also influenced by environmental factors. These factors, although there are many others, might include the amount of time spent in a high chair or infant seat or the availability of furniture on which to pull up. It is the way that these various factors combine that makes each child unique and special. As a result, our intervention with children who have special needs must consider strategies to address both constitutional (for example, therapy to facilitate more normalized muscle tone) and environmental factors (for example, designing an environment where the child can safely move, explore, and practice pulling to stand).

Young children spend most of their time with their families. Children who receive special services may see an interventionist for as little as one hour a month or as much as 30 hours per week. The rest of their time is spent with their families and caregivers. In addition, children's interaction with the intervention system is temporary. Children's teachers or therapists may change from year to year. Families, however, are not temporary. Families' involvement with their children is constant and long-lasting. As a result, they are usually the ones who know their children best. They have seen their children happy, sick, excited, and tired. They know what their children like to do and which nursery rhymes make them smile. This knowledge puts families in the best position to know what effect a child's capabilities or special needs have on that child's ability to experience, participate in, and enjoy life. Since life extends far beyond the classroom or intervention group, it is imperative that the vision of intervention services expand beyond the walls of therapy rooms and offices and into the community in which the child lives.

The Effect of a Child with Special Needs on the Family

Not only does the family influence the child, but the child also has a significant impact on all other family members. Family systems theory emphasizes the interactional relationship between the child and the family (Minuchin 1985; Turnbull and Turnbull 1990). Anything that affects one member or aspect of the family system also affects other members and aspects of the family system.

The birth of a child with special needs can have a profound impact on the family. Although parents of children with special needs report a great deal of fulfillment and satisfaction in raising their children, research indicates that parents of children with special needs experience unique stresses (Crnic, Friedrick, and Greenberg 1983; Garrett 1993). These stresses are not constant over time and vary with the age of the child (Gallagher, Beckman, and Cross 1983). Several critical periods are particularly stressful for families. These times seem to be stressful because they include events that emphasize the differences between their child with special needs and typically developing peers (Farran, Metzger, and Sparling 1986; Fewell 1986; MacKeith 1973; Wikler 1981). The critical periods of stress occur:

- when families first encounter and recognize the child's special needs
- during the early childhood period when children are expected to reach developmental milestones, such as walking and talking
- at the entry into school
- during the adolescent period
- at the beginning of adult life

(Fewell 1986)

The first three of these critical periods occur by the time a child is 5 years old, making the early childhood years a succession of particular stresses for families.

Although the amounts and types of stress differ with each family, child, and the nature of the child's special needs, certain types of stressful situations are frequently reported by families on a day-to-day basis. Families indicate that they experience stress when they attempt to obtain information about their child's condition and as they access and deal with service systems (Featherstone 1980; Schulz 1985). The additional time required to care for a child with special needs can create problems in accomplishing routine tasks, such as housekeeping, grocery shopping, and finding an appropriate babysitter (Dunlap 1979). Finally, the costs of specialized services and equipment may burden families financially (Kornblatt and Heinrich 1985; Butler, Rosenbaum, and Palfrey 1987).

Interventionists should be aware of the effects that a child with special needs may have on the family. In some instances, developmental intervention may be able to help alleviate some of the stress through facilitation of child development and independence. However, many circumstances exist in which developmental intervention can do little to mitigate existing stress and, in fact, can even exacerbate the situation. One mother, now a skilled family advocate, tells a story about a time when her son was young and she was feeling very overwhelmed. The education and therapy staff at her son's special preschool had developed a program for implementation at home. It consisted of specified activities and corresponding data sheets. This mother was supposed to conduct the activities with her son, keep the data, and return the data sheets at her next therapy visit. Though she was very busy, she usually managed to fit the activities into their schedule. The data sheets were another matter. Although she can now laugh about it, she says she can still feel the frustration and guilt she experienced as she stayed up late the nights before therapy appointments "forging" the data sheets—even using different colored pens and pencils to make them look authentic. She said that she would have felt like an incompetent or bad mother if she had told the preschool staff that parts of the home program were too much for her to handle. This type of situation can be avoided if teams adopt a family-centered approach to intervention.

Principles of Family-Centered Intervention

As knowledge grew about the importance of the family in the intervention process and researchers looked at the effects of the child with special needs on the

family, something else also happened. Families and professionals started to discuss and investigate the types of help that were most useful and effective. From these endeavors, the concept of family-centered intervention emerged. Because the term *family-centered* reflects a philosophy, it is subject to different interpretations. There is general agreement, however, that it means expanding the focus of attention in intervention services. It means looking beyond the child to consider the priorities, resources, and concerns of the child's family. This does not mean that families are viewed as the objects of services; rather, they are considered contributing partners in the intervention efforts and full, equal members of the intervention team.

As with any philosophy-based endeavor, family-centered services are shaped by guiding principles. Two of the most significant of these are:

- recognition and respect for the uniqueness of each family
- the right of families to define what is important for them

Recognition and respect for the uniqueness of each family requires appreciation of diversity. Differences are characteristics to be valued and utilized rather than deficits to be managed. Families also come in many different forms. The 1950s stereotype of dad, mom, and two children does not hold true today. Although two-parent families certainly exist, there are also many other configurations, including single-parent, blended, extended, and adopted families. Families are not necessarily defined by family trees, marriage licenses, and birth certificates. Often, people have close ties that extend beyond the traditional blood and marriage definition of family. Some families consider friends, neighbors, and church members to be parts of their family unit. The Individuals with Disabilities Education Act (IDEA) recognizes the importance of these relationships and supports the concept that families define themselves. This means that the family includes whoever the family decides to include. Intervention teams must acknowledge the family support structure already in place and take care not to usurp it. Efforts should be made to help families build on these supports and include them on the intervention team if the family wishes.

Family diversity is also expressed in other ways. Families come from different cultural, ethnic, and socioeconomic groups. Such diversity necessitates ensuring the availability of interpreters and translators when team members speak different languages. Sensitivity to family differences, however, goes beyond consideration of language alone. Families also have different values, customs, capabilities, expectations, and coping styles. They have hopes and dreams for their children that need to be taken into account when planning and implementing intervention programs. Within some teams, the family's values, priorities, and expectations may be quite different from those of other team members. When this occurs, teams should consider the second principle for providing family-centered intervention.

The second guiding principle of providing family-centered intervention involves the right of families to define what is important to them. This guideline also means that families are the ultimate decision makers about what happens to them and their children. Families are in the best position to know what effect a child's capabilities or special needs have on that child's ability to experience, participate in, and enjoy life within their community. As a result, they are in an excellent position to assume a guiding or leadership role as the team determines assessment and intervention priorities. Some families feel very comfortable in this leadership position while others do not. Team actions should be based on the assumption that families have, or can develop, the capabilities to lead the team if they choose to do so. Other team members should support the family as they explore and expand this role within the team.

Fatima is the guardian and primary caregiver to her grandson, Abdul. During their first IFSP meeting, Fatima wanted the process to be led by the professional staff. She felt most comfortable listening to the interventionists' reports and responding to their inquiries. She wasn't really sure about the best way to contribute to the process. She thought that the professional staff should determine the most appropriate ways to help Abdul. As she and her family became more accustomed to the service system and procedures, she began to understand the many ways that her knowledge and perceptions were useful in planning and providing early intervention to her grandson. At the first six-month IFSP review, Fatima felt much more confident in expressing her opinions and asking questions. By the second six-month review, she was comfortable leading the discussion in a variety of areas and guided the team in determining outcomes and strategies that were appropriate for her family.

Another aspect of defining what is important includes the right of the family to decide what roles they will play in planning and implementing services. Anwar's daughter, Yasmine, has cerebral palsy. He wants to be involved in every aspect of her developmental program. He is present at all physical therapy sessions and has encouraged the therapists to train him how to do special exercises and movement activities. Anwar sets aside special time each evening to play "moving games" with Yasmine. It is an enjoyable time for both of them. A computer buff, Anwar has also devised a recordkeeping system for the "moving games." He shares these records with the physical therapist on each visit.

Bryan's son, Kevin, also has cerebral palsy. Like Anwar, Bryan is very interested in his child's intervention program; however, he wants his involvement to take a slightly different form. Kevin has two older brothers and very much enjoys spending time with them. One of Bryan's priorities is to encourage and strengthen this sibling interaction. He works closely with the therapists to determine ways that Kevin's motor program can fit into family activities, such as trips to the grocery store and evenings in the backyard. Although these fathers approached their involvement differently, each makes important contributions to his child's developmental intervention. By defining their priorities and their roles in the process, these fathers have developed strategies that best fit their particular situations.

Building a family-professional partnership is a special kind of team building. It is a process, not an event, and therefore takes time to develop. Just as intervention with a child progresses along a developmental course over time, so does the ability to work well as a team. All members of any developing team must make adjustments to accommodate other members. It is critical that the family not be expected to make the majority of the accommodations on the intervention team. The special team-building process is enhanced when the team "meets the family where they are" and supports them in any changes they want to make. Constructive teams recognize and build on family capabilities to make the desired changes, in addition to helping families develop new capabilities. Finally, as with all teams, family-professional team building occurs best when it is conducted in an atmosphere characterized by mutual respect and honest communication.

An Activity-Based Approach to Family-Centered Services

This section of the chapter provides an example of the compatibility of family-centered services and an activity-based approach to intervention. When the term *intervention team* is used in this example, it always includes the family as full participating members.

Anita is 2½ years old. She has cerebral palsy characterized by low muscle tone in her trunk and high extensor tone in her arms and legs. She was born with congenital cataracts that were surgically removed. Anita wears glasses and is able to see objects and large pictures. Her hearing is within normal limits. She also has a gastrostomy tube. Her adaptive equipment consists of a stroller fitted with a positioning insert and a bath chair.

Anita is an only child. She lives with her mother, Maria, and her father, Luis. Luis teaches at the local high school. Maria is also a teacher but left her position when Anita was born. She had intended to go back to work after six months but has postponed her return to work because of Anita's special medical and developmental needs. Maria takes Anita to a parent-run play group at a local church two mornings a week.

During a recent assessment conducted in her home and at the play group, Anita demonstrated the following abilities. She was able to roll from her stomach to her back. When seated in her stroller insert, she used her arms to bat at objects and held toys placed in her hands. She tried to imitate physical movements such as lifting her arm or moving her foot. Anita smiled when she heard music and used a large switch to turn on a tape recorder. She also used a switch to activate a toy dog and caterpillar. Anita was able to make some vowel-like sounds. These seemed to require a lot of effort and were not produced very frequently. She occasionally moved her head from side to side to indicate "no." Like the vocalizations, this movement appeared to require a great deal of effort from Anita. She responded appropriately to most of what was said to her and enjoyed listening to stories. She followed simple directions when she had the physical ability to do so and looked at large photos of her parents and grandparents when asked to do so. Anita received most of her nutrition through the gastrostomy tube. She was able to swallow puréed food but usually resisted her parents' attempts to place food in her mouth. She enjoyed swinging, rocking, and playing in tepid water. She was hypersensitive to textures and cried when approached with sticky, rough, or gritty materials.

Anita's intervention team, which consisted of her parents, an early childhood interventionist, a physical therapist, and a speech-language pathologist, met one evening to develop an intervention plan. This team had worked together since Anita began receiving services at four months of age. They knew each other well and were comfortable talking with one another. They used consensus as their decision-making process. The team met at Maria and Luis's home. Although the early childhood interventionist acted as general facilitator, all team members contributed to the meeting, introduced issues, and led certain aspects of the discussion. The team decided to use a three-step process for planning. They had used this approach in the past and thought it was an efficient use of their time. The three steps included:

- establishing priorities and desired outcomes
- developing general strategies for achieving outcomes
- deciding on specific activities to implement the general strategies

In order to establish priorities, Maria and Luis reviewed with the early intervention staff the activities that Anita could do and the ones that she seemed to enjoy the most. They told some stories about family activities that they had all enjoyed. They also discussed developmental areas that were of concern to the family. Their primary area of concern centered on mealtime. Luis and Maria were eager for Anita to take more food by mouth. Although past medical issues had caused coughing and choking, Anita's parents and physician felt that those issues were resolved. Still, Anita resisted taking any food by mouth and sometimes started to cry. The family's second area of concern involved communication. Maria and Luis described the frustration they felt in not always knowing what Anita wanted or needed. They said they wished that Anita had a better way of communicating with them. In addition, although Anita seemed interested in the other children in her play group, Maria and Luis felt that Anita's inability to speak kept her from being a true participant in activities.

Based on these priorities, the team agreed to concentrate on two areas for intervention: increasing the amount of food taken by mouth and establishing a communication system. In the past, intervention had stressed motor development. The group decided that the current motor program would continue and special attention would be given to the ways that Anita's motor abilities affected oral feeding and communication skills. Discussion then turned to other factors that might either help or interfere with reaching the desired outcomes. The team talked about the things that would enhance Anita's ability to take more food by mouth. These factors included resolution of the medical problems that had caused the earlier coughing and choking, her ability to manage and swallow small amounts of puréed food, and the appropriate sitting position provided by the stroller insert. Several interfering factors were also identified. These were past episodes of coughing and choking that would make oral feeding a scary experience; difficulty with lip, mouth, and tongue movements; and hypersensitivity to textures and temperatures. The team also discussed how difficult it was for Anita to control her environment because of the effort required for movement and communication. This lack of control might also make mealtime a frustrating and frightening situation. The team decided that, although additional strategies would be needed at a later time, intervention would initially focus on having Anita participate in mealtimes in ways that were pleasant and nonthreatening to her, increasing Anita's exposure to various textures and temperatures, and improving Anita's ability to control her environment by increasing her ability to communicate. These decisions naturally led to discussion of the other priority area—communication.

In the area of communication, the team identified many facilitating factors. Anita seemed to understand much of what was said to her. She initiated interactions with her family; she displayed interest in other children and had the opportunity to interact with them at the play group; and she followed simple directions and recognized large, familiar pictures. Anita enjoyed listening to stories and seemed to anticipate her favorite parts. She used body movements to indicate "no." Anita's ability to use a large switch, imitate some physical movements, and make some vocal noises were also considered strengths. The factor that most interfered with Anita's ability to communicate was determined to be her physical challenges. The team discussed the motor components necessary for speech production. They decided that although her motor skills were slowly developing, her need and desire to communicate greatly exceeded the rate of her motor skill acquisition. The speech-language pathologist suggested developing an augmentative communication system. Luis and Maria asked many questions about how an augmentative system would work, how children in the play group might react, and what effect it might have on Anita's desire and ability to learn to talk. The therapists and educator answered the questions candidly and discussed both the advantages and drawbacks of an augmentative system. Maria then said that she would like more time to think about this issue. The team agreed that it was a good idea for Luis and Maria to have time to consider this option. The family also indicated that they would like to observe a child using an augmentative system and talk with the parents of that child. The educators and therapists supported this suggestion and agreed to help Luis and Maria make the necessary arrangements.

The team decided that the meeting had been very productive but also agreed that, since they had already discussed so many issues, they would schedule another meeting to continue talking about a communication plan and decide on specific activities to meet both priorities.

At the second team meeting, Maria and Luis reported that they had observed several children using different types of augmentative communication systems and had also talked with several of the children's parents. They said that even though they hoped Anita would learn to talk some day, they were now much more comfortable with the concept of augmentative communication. The therapists reminded the parents that all development is interrelated so that some of the strategies that the team had already talked about would also facilitate the development of oral language. For example, the continuing motor program would help Anita build the trunk strength and stability necessary to support speech. In addition, many activities that address the desired outcome of oral feedings can also encourage oral language production. The team then decided upon two initial strategies to facilitate communication: to present opportunities for Anita to make choices and to provide her with a switch-activated communication system. These tactics also complemented and supported the team's desire for Anita to gain increased control over her environment.

The team then turned its attention to activities. Luis and Maria expressed a preference that activities conducted in the home be as natural as possible. They wanted to help Anita but also wanted to do so in ways that fit easily into their daily lives. Based on this preference, the team decided that it would focus on daily activities and routines when planning for Anita. To do this, the team needed to identify the family's daily routines. Led by Maria, the team developed the following outline of Anita's typical day:

- wake up
- eat breakfast
- get dressed
- play group (Anita and Maria attend play group two mornings a week. On other days they do errands such as grocery shopping.)
- eat lunch
- nap
- various activities (On some days Anita plays by herself with her switch toys or music tapes. Other days Maria plays with her or reads a book to her. The intervention team visit also occurs at this time one day each week.)
- eat dinner
- time with dad (Luis and Anita do something together. Favorite activities include rocking together in the big rocking chair and playing on the floor.)
- bath
- story and bedtime

The team examined these activities and the opportunities for skill development that each one provided. Maria and Luis expressed their desire that the team start slowly and capitalize on some of the activities Anita enjoyed. With those considerations in mind, the team decided to concentrate on several daily activities. These were mealtime, dressing/undressing, bath time, and story time.

Meals

Since the team members wanted mealtime to be less stressful for the whole family, they consulted with Anita's physician and decided to initially decrease the emphasis on oral feeding. Anita could sit in her positioning insert and engage in family interactions even if she did not want to eat. Anita's food would be prepared and available to her. She would be offered food but it would not be forced on her. This approach would provide her the opportunity to use the yes/no options of the communication system and, hopefully, to allow her to begin to recognize that she had a measure of control over what happened to her.

Mealtime also provided multiple opportunities to address other priority areas. Maria suggested that she and Luis take Anita into the kitchen during meal preparation. Once again, she could engage in family interaction. Luis suggested that Anita could practice making choices by helping decide what bib she would wear. For example, Luis could hold up two of her bibs and ask, "Which one do you want?" Anita could indicate her choice by looking at or reaching toward one of the bibs. Meal preparation offers sensory experiences such as smelling food as it cooks, as well as the chance to touch or taste some food items.

Dressing

The team felt that choice-making could easily be incorporated into dressing and undressing times. Maria or Luis would hold up two items of clothing and ask, "What do you want to wear?" Anita could indicate her choice by looking or reaching. The family had already incorporated some movement and gentle stretching routines into this activity and felt that the addition of choice-making made this daily routine even more useful.

Bath Time

Taking a bath was a favorite activity for Anita because she enjoyed playing in water. The team thought that bath time might be a good way to introduce different textures to Anita in the form of sponges and bath toys. Luis, who by now was interested and excited about incorporating choice-making into activities, said that Anita could reach or look to choose her washcloth, towel, and bath toys.

Story Time

Listening to stories was another of Anita's favorite activities that offered multiple opportunities for skill development. Anita could indicate her choice of storybook by looking or reaching. The team decided to introduce "feely" books that contained different textures for Anita to touch and feel. Story time also provided an excellent opportunity for using an alternative communication system. The team elected to set up a switch-activated, closed-loop tape so that Anita could tell her parents when it was time to turn the page.

By working together, the team developed a plan that incorporated Anita's goals into the family's daily activities and routines. During home visits, the team will discuss the implementation of the plan and make modifications as needed to fit the family's lifestyle and Anita's abilities.

Too often, home intervention programs are intrusive or burdensome to families. Under these circumstances, it is little wonder that many of these programs are inconsistently implemented. When consideration is given to family priorities and family lifestyles, the team can develop strategies that use daily routines and interactions to promote development. This method results in an intervention program that is comfortable and beneficial to the child, family, and other members of the team.

≣ 5 Planning and Implementing Activity-Based Intervention in Various Environments

Young children spend time in many different places. Home, of course, is the first place that comes to mind, but young children often find themselves in many other environments. Last week, Kim, an 18-month-old girl, could be found at home with her parents and older brother, in a child-care situation with two other children, on the bus with her mother, in the car with her father, at an evening infant intervention group, and at a fast food restaurant with her family. Environments may be formal or informal. They are composed of different people and contain various types of lighting, noise levels, furniture, and materials. All environments, however, contain opportunities for learning. It is the intervention team's job to figure out the best way to use these opportunities in efficient, functional, and pleasurable ways. This chapter presents a planning strategy that can be used to apply an activity-based approach to intervention in almost any environment.

A Strategy for Activity-Based Planning

An activity-based approach to intervention can be applied to any setting by conducting four relatively simple operations:

1. Identify the goals or desired outcomes for the child.
2. Identify and analyze the environment.
3. Identify and analyze events within the environment.
4. Match the opportunities for development and learning with the desired outcomes or goals for the child.

Let's take a look at each of these operations in a little more detail.

Identifying Goals or Desired Outcomes

This operation is actually a prerequisite to activity-based intervention. Goals or desired outcomes are typically determined at IEP and IFSP meetings so that they are readily available to activity-based planners. This step is first in the application process as a reminder that desired outcomes and the family priorities that shape them are the guide for all planning and implementation decisions. For the purposes of activity-based planning, it doesn't really matter how the goals are written. They may be written very specifically, as in the case of behavioral objectives, or they may be more generally defined, as in the case of desired outcomes. It is important for the team to have a good understanding of the abilities, skills, or areas of development that the intervention will address. In addition to identifying goals, the team should also consider factors that facilitate or interfere with goal attainment. In chapter 4, we saw how Anita's team used their knowledge of these factors extensively (e.g., ability to use a switch, enjoyment of books, and effort required to produce vocalizations) as they developed her home program.

Identifying and Analyzing the Environment

This is a preliminary step for uncovering the learning potential within any given setting. At this stage, the team needs to answer several questions:

- What is the setting?
- Why is the child in the setting?
- How often is the child in the setting and how much time does the child spend there?

- Who else is in the setting?
- What is the physical environment like? (Consider space, materials, and furnishings.)
- How amenable is the environment to change?

The reason for the first question is obvious. The team must know what the environment is before it can be analyzed. Answers to the other questions provide important pieces to the planning puzzle. The reason that a child is in a setting can affect the type of activities that are the most natural and functional in that environment. Infant intervention groups, although they serve a variety of purposes, usually exist to facilitate development and typically have some type of structure. This setting, therefore, lends itself well to the inclusion of some planned activities. On the other hand, a child visits grandpa's house for a different reason. In this setting, there is less structure, less emphasis on development, and more emphasis on affiliation. Just like an intervention group, grandpa's house can be a wonderful learning environment, but the activity-based plan would probably highlight spontaneously occurring activities and family routines rather than planned activities.

Chapter 2 discussed how children acquire and master skills. Our knowledge of this process affects how we select environments for activity-based intervention. Children learn to do things well by practicing the skills they acquire. Some children require many acquisition and practice opportunities. The frequency and amount of time that a child spends in an environment determine the number of available opportunities in which to acquire and practice new abilities. As a result, environments in which children spend a lot of time provide more occasions for practice than locales where they spend very little time. Jonathan is learning to use a voice output communication device to ask for certain food items. He eats two meals a day at home and has lunch at his preschool program. His family goes to a fast-food restaurant about once every two weeks. Where is Jonathan going to get the most practice using the device? Although the fast-food restaurant is an excellent place to help Jonathan acquire mastery and generalized use of an acquired ability, by itself it does not provide sufficient opportunity for him to use the device. The home and the preschool classroom are more appropriate settings in which to acquire initial proficiency.

Knowing who else is in the setting with the child is also helpful for team planning. The number of people and their relationship to the child affect the amount and type of interactions that occur in any environment. One of Malika's goals is to improve her ability to engage in associative play with peers. She spends mornings with two neighbor children her own age in a day-care situation. Her afternoons are spent at her Aunt Bernita's house with her 13-year-old cousin. The day-care setting lends itself to activity-based programming for Malika's play skills goal, while at Aunt Bernita's house addressing the same goal would need to be more contrived.

Teams should consider the setup and materials within an environment when making decisions about activities. Preschools, day-care facilities, and nursery school rooms are often designed around centers. Each center serves a particular function and contains an appropriate collection of materials. Frequently these rooms contain an art center where children can engage in sensory exploration as they finger paint, smear whipped cream on the table, or pound clay. No team would ever suggest that a family allow a two-year-old to engage in these activities on the newly installed living room carpet at home. Instead, the bathtub or a kiddie pool placed outside would be suitable spots for "painting" with colored shaving cream.

A final environmental consideration involves the amenability of the situation for change. Some environments need modification in order for a child to participate in activities. If these adjustments cannot be easily made, teams may want to consider alternatives. One of Wendy's goals is to increase her vocabulary. Wendy's family addresses this objective by labeling and talking about things that they see while driving in the car. Wendy's bus ride to her special preschool program takes approximately 30 minutes each way, so she spends about five hours a week on the bus. Can the labeling activity be used during the bus ride? It is unreasonable to think that the bus driver, the only adult on the bus, will be able to engage Wendy in conversation during the ride. The other children on the bus also have limited communication abilities, so that a peer-mediated strategy isn't feasible, either. The team decided that the bus environment was not really amenable to the changes required for this activity and turned to consideration of other places where Wendy spends time.

Identifying and Analyzing Events within the Environment

In this step, teams describe what typically happens in the setting and identify different developmental and learning opportunities. Activity-based learning opportunities can take several different forms. Daily routines such as mealtime, dressing, and toileting provide multiple occasions for developing and practicing skills. Unplanned activities occur when an object, person, or event spontaneously captures a child's attention so that the child initiates or engages in interaction or play. Planned activities, such as those contained in chapter 10, are activities in which someone constructs an environment that increases the likelihood that a child will engage in certain actions and behaviors. Most environments contain a variety of these different types of events that provide opportunities for learning. The trick to using activity-based intervention is to search beneath the surface opportunities of events to identify all of the developmental areas involved. Life is composed of motor, sensory, social, cognitive, and communication components that should not be isolated from one another. The task of activity-based planners is to look for these different elements within activities.

Although by no means comprehensive, the following activity-based outline provides a few examples of the many different developmental components contained in a trip to the playground.

Activity: Trip to the playground

Materials: playground equipment, large and small balls, blankets

Developmental Components

Sensory: feeling grass, sand, and dirt; swinging; sliding; rolling; smelling grass, dirt, and flowers

Gross Motor: rolling, creeping, crawling, walking on uneven surfaces, climbing, moving around and through equipment (motor planning)

Fine Motor: picking grass and dandelions, picking up and releasing balls, throwing balls

Self-Help: putting on/taking off jackets or sweaters before and after going outside, washing hands after playing in sand or dirt

Cognitive: finding objects hidden in the sand, grouping stones by size, grouping flowers by color, building a tent using blankets and the frame from the swing set

Communication: learning concepts of up and down, in and out, more, fast and slow; naming swings, slide, and balls; vocal and verbal imitation; following directions

Social: rolling a ball back and forth (reciprocity), imitating other children, interacting with other children and adults

Even from this brief list, you can see the developmental areas that could be addressed in a trip to the playground. This list also contains a combination of activity types such as routine activities (washing hands, dressing/undressing), planned activities (ball play, tent making), as well as the opportunity to capitalize on unplanned activities (anything else that catches a child's attention). Routines and planned activities can be determined during the planning process. Because the team has carefully considered the children's goals in planning the playground unit, the adults are also in a good position to anticipate, recognize, and capitalize on spontaneously occurring, child-initiated activities.

Matching Development and Learning Opportunities with Desired Outcomes

The final step in activity-based planning is to match the developmental and learning opportunities you identified in your analysis of settings and events with the goals that the team has established for the child. In other words, you will integrate the information derived from Steps 1, 2, and 3.

Two aspects of this type of activity-based planning are especially functional. One aspect is that it is a very efficient use of time because many of a child's goals can be addressed in a single activity. The playground activity described above offered intervention opportunities in all of the developmental domains. A second functional aspect of activity-based planning is that, with some modification, children with different abilities can participate in the same activity. The participation of many children in a single activity is especially important as we move our intervention efforts out of therapy rooms and into natural and integrated settings.

Traditionally, intervention has been conducted in special preschool programs, infant intervention groups, therapy sessions, and home-based programs. Now that we have begun to recognize the value of providing services in environments that include children with special needs and their peers, intervention is occurring more often in formal and informal play groups, nursery schools, day-care centers, and family day-care homes. Activity-based planning always examines the environment. As a result, it doesn't matter whether intervention occurs in a special preschool or an integrated day-care center. It doesn't matter whether the child sees a physical therapist on the playground, in the office, or at home. The planning process is the same. This does not imply that teams should adopt a "one size fits all" approach. Although the planning strategy stays constant, the results of the strategic planning process consist of a customized plan that varies according to the child, environment, and event variables that were identified and analyzed.

Organizational Mechanisms

Despite the technical-sounding name, organizational mechanisms are simply tools that help orchestrate the implementation of intervention. They are strategies that structure and bring order to the environment, and they can be particularly helpful when providing intervention in group settings. With modification, certain aspects of these mechanisms are useful in individual settings as well. This section discusses themes, activity centers, and schedules, three mechanisms that can be used to organize content, space, materials, and time.

Themes

A theme provides a way to organize the content of activities by acting as a thread to tie different activities together. Themes can focus attention on

particular concepts and vocabulary. They can help children recognize relationships that exist between different materials and activities. As themes change, children are introduced to new toys, objects, and materials. This presentation of novel stimuli arouses curiosity, encourages exploration, and promotes the development of expanded play schemes. It also helps prevent children and adults from falling into repetitive, stereotypical patterns. For these reasons, a theme can also be an effective organizer for individual sessions as long as the interventionist makes appropriate modifications in the theme depending on the length and frequency of sessions and the child's individual interests.

Themes can be generated from a variety of sources. Children's interests are frequently used as a starting point and many successful units have been based on characters such as Big Bird and Mickey Mouse. A favorite story or song can also serve as a source for themes. Other times, themes are developed from events that have relevance for the children in the group. For example, babies have been a popular theme in our preschool classes, especially when one of the children has a new brother or sister. Parents are full of good ideas when it comes to themes. Regularly asking families for suggestions provides many innovative ideas. Some intervention teams occasionally use part of their meeting time to brainstorm ideas for thematic units. If inspiration evaporates, you can always refer to curriculum and resource books that can help get the creative juices flowing again. Appendix A of this manual lists some resources for themes and activities.

The types of themes just described are most appropriate for preschool children. For toddlers and younger children, the most successful themes center on items and objects with which they have had direct experience, such as items of clothing or familiar toys. As a result, for this age group, a unit on dogs or cats is likely to be more engaging and functional than a unit on circus animals.

When choosing themes, professionals must be sensitive to the different cultures represented in the group. Themes and the activities they support should reflect the diversity of the children, families, and other adults in the community. This includes recognition and respect for ethnic and racial diversity, as well as differences in family configurations and lifestyles. Books, materials, and activities should present people of different ages, backgrounds, gender, and abilities performing a variety of tasks and engaged in numerous occupations. The detail necessary to adequately and appropriately address the development of an anti-biased curriculum is beyond the scope of this book. Fortunately, many published resources are available that intervention teams can use for information and guidance. One that we have found particularly helpful is the *Anti-Bias Curriculum* by Louise Derman-Sparks and the ABC Task Force (1989), published by the National Association for the Education of Young Children. Appendix A lists additional resources on this topic.

Activity Centers

Activity centers organize materials and the space in which activities occur. Materials that serve similar or related purposes are grouped together in centers. These groupings are often designed around the type of activity that is expected to occur in that area. Rooms typically contain five or six areas. These might include a quiet area for looking at books or listening to music through headphones and a block area for playing with blocks and other manipulative toys. Preschool rooms often contain art centers where children can engage in creative, sensory, and messy play. Most preschools also have a household corner containing dress-up clothes and household objects, such as kitchen and self-care items. Depending on the size of the room, there is often a space for large movement activities and whole group activities as well as an area for snack. Centers are organized to make maximum use of the space available, while also paying attention to lighting, noise levels, and traffic patterns. Centers can accommodate routine, spontaneous, or planned activities. Often, one center will be the site of a planned activity for some children while other centers engage children in child-directed activities.

A home is also composed of activity centers. The kitchen is a center for food preparation and eating, the bathroom is a center for self-care, and the living room is a center for social interaction. Often, families set up mini-centers within a child's room or play area. One area may be designated for looking at books or listening to music. Toys may be played with and stored in a special location. Some families even designate a messy area where children can engage in art activities or play with materials such as clay or glue.

Schedules

A schedule is a mechanism for organizing time. Environments that contain groups of children are busy places. The adults in these environments have a lot to do. Usually, young children do not care for themselves independently, so routines such as toileting or meals can take a significant amount of time. Although routines can provide excellent learning opportunities, child-care centers and preschool classes also want to provide a variety of other meaningful experiences for children. Schedules are a way to balance the amount of routine, spontaneous, and planned activities that occur throughout the day. In addition, if an integrated therapy model is used, a schedule can help ensure that an interventionist is available to facilitate a certain planned activity or interact with a particular child during child-initiated activities.

The schedule's balance is affected by the age of the children in the group. Although preschoolers usually benefit from roughly commensurate amounts of routine, spontaneous, and planned activities, infants and younger children require schedules that include a higher proportion of child-initiated and routine activities.

Implementation

The following section describes how an activity-based approach to intervention can be implemented in different settings. The first example involves a group of children and the second example illustrates an individual setting.

Group Setting

This particular example demonstrates how an activity-based approach can be used to provide intervention for children with special needs in an inclusive setting. The setting is in an inclusive nursery school. The group consists of seven children who attend the nursery school three to five mornings per week. They are all between two and three years old. The adults in this group include an early childhood educator and a teaching assistant. Parents are encouraged to attend the group, so one or two parents are frequently present.

Three of the children, Luree, Leon, and Maggie, have identified special needs. Each has an individualized education or intervention plan that contains their learning goals and objectives. Luree's goals are to improve her eye-hand coordination, improve her ability to cross the midline, increase the length of her utterances, and increase her interaction with peers. Desired outcomes for Leon include increased ability to indicate choices, increased tolerance for various textures, and improved vocal imitation abilities. Maggie is working toward increasing her receptive vocabulary and finding objects when told their function.

Stephen, Sue, Lamont, and Juan are the other children in the group. Even though they do not have identified special needs, each has a unique pattern of development, learning style, and set of abilities. In general, they are involved in activities that help them establish more elaborate cognitive and play schemes, increase their expressive language abilities, and refine their motor skills.

The intervention team for Luree, Leon, and Maggie is composed of each child's family, an early childhood educator, a teaching assistant, a special educator, an occupational therapist, a physical therapist, and a speech-language pathologist. The team meets on a regular basis to conduct planning sessions. These planning sessions focus on creating appropriate developmental experiences for the whole group as well as providing consultation regarding the children with special needs. In addition, individual team members make regularly scheduled visits to the classroom to facilitate activities and provide intervention to specific children during routine and child-initiated activities.

The room is set up with a large common area in the middle and five activity centers along the perimeter. There is a connecting bathroom and two doors leading out of the room. One door opens into an inside corridor of the building and the other leads to a fenced, outdoor play area.

The common area of the room contains child-sized chairs and a table and is used for eating snack. The furniture can be moved out of the way so that the area may also be used for large motor play when the weather prevents the group from going outside.

The five centers in the room have been designated Quiet Corner, Block Play Area, Art Center, Sensory Corner, and Dress-Up Area. The Quiet Corner is furnished with beanbag chairs and pillows. It contains books and a computer that can be accessed through a switch and other peripheral devices. The Block Play Area is a section of the room that consists of shelves and floor space. The shelves contain blocks, toy sets, and other small, manipulative items that can be used in play. The Art Center contains several easels and a small table. Children can play with paints, crayons, paper, glue, and other craft supplies. In the adjacent Sensory Corner, there is a sand and water table as well as tubs containing beans, rice, and other textured materials. The Dress-Up Area includes a model kitchen, a large mirror, a variety of children's and adults' clothing items, and costumes. Some of the materials in each center are changed periodically to correspond to the different themes used throughout the year.

The classroom staff has established a schedule that helps organize their time.

9:00-9:15 Arrival/Bathroom

9:15-9:30 Hello Time

9:30-10:15 Centers

10:15-10:45 Snack

10:45-11:00 Bathroom

11:00-11:30 Outside Play

11:30-12:00 Story Time and Goodbye

The times indicated on the schedule are approximate. Modifications are made in the schedule as needed in order to accommodate the interests or requirements of the group. Sometimes transitions between centers or activities take longer than anticipated. For instance, snack or bathroom time may exceed original estimates. Other times, children who are engaged and participating in productive activities are allowed to continue and adjustments are made in other areas of the schedule.

Activities in this group are developed around themes. The theme for this month is "Things that Go." The staff has equipped each of the centers with items appropriate to the theme. Books about cars, buses, and bicycles have been placed in the quiet corner.

Theme-related software has been loaded onto the computer. Vehicle-related manipulatives are on the Block Area shelves and bus drivers' hats have been placed in the Dress-Up space.

On this particular day, two activities have been planned for activity centers. In the Sensory Corner, small toy vehicles have been buried in the sand table and in the tubs of rice and beans. In the Art Center, children will have the opportunity to make designs by rolling toy trucks through "mud puddles" of paint and then driving them onto paper "roads." In the other centers, the children will engage in spontaneous play with the toys and materials available.

After arrival and bathroom time, the children and staff meet in the Quiet Area. They have an established routine in which they greet one another and sing a good morning song. The children know several good morning songs. One student chooses the song for the day either verbally or by pointing to pictures that are associated with the song. Opportunities to make choices are appropriate for all children and specifically address one of Leon's developmental objectives. After the greeting and song, the teacher introduces a new toy. It is a switch-activated school bus. The children explore the bus and are given time to figure out how it works. They also talk about the different parts of the bus and the purposes of those parts. This exploration and discussion address both of Maggie's receptive language goals. The children then "drive" the bus to the Block Play Area, park it there, and transition to center time.

Children choose the centers where they want to play and move freely among the different areas. A parent volunteer facilitates the planned activity in the Sensory Corner. Three children are digging into the materials and finding the vehicles. As they "drive" the discovered vehicles through the varied mediums, they imitate each other's actions and vehicle noises. This facilitates attainment of two of Leon's goals: to increase tolerance of textures and to improve vocal imitation abilities.

In the Art Center, Luree and Stephen are making "mud tracks" with their trucks. This activity addresses Luree's eye-hand coordination and midline goals. The teaching assistant is also making mud tracks and is describing what he is doing. Luree looks at him, points to a jar of paint, and says, "more." The

teaching assistant guides Luree in expressing this request to Stephen, who is closer to the jar of paint, and expanding the utterance to "more mud." This brief exchange addresses two more desired outcomes: increasing the length of utterances and increasing interaction with peers.

The teacher is moving among the other centers and interacting with the children. She is facilitating, supporting, and helping children expand their interactions with the environment. She encourages and guides children who tend to get "stuck" in a single center or activity scheme. She also monitors traffic patterns and congestion within the centers. Because she is aware of the developmental goals for all of the children, she is alert to child-initiated opportunities for learning and is ready to support and expand these spontaneous activities.

The theme is a unifying thread throughout the day's schedule. At snack, children eat crackers baked in the shapes of cars and trucks. During outside play, riding toys and wagons are available to the children. In addition, the bus drivers' hats from the Dress-Up Area have been brought outside for the children to wear as they ride around. The story for the day involves a little boy who rides a big yellow bus to school, and the closing song is "Wheels on the Bus."

By using an activity-based approach to the curriculum, this nursery school provides learning and social experiences that are appropriate for all of the children. Throughout the planned, routine, and child-initiated activities that made up the day, all the children developed skills in multiple areas as they interacted with the environment. In addition, the developmental goals of Maggie, Leon, and Luree were easily integrated into these activities, which made intervention not only efficient and functional but fun for them, too.

Individual Setting

Activity-based intervention also fits into an individual therapy session, as in the following example.

Emily is a four-year-old girl. Kimba, an occupational therapist, comes to her house for one hour each week to provide therapy. Emily's goals are to improve her ability to pick up and manipulate small objects and improve her motor planning abilities.

Emily's intervention team is composed of her family and Kimba. The team uses a triadic approach to intervention, and Emily's mother, Anne, participates in each session. Anne and Kimba like to develop activities that take advantage of Emily's interests and use toys and materials that she has at home. The mother and therapist talk briefly on the phone a day or two before each session to develop a general plan. This prior planning also helps Anne prepare Emily, who was initially shy, for what will happen during therapy.

During this week's planning call, Anne tells Kimba that Emily is very excited about a set of toy dishes that the family purchased at a yard sale last Saturday. They brainstorm some activities that could use the dishes to address Emily's outcomes. In less than ten minutes they decide to conduct the therapy session around a picnic theme.

Because it is raining on the afternoon of the session, the picnic is held on the kitchen floor. Emily practices motor planning during many of the picnic activities. She helps spread a blanket on the floor. She goes to her room to get the dolls and stuffed animals who have been "invited" to the picnic and places them in appropriate spots around the blanket. She arranges the dishes for each participant, including Kimba and Anne, and figures out how to serve each one the pretend food without stepping on the blanket, the dishes, or the guests. Throughout these activities, Emily is also manipulating the small dishes and utensils as she "prepares" the food and feeds the stuffed bear who is "just a baby and can't feed himself yet." She also manipulates objects as she cleans up after the picnic and washes the dishes. All through the picnic, Kimba and Anne encourage, support, and facilitate Emily's development, using verbal directions and physical guidance when necessary.

Even though Emily's goals focused on her fine motor abilities, the picnic provided opportunities for skill development in many other areas as well. A few examples include:

Sensory: playing in the soapy water while washing dishes

Gross Motor: moving around while carrying objects

Self-Help: eating and washing

Cognition: sequencing the tasks of food preparation or dishwashing; talking about concepts such as wet/dry and cool/warm

Communication: following directions; making requests; talking about attributes such as color, shape, and size; defining the functions of objects

Social: engaging in appropriate mealtime conversation and behavior

As you can see, this hour of therapy was very productive. It centered on Emily's current interests so that she was enthusiastic and engaged throughout the therapy session. Because it used her own toys and other items from the home, the activity can be easily replicated, giving Emily more chances to practice and refine skills. Anne's involvement in the session allowed her to learn some of Kimba's techniques and strategies for use at other times. Most important, the therapy was conducted during meaningful activities in a functional setting so that maintenance and generalization of acquired skills was enhanced.

≡6 Adapting Activities to Children's Ages and Abilities

Activities are easiest to plan, at least initially, when all participants are functioning at about the same level. However, in a typical classroom or play group, children will present very different abilities and needs. The group of adults caring for the children will also have individual differences in what they do very well and what they do not do well. When all of these individual abilities are combined, the talents balance out and there is usually someone who is good at whatever needs to be accomplished.

This chapter examines ways to adapt basic activities to meet the various needs of children at different ages and ability levels. It looks at ways to modify goals or expectations, ways to adapt the activities, and ways to use the children's diverse abilities to facilitate desired outcomes.

Modifying Goals or Expectations

Families take children of all ages to the zoo, but their expectations for the children's behavior and for what they may learn from the experience vary greatly with the age of the child. An infant may accompany the family to the zoo in a baby backpack or stroller and simply be expected to come along for the ride. The baby may enjoy the movement; the new sights, sounds, and smells; and perhaps a taste of some new food, such as a snow cone. A toddler may begin to recognize some of the animals and to associate sounds with them. The same toddler may spend some of the time exploring the sidewalks, climbing on railings, or playing on the grass, as well as riding in a stroller. A preschooler may begin to compare the characteristics of different animals and to categorize them: zebras are like horses; lions and tigers are like big cats. The preschooler may also enjoy motor

explorations almost as much as looking at the animals. An elementary or middle school child may want to make a special trip to the zoo to study a particular animal or group of animals that is of interest. The family's expectations of each child for an activity, such as a trip to the zoo, vary considerably, although overlap exists among the different age groups.

This same concept holds true for planned activities in an intervention program. Modifications in individual goals or expectations for some activities seem more obvious than for others. Let's take a look at a couple of obvious examples and then we will look at modifying expectations for some activities in which the adaptations are not so obvious.

Water Play

Water play is one example that comes quickly to mind. Young children from infancy on up enjoy playing in water. Initially, infants tend to just splash. Through splashing they are learning about cause and effect. They are also learning how to move and to control various body parts. If they are sitting independently while splashing, they are probably also challenging their balance. The caregiver facilitating the activity is probably also providing the infants with language about the body parts being used, the names of their actions, and other descriptive words; for example, "You're hitting the water with your hand hard. You made a big splash. I got all wet."

Besides splashing, children beyond infancy often enjoy playing with floating toys in the water. As they explore the dynamics of which objects sink and which float, they are also learning about the physical properties of objects. They may try to fit objects together; for example, putting a sailor in a boat or fitting a boat to a dock, which expands their knowledge of spatial relationships. They may also learn some of the social rules for relating to objects: pour water from a cup into the tub, not onto the floor; cups are for drinking and pouring, not throwing. For children who are ready, letting them attempt to catch floating objects with a large spoon or toy fishing pole facilitates their ability to use tools as extensions of their bodies for accomplishing tasks. The addition of bubbles to a bath can facilitate the child's understanding of object permanence as the toys disappear beneath the bubbles and later reappear. Older children may engage in more complex motor play and may add a dimension of pretend play to their activities; for example, acting out going fishing or pretending to be a fish.

Preschool Intervention

A planned water play activity in the classroom, play group, or during an infant intervention session can easily incorporate all of these developmental levels. Let's take the example of a preschool classroom made up of seven two- and three-year-olds with a range of developmental disabilities. Sarah and Lakesha have Down syndrome. Lakesha has been walking for some time, but Sarah is just beginning to take some steps while holding onto an adult's hand. In addition, Sarah has a moderate degree of tactile hypersensitivity. Roberto has cerebral palsy. He is beginning to use words to communicate but still requires a lot of support to maintain any upright positions against gravity, including sitting. Paul has been diagnosed with pervasive developmental disorder. His attention wanders and he tends to wander with it. Ben and Jeff are twins with generalized developmental delays and specific delays in both receptive and expressive language. Leah has cerebral palsy. She is more affected on her right side than her left and one of the main goals for her is to increase her awareness and use of her right side.

It is springtime. The weather has been warm for several weeks and the interventionists have decided that the class is ready for water play. Since Sarah has some tactile hypersensitivities, one of the goals for her during the water play activity is to accept some different kinds of tactile stimulation. One goal for Paul is to increase the length of time he remains focused on the activity. Ben's, Jeff's, and Roberto's language goals will be reinforced during the water play activity. In addition, Roberto will be positioned in the pool so that he will be partially supported but will have the

opportunity to work on his sitting balance. Lakesha is beginning to develop the idea of representational play.

The intervention team, consisting of an occupational therapist, a physical therapist, a speech-language pathologist, the classroom teacher, and the teacher's aide, have provided several sizes of paintbrushes and sponges. The children are encouraged to "paint" and sponge each other as well as the outside wall of the classroom. This part of the activity addresses Sarah's need for tactile experiences, Leah's need to increase awareness and use of her right side, and Lakesha's need to practice representational play. It also provides ample opportunity for language development for all the children. Thus, each child has individual goals that the interventionists may facilitate differently, but all participate in one activity together.

Infant Intervention

Let's take the same activity, water play, and explore how it might be used with a younger group of children. An infant intervention team meets weekly with a group of six children up to two years of age and their parents. They have chosen water play as the main theme for the evening because several of the parents have asked for suggestions for summer activities. Rhonda, new to the group, is a two-month-old baby with Down syndrome. Lance and Larry are presently the "stars" of the group. They are 20-month-old twins with developmental delays of unknown origin who have just begun to walk. Tonya just celebrated her first birthday, although her age, when adjusted for her prematurity, is just nine months. María is another baby with a history of prematurity. Her adjusted age is 16 months. Finally, there is Martin, a very sensitive 11-month-old who spends much of his awake time crying. How can this group use water play effectively?

The team decided to use a water table rather than a pool to introduce water activities. Lance and Larry are encouraged to play with floating toys while the physical therapist facilitates more advanced standing balance and weight shifting. Meanwhile, their play with nesting cups helps them learn about spatial relationships and lays the groundwork for higher-level observation skills. The activity also helps them develop fine motor skills, eye-hand coordination, and an understanding of the social rules related to this type of play, such as keeping the water in the table, not on the floor. Tonya still tends to be stiff and to resist positioning on her stomach. Her mother sits in a chair and holds Tonya in prone on her lap, encouraging her to splash in the water and to look at the effects she is creating. María needs to expand her ability to use tools. She also needs to develop standing balance. She is positioned in standing on a small stool next to Lance and Larry so that she might be motivated to imitate their somewhat more advanced motor skills. She uses a kitchen strainer to scoop up water and to sink toys that float by. Rhonda is positioned in sidelying in her mother's lap so her hands can just touch the water at the edge of the water table. Her mother talks gently to her about how the water feels. She and Martin are given one end of the water table to themselves to minimize splashing from the older children. Martin is wrapped in a blanket to help calm him. The occupational therapist holds him in prone and pats him rhythmically. Soft, calming music plays in the background. The goal for Martin is to help him organize himself and then to maintain a calm, alert state when confronted with a variety of sensory stimuli. Once again, each child has individual goals based on individual needs but they are able to participate in a single activity together, facilitated by adults who are aware of all of these different goals.

Cooking

Cooking is another activity that lends itself naturally to adaptations for children of various ability levels. Mothers have probably been adapting cooking activities for the developmental level of their children since cooking was discovered. Young babies enjoy simply playing with the ingredients—tasting, touching, spreading, smelling, rolling, and splashing. These activities encourage the integration of sensory experiences; for example, this is what flour looks like, smells like, feels like, tastes like, and these are the things I can do with it. They also lay the foundation for later conceptual understanding: some foods are made up of different components, which are called flour, sugar, and butter; some foods are cooked; some foods are eaten just as they are; some things are not foods; apples, oranges, cherries, peaches, grapes, and plums are all foods called fruit. At the same time, the baby is practicing fine motor skills and eye-hand coordination by poking, pinching, grasping, and releasing. If the caregiver is talking to the baby about the experience, the baby is learning to associate words with the items being manipulated and the specific manipulations used.

At a later stage, toddlers can practice imitation skills as they try to copy the adult's actions in cooking and cleaning up. At the same time, they are refining their motor skills as their imitations come closer and closer to performing the actual activity. Their language skills are continuing to grow as the adults describe characteristics of items and activities; for example, "We need to take the red skin off the apple;" "Oh, stir slowly so you don't splash." They are also learning to sequence events—peel the apples, cut the apples, cook the apples, eat the applesauce. As the children mature, they use these experiences as the basis for pretend play of increasing complexity, initially playing out the basic cooking sequence but eventually incorporating it into an elaborated play scheme involving going to work, working, coming home, and preparing a meal.

Preschool Intervention

Let's imagine the same two groups we just looked at during water play activities, but this time involved in cooking activities. The intervention team for the preschool group has planned to make milk shakes with the class. The milk shake activity involves cutting up some fresh fruit and putting it into a blender along with milk, ice cream, ice cubes, vanilla, and sugar. The children are seated around a low table for the activity.

One general goal for all of the children in this activity is to improve both receptive and expressive language skills. Specific language goals for each child differ considerably. Ben, Jeff, and Sarah are still at the stage of identifying objects, so one of their goals is to point to the named object when asked. This goal also incorporates a very early form of following directions. Another goal is to imitate some of the names for the objects. Roberto is already using single words. One goal for him is to begin combining two words. He will need to be well supported in his chair in order to accomplish this goal; otherwise he will not have enough energy or breath support for two-word combinations. Lakesha has begun to use a few words and many signs to communicate. For her, too, one goal will be to begin combining words or signs. For Paul, the primary goal is to capture his attention for an increasingly longer period of time. This can be considered a language goal as well as a cognitive goal because without the ability to attend to an activity, Paul will be unable to develop other skills and concepts associated with the activity. Additionally, Paul's speech-language pathologist has begun to experiment with facilitated communication for Paul since he does not seem to be developing verbal language despite consistent efforts to support it both at home and at school. For this activity, Paul's goal is to point to captioned pictures representing the ingredients as they go into the milk shake, using facilitation. This goal also incorporates the concept of sequencing, another important language and cognitive goal. Leah will share in a similar goal, but without the use of facilitation. Since her language appears to be developing on target, she will be encouraged to point to the picture cards in sequence using her right hand. This goal facilitates her continued language development while addressing her motor needs. She will also be encouraged to name objects and actions throughout the activity, providing a peer model for the other children.

The milk shake activity also addresses motor goals for several of the children. Leah's need to increase her awareness and use of her right side is incorporated not only in the picture-sequencing activity, but also as she is encouraged to add ingredients to the blender using her right hand. Roberto, too, is encouraged to grasp and manipulate the cooking utensils as the ice cream is scooped out and put into the blender and as the vanilla and milk are measured and poured. Sarah, Lakesha, Ben, and Jeff are also refining their fine motor skills by cutting fruit, manipulating the small and slippery pieces, and dropping them into the blender with control.

Sensory and oral-motor goals are also incorporated in this activity. Children with tactile hypersensitivities, like Sarah, are exposed to different textures in a motivating group situation that may encourage them to explore just a little more than they would otherwise. Some of the ingredients used are cold and can stimulate muscles in the face and mouth, increasing the children's awareness of and ability to use these muscles with more control. The thick liquid facilitates drinking and straws can be introduced for those children who are ready for the challenge. All of the children are participating in the same activity, yet each has different goals.

Infant Intervention

Making milk shakes can also be an appropriate activity for the infant group, but for purposes of illustration we will imagine that the intervention team for this group has chosen a more basic activity—making instant pudding. For Lance, Larry, and María, many of the goals are similar to those just outlined for the preschool group. Language goals include identifying objects and actions and beginning to use single words to communicate. These goals also incorporate early levels of following directions and sequencing. For Tonya, the language goals are a bit simpler—the beginning association of words with people, objects, and actions. Expressively, Tonya may be expected to use gestures paired with vocalizations to communicate.

The motor goals for these four children are similar also. Opening the pudding packet, stirring, pouring, and using the eggbeater all require some shoulder girdle strength and stability, as well as the use of both hands together. Proper positioning of the ingredients and utensils can facilitate trunk rotation as the children turn and reach for the needed items. The children are encouraged to imitate the adults as they demonstrate each step of the activity. Touching the different ingredients provides a tactile component, while smelling the pudding adds yet another sensory component for the children to incorporate and use in integrating the total experience.

But what about Rhonda, the two-month-old? How can she benefit from this activity? Because of her low muscle tone, she tends to be rather passive, moving less than other babies. Positioned near the other children and stimulated by the sights and sounds of the activity, she can be motivated to follow a large cooking spoon with her eyes as her mother moves it slowly through a horizontal arc. In sidelying, she can be encouraged to look at her reflection in the shiny metal cooking bowl or possibly bat at a set of measuring spoons dangled near her hands.

The interventionist working with Martin continues to help him organize his responses and to maintain that organization. Since he enjoys sweet foods, the taste of the pudding helps him to get organized for part of the session. Putting dabs of pudding on his fingers and helping him suck it off helps him learn how to get his fingers to his mouth, which also helps him to get organized and to maintain his level of organization. In this example we again see that by modifying the goals or expectations for each child, often they can all participate in the same activity at an appropriate level.

Dress-up

Let's look at one final example of ways to modify goals and expectations so that all children in a group can participate in a single activity. Unlike water play or cooking, dress-up is an activity that may seem appropriate for a more restricted age or ability range. Let's look at the Winter Clothes activity from January's sample activities (Week 3, Activity 2) and see how it could be used with the two groups we have been discussing so far.

Preschool Intervention

For the preschool group, Sarah's goals for the activity might include:

- touching and wearing different textured items
- walking to the mirror or to specific items
- putting on different clothing with help and removing the items independently, except for buttons or hooks
- finding items as an interventionist names them
- naming some items spontaneously or in imitation
- imitating the actions of other children or adults
- indicating which of two items she wants to wear
- indicating how to wear different items (hats on head, boots on feet)

Lakesha's goals might include:

- putting on different items independently
- asking for help with items if needed
- combining words or signs (more shoes, pretty hat)
- finding specific items when asked
- identifying items that belong together
- using words and/or gestures to interact with peers
- putting items on dolls

Goals for Roberto might include:

- pushing his arms through sleeves with assistance
- maintaining an upright position with facilitation
- indicating which of two items he wants to wear
- pointing to items when named by an interventionist

- combining two words when well supported in sitting
- asking for specific items he wants or activities he wants to do

For Paul, goals might include:

- staying in the area of the activity for at least ten minutes
- indicating which of two items he wants to wear
- putting on and taking off items with assistance
- asking for help if needed
- dressing and undressing the dolls with assistance
- indicating the appropriate use of each item
- finding items named by an interventionist

Leah's goals might include:

- putting on and taking off items with assistance (including adaptive approaches to accommodate her more involved side)
- increasing awareness and use of her right side
- describing items and activities ("I wear big boots," "Ben wear hat")
- dressing and undressing the dolls
- incorporating the dolls into play routines ("Dolly got raincoat. Go outside.")
- asking for help if needed
- using language and gestures to communicate with peers

Goals for Ben and Jeff will be similar since they are functioning at about the same level. Their goals might include:

- indicating the appropriate use of each item
- putting on and taking off items independently
- finding items when named by an interventionist
- naming items spontaneously or in imitation
- using gestures to interact with peers
- putting on simple items, such as hats on the dolls
- indicating which of two items they want to wear
- taking turns with certain items

By focusing on different goals to address the various needs of each child, the interventionist has enabled all the children to participate in the same activity together, each at an individual level. Now let's see how this activity could be used with the infant group.

Infant Intervention

At 20 months, Lance and Larry will have goals similar to some of the preschool children. These might include:

- indicating the appropriate use of items
- finding items when named by an interventionist
- naming some items spontaneously or in imitation
- walking to the mirror and to different items
- imitating actions of peers or adults
- putting on and taking off items with assistance

María's goals might be similar to those for Lance and Larry. Goals for Tonya might include:

- manipulating a variety of textured items while positioned in prone
- putting on and taking off hats with assistance
- taking turns with an adult putting on a hat and taking it off
- playing peek-a-boo with a hat
- finding items hidden in an old purse or in pockets or shoes
- maintaining good sitting balance and postural quality

Goals for Rhonda might include:

- responding as different body parts are rubbed with various textures
- visually attending to and tracking different items
- holding her head up in prone while positioned on different textured items
- responding to different voices and sounds coming from different directions

The main goal for Martin continues to be helping him to calm and organize himself and to maintain that state for increasingly longer periods of time. The interventionist combines rhythmic motion with swaddling in a light blanket. As Martin calms, the swaddling is gently loosened. As Martin maintains his calmer state, he is given some textured materials to touch. Again we see how this activity can be appropriate for the entire group when each child's goals are modified as needed.

Modifying Activities

Even though the emphasis in the previous section was on illustrating how to adapt activities through modifying the goals or expectations for each child, you probably noticed that sometimes the activities themselves were modified, too. This section focuses on modifying the activities as another effective means to allow a group of children with various ages and abilities to interact together in a naturalistic environment.

Let's look at some of the ways in which the activities described above were modified to meet the needs of the individual children involved in them. For Martin, modifying goals and expectations to some extent also meant modifying the activities. While the other children participated directly in some aspect of the activity, Martin was at the fringes, trying to organize himself and the various sensations to which he was exposed. For Martin, the activity frequently consisted of being swaddled in a light blanket and patted or moved rhythmically in the vicinity of whatever the rest of the group was doing.

During the cooking activity with the preschool group, Paul's speech-language pathologist modified the activity by incorporating facilitated communication using captioned pictures. With the infant group, the cooking activity was also modified for two-month-old Rhonda. While the older children manipulated cooking utensils and explored with ingredients, Rhonda developed her visual tracking skills by following a cooking spoon. She improved her understanding of cause-and-effect relationships and increased motor skills by batting at a set of measuring spoons and practiced visual attending skills by looking at her reflection in a metal cooking bowl. Items from the group activity were used to facilitate her specific goals so that she was at least partially involved into the activity. In a similar way, Martin's interventionist incorporated the pudding from the cooking activity into an activity designed to help him develop the ability to calm himself.

These examples illustrate two different ways of modifying activities to incorporate children at different age and ability levels. In Paul's case, the group activity was modified by introducing a specialized activity within the main activity. For Martin and Rhonda, elements of the group activity were incorporated into individualized activities that took place on the fringes of the overall activity. Other possible ways to modify activities include using parallel activities, substituting materials or components of activities, and modifying the type or amount of facilitation provided. Modifications for children with physical challenges are mentioned briefly here and addressed in detail in chapter 7.

Using Specialized Activities

It is usually not difficult to incorporate specialized activities, such as facilitated communication, into ongoing group activities. Sign language and augmentative communication devices of all types are becoming increasingly common in early intervention settings. The resource list in Appendix B provides sources of information about alternative communication techniques.

Some behavior management programs might also be considered specialized activities that can be incorporated into ongoing group activities. For example, suppose there was a child in the group who engaged in self-abusive behavior. This child would participate in the regular activities of the group but the activities designed to prevent the self-abusive behaviors would be incorporated into the overall activities for this child. Likewise, a child who required a specialized program to increase appropriate behavior while decreasing aggressive behavior would be incorporated into the group activities. The specialized behavior program would be used during these group activities as needed. An interesting group activity can often be used as a motivator, or a distractor, for children who need to learn to keep their glasses on or wear their hearing aids.

Using Elements of the Overall Activity in Individualized Activities

However much we may advocate for all children in a group to participate in the group activity, there will be occasions when it just doesn't work. These situations are infrequent, but it is important to be able to plan for them appropriately when they occur. Martin's case, in the previous example of the infant group, was one such occasion. Rhonda's case, less dramatically, was another.

In situations where it really is inappropriate for the child to participate in the group activity, the child can still be brought into the group by incorporating elements of the group activity into the child's individualized activities. In Rhonda's case, she was too young to participate in making pudding. By keeping her physically near the group and using some of the same utensils that the group was using in their activity, she was incorporated to some degree into the group activity.

A two-month-old would not be ready for some of the suggested activities described for the first week of March (see chapter 10); however, the decorated bags from Activity 1 could be used to facilitate visual tracking, reaching, and batting, as could the balloons in Activity 2. The balloons could be loosely tied to the baby's wrist or ankle to develop beginning understanding of cause and effect as the baby's arm or leg movements caused the balloons to move. Likewise, a two-month-old could participate in the Rhythm Band activity (July, Week 1, Activity 1) by activating wrist or ankle bells and by responding to different sounds or increases and decreases in volume.

In a different scenario, let's take the example of a four-year-old with multiple disabilities who is deathly afraid of animals. It is pet week in the classroom and different animals are visiting daily. This little boy's response to each of these animals is to scream, cry, thrash himself about, and bang his head on the floor. The intervention team is understandably reluctant to have this child participate with the group when the animal of the day is introduced because both the child and the rest of the class are traumatized by the child's response. Instead, the team has agreed to let the speech clinician work with the child on an individualized basis during this time. They play together in a corner of the classroom, as close to the circle as they dare, with various representations of the animal of the day, such as stuffed animals, plastic figures, illustrations, or photos. They imitate the way the animal moves and the sounds it makes, and talk about the animal's characteristics.

Using Parallel Activities

Another way to modify activities to meet the needs of individual children in the group is through the use of parallel activities. Some group activities can be planned to incorporate parallel components from the beginning, while others may need to be modified in midstream. For example, the Red Toys activity (February, Week 1, Activity 3) incorporates a variety of manipulatives to be used in a parallel fashion by the children in the group. So does the Farm Animal Toys activity (July, Week 3, Activity 3). But suppose your activity is Family Portraits (February, Week 3, Activity 4) and you have a child in your group who still needs concrete representations and doesn't do well with pictures. An interventionist could use dolls to help that child make a more concrete family portrait while the rest of the group uses pictures. Or suppose your activity is Potato Print Flowers (April, Week 4, Activity 3) and you have a child in your group who really is not ready to grasp and manipulate another object as an extension of the hand. That child could make hand prints while the rest of the group makes potato prints.

Substituting Materials

Closely related to parallel activities is the idea of substituting materials or components of activities as a way to accommodate children of different ages and ability levels within a group. This approach is often one of the easiest to put into effect and can be done on the spur of the moment if a planned activity unexpectedly turns out to be inappropriate for one or more children in the group. Suppose you have planned to make peanut butter dough and discover that one of the infants in the group is allergic to peanut butter. In fact, she is so allergic to peanut butter that her mother doesn't even want her to touch it. This child can still be included in the group by giving her regular play dough to manipulate and substituting fruit or a graham cracker for her snack. Likewise, a child who has difficulty manipulating small blocks can be given larger blocks, magnetic blocks, or Velcro® blocks. These are examples of ways that interventionists can substitute materials in an activity to better adapt them to a specific child's needs.

Now let's look at some examples of ways to substitute components to better adapt an activity for an individual child. Let's say that the group has planned a beach activity (July, Week 2) but one of the children is recovering from surgery and cannot get into the pool. Depending on the situation, the child could be positioned next to the pool and allowed to play in the water with his hands, positioned with a small basin of water, or placed at the water table, or he could just use the sand (or beans if sand was contraindicated as well). As another example, let's take an obstacle course activity (February, Week 1, Activity 1). Suppose that most of the children in the group are learning to climb up the slide and slide down it but one child is not yet able to climb, even with facilitation. That child could be assisted to slide down the slide, waiting her turn in line with the interventionist who is assisting her. Or suppose there is a child who cannot crawl through the tunnel. That child could be rolled while in the tunnel or pulled through the tunnel on a blanket.

Modifying the Facilitation

Activities can be adapted by modifying the amount or type of facilitation used with a child. Some children may complete an activity independently, some may require frequent verbal cues, and others may require total physical support. The types of facilitation that can be provided range from physical guidance (hand-over-hand) to physical prompting and verbal prompting. Modeling can also be used to facilitate a child's response. The level of facilitation can range from complete assistance to minimal assistance. Let's take Planting Flowers (April, Week 4, Activity 1) as an example. An interventionist might model the activity for the preschool group described earlier in the chapter. Lakesha might then begin to dig in the dirt with her spoon, requiring some physical guidance from time to time to get the dirt into her cup. Roberto requires total physical support to complete the activity. Paul, who is interested in the activity, might be able to complete it with minimal physical help and an occasional verbal prompt. Leah, likewise, needs some physical guidance to use her right hand to stabilize the cup. Ben and Jeff require moderate physical prompting, while Sarah requires moderate physical guidance. This activity has essentially been individualized for each child by adjusting the type and amount of assistance provided.

It is important to note, however, that children learn best through active participation. If the planned activities always require total physical support for a child to participate, they are not being planned appropriately. Roberto, in the example above, gives every indication of understanding the activity and is prevented from participating more actively by his motor dysfunction. In this situation, it is appropriate to give him the physical assistance he needs to plant flowers; yet it will also be important to include activities that he is able to complete independently, as well as activities that he can complete with minimal to moderate assistance. Chapters 7 and 8 provide more suggestions for adapting activities to meet the needs of children with disabilities.

Using the Children's Differences

We have talked about ways to adapt basic activities to meet differing individual needs by modifying the goals and expectations that we have for each child and by modifying the activities themselves in a variety of ways. Another way to adapt activities to meet individual needs is to take advantage of the differences among the children within the group. In the example of the infant group during water play, María, a younger child, is positioned next to Lance and Larry, older children with more advanced motor skills, to encourage her to imitate some of their motor behaviors. Leah, during the preschool cooking activity, provides a language model for the other children. These are two examples of how interventionists can capitalize on the differences within a group to enable peers to facilitate behaviors in each other. Let's look at some other examples.

In the Going Shopping activity (June, Week 1, Activity 1), children who are walking can push others in boxes or on riding toys. In the Fishing activity (June, Week 3, Activity 1) children who are more skilled with using both hands together can take the "fish" off the poles for those children who cannot yet do so. Children who are able can rock the boat for those who cannot. For some children, the social and cognitive "leap" to pretend play may be particularly difficult. In activities such as Winter Clothes (January, Week 3, Activity 2) children who are already pretending with dolls can model the behavior and help to facilitate this type of play with those children who have not yet developed it. Along similar lines, children who have begun sequencing play acts can model this behavior in their play with children who have not yet begun to do so. This type of peer modeling is sometimes more effective than similar adult modeling.

A word of caution about using children's differences to facilitate behaviors is in order here. It is sometimes easy to feel that children who are modeling more advanced behaviors are more capable or mature than children who have not yet developed these behaviors. The same children who may be more advanced in one area may be delayed in another. Leah, from our preschool example, is such a case. While her language abilities served as a model for the other children in the group, her motor skills were delayed. The same child should not always be expected to be the role model for the group. It is important to remember that every individual has a unique pattern of strengths and weaknesses and that, as a group, these probably balance out. Interventionists should look for and appropriately incorporate the individual contributions of each child.

7 Adapting Activities for Children with Physical Challenges

All individuals have unique abilities and needs. Some children will have multiple challenges, some will have a specific physical challenge, and some may have both physical and mental delays. It may be necessary to modify activities to accommodate different areas of need within the same individual. For example, a child with cerebral palsy may have specific motor needs and also require an augmentative communication system.

This chapter assumes that readers have some basic familiarity with physical challenges and motor delays and dysfunctions. It is not intended to provide introductory information about this area of intervention. The resource list in Appendix A gives suggested sources for those who need additional information about this topic.

Several approaches may be considered for adapting activities for children with physical challenges. These approaches include adapting the environment, using adaptive equipment, and modifying the activities. Although the previous chapter discussed at length ways to modify activities, this chapter will review some of those ideas and give specific attention to addressing physical challenges.

Adapting the Environment

Adapting the environment to eliminate certain obstacles or to facilitate certain behaviors can sometimes be one of the simplest kinds of modifications to make. This has been evident in the adult population where the simple addition of ramps has made countless buildings and the activities that occur in those buildings accessible to people whose mobility is dependent upon wheelchairs (Smith and Smith 1978). Similarly, adapting the environment in homes, classrooms, play groups, and infant programs can make important differences in children's functioning.

Let's first consider some familiar examples from the home. Most families whose homes include stairs use some type of gate or other barrier to keep babies and toddlers away from the stairs until their motor skills and judgment have matured to the point where the children are considered safe on the stairs. Safety plugs block electrical outlets and prevent injury. Safety latches serve a similar purpose in keeping young children out of drawers and cabinets. Moving breakables out of reach is a simple form of "babyproofing" that may eliminate one arena of struggle between baby and parent. These are all examples of environmental modifications that promote safety and reduce conflict between parent and child. How can environmental modifications be used to improve functioning in children with physical challenges?

At home, furniture might be positioned so that a child can practice pulling up to stand, if that is a desired goal, or so that a child has good back support, for example, against the couch, for sitting or sidelying. If the child watches television while sitting on the floor, the TV might be moved to a lower shelf to facilitate good sitting posture, including chin tuck, instead of encouraging the more typical neck hyperextension and elevated shoulders posture typically seen in children with low tone in the trunk. Encouraging play on a low table rather than putting toys on the floor may also help to facilitate more functional posture. On the other hand, sometimes putting children on the floor rather than in walkers or other pieces of equipment encourages more advanced motor and play skill development.

These ideas apply to the classroom, day-care center, or early intervention setting as well. In addition, child care and early intervention programs are often able to specialize their environments in ways that are not practical for most families. Child-sized tables and chairs and low, shatterproof mirrors encourage babies and young children to interact, pull up, stand, shift weight, and reach up while participating in various intervention activities. Child-sized railings and grab bars may help children who are still developing their balance and coordination. Removing obstacles from a child's path may enable the child who still uses rolling to get from place to place more efficiently. Providing natural pathways between activities, with critically spaced furniture at the right height to support children who are cruising or walking with support, is another environmental adaptation that may facilitate motor development in children with physical challenges.

Using Adaptive Equipment

When we think of modifications to meet the special needs of children who are physically challenged, adaptive equipment probably comes to mind first. There are several types of adaptive equipment to consider. The first, positioning equipment, is probably most commonly used. Augmentative communication, mentioned in the previous chapter, can also be considered adaptive equipment. Capability switches, which enable an individual to activate battery-operated devices and toys through a variety of simple movements, are another type of adaptive equipment. Finally, there are physically modified toys, tools, and utensils. This chapter is intended to provide a brief overview of these kinds of adaptive equipment. The next chapter discusses in more detail how to use some of the newer technology, such as capability switches, computers, and augmentative communication devices, but it is not meant to be exhaustive. The resource lists in Appendix A provide sources of additional information on these types of adaptive equipment.

Using Positioning Equipment

Most professionals in the early intervention field are familiar with some types of positioning equipment. Positioning equipment is intended to provide appropriate support to maintain functional postures and support functional movement. The equipment can be used to assist individuals in sitting, sidelying, prone, or standing, and can be as simple as a covered paper towel roll placed behind the child's neck or as complex as a wheelchair that costs several

thousand dollars. When using positioning equipment in an activity-based program, several guidelines apply:

- The equipment needs to provide developmentally appropriate positioning for the activity. This means that if the group is playing in the sand while standing around the sand table, it is appropriate to position a child in a stander. If the group is sitting on the floor for circle time, it is not appropriate to use a stander.

- The equipment should be the simplest available to do the job adequately. You don't need to use a therapy roll if the therapist's leg is the right size.

- The equipment should be easy to use. Some chairs or other pieces of equipment require so many adjustments that by the time the child is positioned, the activity is over.

- Children should be repositioned on the average of once every 20 minutes. The human body is designed for movement. If children cannot shift from one position to another on their own, interventionists should shift their positions for them. This may mean planning activities so that a child is not left sitting in an adaptive chair for an entire hour during the intervention session.

Children can be positioned on the floor in supine, prone, sidelying, or sitting. Adaptive chairs and standers of various sizes can be used to position children at the same height as their peers. It is important to plan ahead when using adaptive equipment in an activity so that the right piece of equipment will be available when it is needed, the equipment will be adjusted for the child who is to use it, and adequate time and staff will have been allotted to position the child without disrupting or delaying the activity.

Let's look at how some interventionists have incorporated adaptive equipment into their activities. In one evening infant group is a 15-month-old child named Walter who has moderate to severe cerebral palsy (spastic quadriplegia). The evening's activities have been planned around a winter theme. The first activity is a variation of the basic obstacle course idea (January, Week 3). The physical therapist has planned to accompany Walter during this activity. Since it is a dynamic activity focusing primarily on Walter's motor goals, no positioning equipment is used. During the next activity, a variation of dress-up, Walter is positioned on the speech therapist's lap and assisted with feeling and trying on the different items of clothing. Since the therapist's body is assisting with

Walter's positioning, no other equipment is needed. During the fine motor free play period, the occupational therapist positions Walter in prone across her leg and helps him pull pegs from a peg board. Again, the therapist's body is used instead of a bolster or other equipment.

The team agreed that Walter should also spend time during each session in his new adaptive chair. Although the chair positions him well, it takes several minutes to get Walter properly adjusted. Also, because the chair is new to him, Walter tolerates staying in it for only 10 to 15 minutes before he begins to fuss. As the team planned how to incorporate Walter's new chair into the group's activities, they decided it would not be wise to try to position Walter in the chair more than once during the evening, at least initially. They wanted to use the chair for activities that required good support and that could best be facilitated from a static position. One of their goals was to increase the amount of time that Walter would accept positioning in the chair without fussing. Since Walter's favorite activity was snack, the team decided to use the chair for the activity immediately before snack and planned to leave Walter in the chair during snack. This position was appropriate for the activity planned, scribbling on paper with chalk for this particular session, and for feeding, especially since all the other children would be seated for these activities, too. While the teacher, speech-language pathologist, and parents helped the rest of the group sit and begin the scribbling activity, the physical therapist and occupational therapist positioned Walter in his chair. He was then placed at the table with the rest of the group and the teacher helped him with the scribbling activity. The group then transitioned to snack while Walter, and everyone else, remained seated in the same chairs as for the scribbling activity. Walter was also naturally reinforced by the snack to stay a little longer in his seat without fussing.

As another example, let's consider a preschool group with three of the seven children who are present needing some type of adaptive equipment for independent sitting. In addition, the physical therapist would like for them to be positioned in standing for at least 30 minutes each morning. The theme of the morning's activities is flowers (April, Week 4). The opening activity, Planting Flowers, is designed to orient the children to the theme of the day while focusing on the children's sensory needs. Although this would be an appropriate activity for standing, the

team has decided to defer that positioning until later in the session. This decision was based on several factors: the need to physically prepare the children for standing with some therapeutic intervention, the need to allow the children to warm up to the preschool setting before introducing relatively intrusive intervention such as positioning equipment, the need to begin the opening activity promptly (taking into account the amount of time it can take to get three children positioned in standers), and the fact that a later activity is also suitable for standing. The physical therapist and occupational therapist work with two of the three children during the opening activity. During the Flower Walk activity that follows, the three children who are not mobile ride in strollers pushed by the children who are walking. The interventionists make sure that these three are the first ones to return from the walk and that they are positioned in their standers while the other children remain outside. When the rest of the group arrives, the Potato Print Flowers activity begins. The three children in standers, who also require adaptive seating, complete the potato print activity first and are placed in their chairs while the rest of the group cleans up. Then the whole group, seated around a low table, can begin the cookie-making activity, followed by snack at the same table.

By planning carefully, the interventionists have ensured that the transitions between positions are as smooth and unobtrusive to the flow of activities as possible. They have also made sure that positioning is appropriate for the activities and that position changes occur several times during the course of the session.

Using Augmentative Communication

This section is not intended to provide an in-depth discussion of augmentative communication, but instead to serve as a reminder of how such approaches can be incorporated into planned group activities. Appendix A contains a list of resources that provide more information about a variety of augmentative communication systems.

In one of the examples cited in the previous chapter, Paul's speech-language pathologist incorporated facilitated communication into the classroom cooking activity. Many speech-language pathologists and special education teachers are familiar with the use of sign language in the classroom to facilitate language for children with Down syndrome and other developmental delays, as well as with children who have hearing impairments. Picture communication boards are also familiar in many early intervention settings. Other types of communication devices, such as the Wolf communicator or the Touch Talker, are being used with increasing frequency.

Incorporating many of these communication systems into ongoing activities is often almost as simple as remembering to have the system available. But some planning also needs to be done ahead of time. It is important, for example, to have vocabulary available in all augmentative systems that is related to the planned activities. Sometimes this preparation requires programming devices or adding pictures to a communication board or book. For maximum effectiveness, this preparation needs to be done ahead of time. Often, even verbal children enjoy using augmentative communication devices and they can be shared with all the children in the group. Such sharing sometimes helps to remove the stigma that a child might feel about needing to communicate differently than the other children. For example, if the class is baking cookies, a child's Wolf Communicator could be programmed with the ingredients going into the batter. Children could take turns naming the ingredient being added, using the Wolf if they choose. A communication device could also be used to reinforce the idea of taking turns so that each child would await his or her turn to point to the picture or touch the spot corresponding to the desired activity before being allowed to participate.

Using Capability Switches

This section provides only a very brief overview of how to use capability switches in activity-based intervention. Capability switches are discussed in more detail in the next chapter. Appendix B includes a resource list that provides more information about types of switches available as well as how to use them.

Very often, children with significant physical challenges and motor delays are not able to manipulate objects the way that others do. They may not be able to grip tightly enough, control their fingers carefully enough, or move their arms where they would like

them to go. Children in this situation may want to play with the same toys their peers have but are not able to do so effectively. Capability switches give them vastly increased opportunities to make toys move or to activate objects.

Capability switches enable people to activate electronically powered devices. These can include battery-operated toys and devices as well as plug-in electronics. One component of a capability switch interrupts the flow of electricity to the toy or other device. The other component allows the individual operating the switch to complete the circuit by putting pressure on a hand or foot plate, by breathing heavily on a sensor, by changing head position, by making a particular sound, or through a variety of other methods, depending on the controlled movements in the individual's repertoire and the creativity of the facilitator. Devices can also be plugged into household electronics, such as the TV, radio, or lamp. A capability switch is then plugged into the device and used to activate the TV or other appliance. One form of capability switch that almost everyone is familiar with is the remote control for the TV and VCR. For individuals who lack precise motor control, these devices often have too many buttons that are too small and too close together. Adaptive capability switches work like remote controls but with only one or two buttons that can be operated by whatever action the individual has under the best motor control.

During cooking activities, a capability switch could be used to enable children to turn a blender or mixer off and on. During circle time, children could activate the record player or tape recorder using this device. In the Fan activity (March, Week 1, Activity 3), such a switch is used to allow the children to turn the fan on and off to make the streamers attached to the fan blow or stop.

Capability switches attached to battery-operated toys can be used to help children develop an understanding of cause-and-effect relationships and to develop a sense of their own effectiveness in making things happen. Children who may not have the motor control to bang a drum or push a car across the floor can use a simple pressure switch to make these things happen.

Capability switches enable children to play games when they are not able to manage the small pieces of a board game. They can be used to animate objects for pretend play (make the bunny hop to the garden and eat lettuce; cook dinner on the toy stove) or for solitary entertainment and play. They can also be used as training devices to help children develop the skills they will need to operate more sophisticated devices, such as communication aids and computers, when they are older. The next chapter discusses these possibilities in detail.

Using Modified Toys and Tools

Modified toys and tools are among the most readily available adaptations for children with physical challenges. Puzzles with knobs help children remove and replace pieces easily. Built-up handles on spoons provide an easier grip and curved handles help children who have difficulty rotating their wrists to bring the spoon to the mouth. Some adaptations can be easily made by interventionists or parents. A wide variety of adapted toys and tools are also available commercially.

Plan to use modified toys or tools during the intervention session if doing so allows children with physical challenges to participate in activities they could not manage otherwise. Choose adapted items that are as much like the nonadapted materials as possible. Use the minimum adaptation necessary to enable the child to feel successful. Occupational therapists, in particular, generally have a good background in adapting items or selecting commercially available items.

Activities with a significant fine motor component are the ones most likely to be suitable for adapted items. Let's look at an activity such as Red Toys (February, Week 1, Activity 3), for example. Bristle blocks are often useful without modification because they can stick together without precise stacking. Magnetic blocks or Velcro® blocks can stick together without the child aligning them precisely or using refined release patterns to let go of them once they are aligned. These items could be substituted for plain wooden or plastic blocks. A piece of small plastic tubing or a pipe cleaner can be substituted for the shoelaces typically used in bead-stringing activities. Pegs with knobs at the top are sometimes easier for children to manipulate than straight pegs.

Sometimes merely using a different-sized item can make a significant difference in the child's ability to manipulate it successfully. Larger pegs that fit loosely into their holes are more likely to produce success for children than smaller, tight-fitting pegs. Children may find it easier to stack larger blocks or to string small empty cans with both top and bottom removed onto a plastic tube than to use the standard preschool-sized items.

Paper dolls with Velcro® on their clothes could be used with children whose motor skills interfere with their ability to dress and undress paper dolls. A child could pick up the clothes using a Velcro® strap wrapped around a hand. Adults can construct "play boards" with grooves for miniature people, cars, and scenery to move along. The figures can be manipulated using extensions underneath or on the sides of the boards.

Children's clothing, too, can often be adapted to make it easier for children with significant physical challenges to put on and take off. Velcro® instead of buttons, snaps, or zippers is sometimes all that is needed. Changing openings from the back to the side or front is also helpful. The occupational therapist will have a variety of ideas for adapting clothing so that it is functional for children with physical challenges.

Modifying Activities

The previous chapter discussed ways of modifying activities to accommodate children of differing ability levels within a group. Let's look again at some of these ideas, this time with an emphasis on addressing specific physical differences. Specialized activities might be incorporated into overall group activities if, for example, the child's motor goals can be addressed while the child is engaged in another activity with the group. For example, one physical therapist worked on improving Alice's balance and equilibrium responses and on facilitating more use of the left side by placing her on a therapy ball during snack. Alice was more interested in snack than in the subtle changes the therapist was eliciting in her posture, which was as the therapist hoped.

In other situations, children might require individualized activities. They could feel more included in the overall activity if the elements of the group activity were incorporated into their individualized activities. For example, four-month-old Charlie needs to work on developing head control. The rest of the group is sliding down the slide, an activity that is not appropriate for him. By positioning him where he can see the activities of the other children by raising his head, the physical therapist has included him in the group activity and used the activity as a motivator to accomplish an important motor goal.

Parallel activities can also serve as the means to accommodate an individual's specific physical needs. During the Parade activity (July, Week 1, Activity 3), children who are nonambulatory ride in wagons and strollers pushed by the children who are walking. For the walkers, the activity is one of improving gait, weight shifting, processing proprioceptive input, and strengthening shoulder girdles. For the riders, the activity may be one of improving balance and equilibrium, maintaining an upright posture against gravity, processing vestibular input, and perhaps improving head or trunk control.

We have already seen how substituting adapted materials can allow a child with physical challenges to participate in an activity with the rest of the group. It is also possible to substitute one action component for another, again allowing a child with physical challenges to participate fully in a group activity. For example, let's say the group is seated in a circle playing a ball game. The children are throwing the ball to one another as the interventionists name who is to catch the ball. Mimi can't throw the ball. She can, with facilitation, roll the ball, and that is what she is encouraged to do when it is her turn. John, on the other hand, has very little use of his arms but more control with his feet. He kicks the ball when it is his turn.

The previous chapter's discussion on adapting activities by modifying the type and amount of facilitation focused on differences in children's motor skills. We will not repeat that discussion here. We will, however, repeat the caution that a child who is completely facilitated through 100% of an activity may not be fully participating in the activity. The amount of learning that occurs under these circumstances is questionable.

Case Examples

This chapter has provided a brief overview on how to adapt activities to meet the physical challenges of some individuals. These included adapting the environment, using adaptive equipment, and modifying

activities. Let's summarize the information by looking at ways that one team of interventionists adapted a session's activities to meet the physical challenges of the children in their group.

The afternoon preschool group consists of three-year-old Darryl, who has a diagnosis of cerebral palsy and a seizure disorder; 3½-year-old Sarah, who has a rare genetic disorder; 2½-year-old Missy, who has a severe sensory integration dysfunction; Glen, a three-year-old with Down syndrome; Tonee, a three-year-old with cerebral palsy; and George, a 2½-year-old with fetal alcohol syndrome. The intervention team has planned activities around the Eggs theme (April, Week 2). Although the entire team participated in planning the activities, only the physical therapist was scheduled to be in the classroom on this particular day along with the teacher and teaching assistant.

The first activity is an obstacle course with plastic eggs hidden throughout it. Small treats have been hidden inside the eggs. Missy, Glen, and George are all walking independently. Tonee is beginning to walk using a walker. Sarah is beginning to roll from one place to another. Darryl still requires total support and is not independently mobile. The physical therapist has taught the classroom assistant how to help Tonee use her walker. She helps Tonee follow the obstacle course using her walker. She hangs a basket on the walker for Tonee to carry the eggs she finds. The occupational therapist has shown the classroom staff how to help Missy organize her activities and thus improve some of her motor planning skills. The teacher gives Missy assistance from time to time, while concentrating mainly on pulling Darryl through the obstacle course on a blanket. At each station, the teacher gives Darryl a choice of whether to participate or not using his communication board. Darryl's basket for his eggs rides on the blanket with him. Meanwhile, the physical therapist helps Sarah use the challenges of the obstacle course to improve her motor skills.

After the children have gathered several eggs, Missy discovers that there are treats hidden inside the eggs. The children quickly lose interest in the gross motor equipment and begin to explore the eggs more seriously. Missy and George are able to get their eggs open. Once they have eaten the cereal they discover inside, they hurry to "help" the other children. From this point, each child requires a different level of facilitation. Once Glen understands that he needs to hold the eggs tightly and pull each end, he is able to open them, too. Darryl needs help with all aspects of the task but is able to eat the cereal pieces once they are placed in his mouth. Tonee holds one side of the egg and pulls but needs help holding the other half of the egg. Using her more functional hand, she is able to bring the cereal pieces to her mouth and eat them independently. Sarah, like Darryl, needs total assistance in getting the eggs open but can eat the cereal pieces independently once she finds them.

Now the interventionists bring out boxes of cellophane grass in which to hide the eggs. They put more treats inside the eggs, this time graham cracker bears, and hide the eggs in the boxes on the floor while the children watch. The physical therapist positions Darryl in prone over a roll for this activity so he can work on weight bearing on all fours, weight shifting, and head control. Sarah is supported in a floor sitter for this activity. The other children sit, kneel, or squat independently. They are given the same level of assistance as before with opening their eggs and eating their treats.

The next three activities could all be done in sitting. The first two could also be done in standing. In order to provide for more position changes, the team decided to let the children stand to dye eggs. Darryl and Sarah are placed in their standers. Tonee supports herself against the table. The physical therapist uses this opportunity to work with Tonee on improving weight bearing and weight shifting in standing. Darryl uses his communication board to choose the colors he will use for his eggs. Sarah works with the teacher to indicate her choices, using facilitated communication. The classroom assistant helps

Darryl and Sarah dip their eggs in the dye, using a bent spoon with a built-up handle that is easier for them to grasp.

Since the egg-dyeing activity has gone very quickly, the team decides to let the children continue standing for the collage activity. Darryl and Sarah share a table-top easel to put their work at an angle to make it easier for them to participate. Tonee has gotten tired of standing and is placed in her chair for this activity. Each child requires, and is given, a different amount of facilitation for the tasks involved. All of the children help clean up and are seated for the snack activity.

Darryl and Sarah require adaptive seating. They use their augmentative communication systems to identify the ingredients for the egg salad, and Darryl shows the order in which the items are added. He uses a capability switch to activate the blender for mixing some of the egg salad while the other children mix egg salad with their forks. The other children are interested in the blender and take turns using the capability switch, too.

While this scenario does not illustrate all of the different types of adaptations presented in this chapter, it shows how many of these adaptations can be interwoven into an ongoing program while addressing the varied needs of the whole group. The children with physical challenges are incorporated into all of the group activities and receive individualized physical therapy while participating in these activities. The adaptations provided are appropriate to both the children's needs and to the ongoing activities. Adaptations are not offered where they are not needed.

8 Incorporating Technology into Activity-Based Intervention

by Nicole A. Pellicciotto, M.Ed.

Technology is anything that makes life easier. We all use technology in our daily lives. Remote controls, answering machines, microwave ovens, and computers have made our lives easier. Assistive technology has allowed children with disabilities to have greater control in their lives; to participate and contribute more in activities in their homes, schools, and communities; to interact more with children who do not have disabilities; and to have opportunities that are taken for granted by typical children.

Augmentative communication has allowed many children to communicate for the first time (Blackstone 1989; Musselwhite and St. Lewis 1988). Children are becoming independent with toileting through using prototypes of ultrasonic bladder sensors (Mineo and Cavalier 1987). Infants with physical disabilities can increase their sensorimotor exploration by using capability switches (Brinker and Lewis 1982). Other infants and young children with disabilities use microswitches with adaptive toys to help them learn about cause and effect, choice making, identification, and classification. These are just a few examples of ways that technology can enhance children's independence and enable them to participate in mainstream society.

Technology is an integral part of most early intervention programs. Infants and preschoolers are learning to run computer programs, use switches for play, and communicate with electronic devices. The goal of this chapter is to provide practical information on using technology in an activity-based early intervention program. The chapter is divided into three parts: setting up computers in the classroom, using capability switches and battery-operated toys, and using augmentative communication systems. It is intended to build upon ideas and equipment that are found in most early intervention programs.

Setting Up Computers

When talking about computers, the term *user-friendly* comes to mind. User-friendly means that something is easy to use. This term certainly applies to the computer in the early intervention program. Work spaces need to be set up so that a child can work on the computer effectively. Let's look at how we might accomplish this.

Placement of Equipment and Positioning of the Child

The placement of equipment is the first thing to consider when creating a user-friendly environment. We will be looking at the position of the monitor, the input device, and the child. Classroom computers tend to be positioned for adult use. Computer carts and stands are great for storing a lot of equipment and they can be rolled from room to room; however, they are not functional work stations for children. Children who sit at these work stations are straining their necks to see the monitor while their feet are dangling. The monitor needs to be at the child's eye level. This means that the teacher might need to move the monitor from time to time to meet the needs of different children. A child in a wheelchair needs a different monitor placement than a child who is mobile. It takes a creative mind to find a good place for infants and toddlers to work at the computer. Computer equipment is often big and heavy, so preschool-sized tables might not be strong enough to support its weight.

Even something that seems inappropriate might be a perfect computer stand. One piece of equipment that is sturdy, adjustable, and functional for infants and toddlers is an aerobic step. The step is strong enough to hold the weight of a monitor. It can be used on the floor for independent seating or with inserts to adjust the height. There is even a nice space for a seat to fit under.

Input devices, such as switches, the Power Pad (Dunamis, Inc.), keyboards, and Muppet Learning Keys (Sunburst), must be placed on stable surfaces. A stable placement prevents the device from moving. Hook-and-loop fastener, such as Velcro®, and clamps are effective for stabilizing input devices. The floor, a table, or a tray is suitable for placement. The input device must be positioned correctly for the child to use. For example, a child in a wheelchair might need the keyboard tilted to access the computer. The input device placement will vary from child to child. After finding a proper placement, that placement should be consistent. Marking the table or tray with tape is a great reminder of proper placement.

Improper positioning can limit a child's ability to accomplish a task. There is no need to worry about software and instruction if a child cannot physically work at the computer. Physical and occupational therapists can help determine an effective position for a child. A child working with the computer should be in a position that is relaxed, energy-efficient, enhances good muscle control, and prevents fatigue (chapter 7 provides a more in-depth look at positioning). A variety of positioning devices can be used with the computer, such as lap straps, trunk supports, abductor cushions, foot rests, and straps.

Environmental Concerns

The environment must also be considered when setting up the computer. Here are some practical tips.

- Place computers near electrical outlets and use surge protectors to prevent electrical surges and voltage spikes.
- Keep computers away from windows and avoid heat exposure.
- Keep computers away from water. (Water and sand centers can cause problems.)
- Tape down all electrical cords to prevent falls.
- Do not use computers during electrical or thunderstorms.

- Keep software in a closed container to avoid moisture.
- Choose a quiet area with minimal distractions for the computer.

Organization for Efficiency

Cluttered computer areas, lack of familiarity with the software or input devices, and not having established rules for computer use can impair the child's experience on the computer. There are a variety of ways to organize materials to make the computer experience more worthwhile for children. The computer area should contain only the essential elements for the activity. As previously mentioned, computer carts are wonderful for storing equipment but are not effective for instruction with infants and toddlers. Too much clutter causes idle hands to wander and touch things that should not be touched. Extra visual stimuli can distract the child from the task. These problems can be addressed by planning ahead, knowing what input devices are used with the software, and having only what is needed available at the work station.

With so many input devices and so much software, it is difficult to remember that, for instance, the "Dancing Man" (public domain) uses a switch and the "Wheels on the Bus" (UCLA/LAUSD) uses a Power Pad (Dunamis, Inc.). Color coding is an effective means to combat this problem. Assign a color to each input device. You can place a colored dot on the corner of the computer disk to coincide with the proper input device. Make a summary chart to keep track of the color-coding scheme (see table 1).

TABLE 1

Color Coding Software with Computer Input Devices

Input Device	Color
Keyboard	Purple
Muppet Learning Keys (Sunburst)	Green
Joystick	Orange
TouchWindow (Edmark)	Yellow
Power Pad (Dunamis, Inc.)	Blue
Switches	Red
Multiple Input (may use two or more of the devices above)	Brown

Now the teacher does not have to remember what software goes with which device. Anyone can pull the software from the disk box and follow the hassle-free color-coding system. Once a color-coding system has been established, the teacher can select software.

Software Selection

Software selection will vary from child to child. The selection will depend upon the child's goals, objectives, and physical capabilities. For example, even though one piece of software is great for letter identification, it does not use a switch input device; therefore, it would not be functional for a child who could activate the computer only by using a switch. The therapist should match the software objectives with the child's ability to access the computer.

An easy way to make this successful match is by color-coding software, as discussed above, and creating an index file card box. Each piece of software should have a corresponding index card that states the title of the software, system requirements, objectives and goals, coding system, and any special information (see figure 1).

Title: Jokus Face (Don Johnston Developmental Equipment, Inc.) **Color Code:** Red

System Requirements: Macintosh LC or higher, color monitor, 2MB RAM, System 7.0 or higher

Objectives/Goals: switch use, beginning cause and effect, visual attention to task

Themes: faces, expressions, people

Special Information: press "Apple and Q" to stop program

Figure 1. Completed Index Card for Software Selection

The interventionist can arrange the file card box by title, objectives, goals, themes, or color coding. This planning allows anyone to be prepared for even the most diverse group. This effective system also allows for a clutter-free environment. The interventionist does not need the computer manuals to remember system requirements or themes of the software. All of the information is stored on the index card for

quick and easy reference. All of the intervention program staff will benefit from the use of this system. Let's look at an example.

The theme of the week is animals. The classroom teacher needs to set up the computer for two children in the afternoon program who have different needs. The first child is Jermaine, who is three years old and has cerebral palsy. He is seated in a Rifton chair to use the computer. Because of his limited motor movement, he is able to access the computer only by switches. Two of his goals are to activate the switch independently and to make choices. First, the classroom teacher scans the top of the index cards in the file box to see all of the programs with a red color coding (remember that the color red indicates the software that uses switches). The teacher wants to stay with the theme of animals, so any software that does not fall into the animal theme is disregarded. Finally, the teacher considers Jermaine's goals and objectives. Two programs that would be appropriate for Jermaine are Frog and Fly (public domain) and Zoo Time: Level 2 (UCLA/LAUSD). Since the teacher knows that children who can direct their own learning are more motivated to learn, two pieces of software are selected for Jermaine to choose from. The importance of having children direct their own learning is one of the premises of the activity-based approach.

Rachel is also three and has developmental delays in speech and fine motor skills. Her input device for the computer is the Power Pad. Currently, the TouchWindow and the keyboard are too difficult for her and switches do not provide enough challenge. Some of Rachel's goals lie in the areas of classification and identification. The classroom teacher follows the same process to select software for Rachel as she did for Jermaine. After selecting the index cards with a blue color coding that indicates the use of the Power Pad, the teacher sifts through the group to find animal themes. Finally, the teacher looks at the objectives and goals to match the software with Rachel's objectives. Once again, the teacher selects two software programs that Rachel can choose from: Zoo Time: Level 2 (UCLA/LAUSD) and Old MacDonald's Farm 1: Level 3 (UCLA/LAUSD).

It is also important to learn about the types of software that are available in the classroom. This information will allow you to know what software can be changed and distributed within your program. Four types of software are available: public domain, freeware, shareware, and commercial software. Public domain software is software given to the public by the original author. The programs may be copied, passed on to other users, or modified to meet a specific user's need. Most of the programs are not copyrighted and they can be found in computer club libraries, on-line services such as CompuServe or Prodigy, and in computer magazines. Freeware is software that the author allows others the right to copy and distribute but typically requests that no modifications be made. Freeware is copyrighted. With shareware, the author allows the user to copy and distribute the programs but provides certain restrictions. Generally the author will grant a time period that a person can use the program after which the user is then asked to pay for the program. The price is usually much lower than that of commercial software and this type of software can be among the most innovative. Just remember that if you use the software, make sure you pay for it. These fees support the authors and help them to continue to write programs in the future. Finally, commercial software is copyrighted and is illegal to copy. There are restrictions on commercial software that specify the number of back-up copies that can be made and the number of computers to run the software. Commercial software can be purchased from retail computer stores, catalogs, and directly from software companies.

Ground Rules

All classroom activities have ground rules. For example, water and sponges remain in the tactile area; blocks are for building, not throwing. Ground rules also need to be established for computer use. These rules improve the organization and efficiency of the classroom. Some areas that need to be addressed include operation times, length of session, number of children present, and choice-making by the child.

Most classrooms and intervention programs have an established routine. For example, activity on the playground occurs after snack time and each child knows to transition outside after snack. Research shows that children with special needs function more productively if a classroom routine has been established (Johnson-Martin, Jens, and Attermeier 1991). As with other activities, the computer sessions need to be built into the routine of the intervention program. Every program routine will differ because every program is different. Interventionists need to establish a routine that works for their group.

Operational Times

One of the real challenges of establishing a routine involves helping children know when it is their computer time. For instance, the teacher will start to become frustrated because she has told Jenny seven times that it is not her turn to use the computer. Jenny is also frustrated because she loves to play "Wheels on the Bus" and is sure that her mom will come to take her home while Nawal is still having his turn.

One way to designate children's turns on the computer is to use stuffed animals to identify each child's time. Assign each child a stuffed animal. All of the animals are then lined up in front of the classroom to show the order of the computer use. When it is time for the child to work on the computer, the appropriate stuffed animal will be placed on top of the monitor. Now Jenny knows that Dinosaur Dan is after Crazy Cat and that when Dinosaur Dan is placed on top of the monitor it is her computer time. This system works well for children with a variety of cognitive functioning levels. Even if Mia does not recognize Buzzy Bird, another child will keep track of her turn. If there is a group that perhaps has no children who have the cognitive ability to recognize their stuffed animals and take their turns, the interventionist should guide the students. With this system, the interventionist does not need to answer the same question over and over and the children have special friends to show them when it is their computer time. This system works best when the stuffed animals are used only with the computer.

Session Length

Session length also needs to be established. Since each student has different physical and hardware needs and software objectives, the length of each session will also vary. Each child will not have equal computer time. The time allotted should be based on the needs of the individual child and take into account the child's attention span, the goals and objectives of the software, and the child's endurance.

Even though the team addresses these areas when planning, difficulties may arise. For example, Jim has been on the computer for 15 minutes and refuses to stop playing. He has difficulty staying on task and is angry because he cannot finish the math maze. Meanwhile, Amid is holding onto Dancing Dog and his face is turning red while the classroom teacher is trying to get Jim off the computer. The use of a stopwatch or timer is effective for combating this time management problem (Hoffman 1988). A simple, inexpensive kitchen timer can help enormously with structuring a child's computer time. The ding of the timer indicates the end of the child's turn and leaves no question as to when the time is up.

Number of Children Present

Depending on the setup of the computer and the software, the teacher might decide to have the children work in pairs or groups. Grouping is very helpful when a lot of children are present and not enough individual time slots are available for each of them. Time can also be a factor if classrooms or groups share computers.

Working in pairs on the computer has advantages and disadvantages. One advantage is efficiency. More children will be able to work on the computer together than would be able to independently. Children with different cognitive functioning levels may be paired together for cooperative learning. The higher-functioning child may act as the model, but it is the team that is praised. Cooperative learning makes the team successful. Finally, working in pairs on the computer encourages turn taking and cooperative play.

One disadvantage of pairing concerns the setup of the computer. Every child needs the equipment positioned successfully for play. A child in a wheelchair would need the monitor placed higher than a child who is ambulatory. One child might need to use a switch, while the other is able to access the computer via the keyboard. These structural differences can be downfalls for many computer pairs. Software may also be a disadvantage. Not all software is created for more than one player. This type of software may be extremely difficult to use in pairs when turn taking is not a part of the software program. Another software difficulty can lie in the area of goals and objectives. It might be difficult for the team to find a software program that will meet the goals and objectives for two

children at the same time. It is helpful if the software has an adjustable level but, unfortunately, not all software programs have this feature. The interventionist has to make sure that the program is not too hard or too easy for either child.

Choice-Making by the Child

The last rule to be discussed is choice-making by the child. Although this is not one of those "golden rules" previously discussed, it can be seen as a rule for the interventionist to follow. Children need to be able to make choices that affect their learning. Research shows that children learn more and are more motivated to learn if they are able to make choices (Brown et al. 1993; Dyer, Dunlap, and Winterling 1990). This understanding underlies the whole concept of activity-based intervention. Allowing the child to direct the activity increases the child's independence and self-esteem. Having the child make choices at the computer can be easy and quick with the organized software index card box. Before the child's turn on the computer, pick out two or three appropriate software programs. Let the child choose which one of them to use. For example, Linda is ready to work on the computer and her objectives lie in the area of cause and effect. Linda needs to access the computer with the TouchWindow. The interventionist goes to the index card file, scans the color code on the corner of the cards and finds the software for the TouchWindow. Then the interventionist scans the objectives and goals section for cause and effect. Two pieces of software are found, Camelephant and Jokus Faces (Don Johnston Developmental Equipment, Inc.), from which Linda can make a choice. This process gives Linda control of her learning and helps motivate her to work.

In this section, we have discussed setting up the computer in the early intervention environment. The key to success is being organized. Organizing the hardware and software allows for easy setup for each child. Establishing classroom rules regarding the computer lets the child transition successfully to and from the computer. Finally, knowing the proper computer placement for each child in your group, including input and output devices, allows for easy individualized setup. In the next section we will discuss capability switches and battery-operated toys. Areas that will be addressed include types of switches, switch placement, the variety of battery-operated toys, and expanding the use of battery-operated toys in thematic units.

Capability Switches

The use of switches allows infants and toddlers with disabilities to:

- have access to play
- experience enhanced learning
- be more independent in their activities
- have increased access to new experiences
- have access to powered mobility
- communicate

A variety of commercial switches are available. Table 2 provides examples of these switches. AbleNet, Don Johnston Developmental Equipment, Inc., Steven Kanor, Ph.D, Inc., Prentke Romich Company, and Zygo Industries all supply commercial switches. See Appendix B for further details. Burkhart (1980, 1982)

also has two wonderful books on making your own switches for the classroom.

Switch Placement and Selection

Capability switch placement depends on the motor abilities of the child. Once again, a team approach can help to identify the gross motor, fine motor, visual, and auditory capabilities of a child. Consult with physical and occupational therapists for ideas and resources. A variety of issues need to be considered when determining switch placement. Improper switch placement will result in children not being able to manipulate their environment. This can be frustrating for the children and the interventionists.

The most important issue that needs to be addressed is motor ability. The child needs to have one consistent movement pattern; for example, turning the head to the left or sipping air from a straw. The child also needs enough force in the movement pattern to activate the switch. A child may have enough force

TABLE 2

Commercial Switches

Types of Switch by Input	Description	Examples
Contact	Activation requires contact between two objects (no pressure needed)	Touch plate Cyber glove Cyber plate Cylindrical touch
Pressure	Activation requires pressure on a surface causing contact between two points	Light touch switch Paddle switch Plate switch Flat switch Reed switch Leaf switch
Pneumatic	Activation requires changes in air pressure	Air cushion Sip and puff
Sound	Activates by sound or voice	Voice-activated switch Whistle switch
Light	Activates to various types of light	Light pointer Head pointer Infrared switch Photo cell switch
Myoelectric	Activation to muscle movements	P-switch Sensor switch
Mercury	Activation results in movement of mercury to base of tube	Mercury switch Tilt switch

to activate a switch once or twice but not enough force to maintain the use. The therapist should consider whether the child is able to repeat the motor movement over time. This consistency is crucial when a switch is used with an augmentative communication system or powered mobility system. If a child cannot activate the switch repeatedly over time, the child will become fatigued. If a child is exerting too much energy to activate the switch, the child's performance and accuracy rate will decrease. Accuracy rate will also depend upon the target size. A child may have enough force to activate a pressure switch but may need a big target. A small target, such as the Jelly Bean switch (AbleNet), might be too small for the child to hit, while a larger target, such as the Big Red switch (AbleNet), would be more effective. The following is an example of two children with different switch placement needs.

Sally is 2½ years old and has developmental delays in all areas. She is able to sit up and roll, and is starting to creep, but her extremely low muscle tone is affecting motor movements. She is easily fatigued and takes frequent naps when tired. Sally is nonverbal and communicates through body language, gestures, and some eye gazing. She generally plays with toys in her left hand; this is her most consistent movement pattern. Due to her low tone, Sally does not have enough force to activate a pressure switch. Voice-activated switches are out of the question because she is mostly nonverbal. Light switches could be an option but she does not sustain her eye gaze long enough to activate the switch. The switch placement and switch selected for Sally is a contact switch mounted next to her left hand when she is seated in her highchair. The highchair gives her enough stability to sit and play and the contact switch does not need force for activation. This is a wonderful placement for Sally and she is able to play without becoming easily fatigued.

Ming is four years old and has cerebral palsy and developmental delays. He wears glasses to correct his strabismus and he had a tracheostomy that makes him nonverbal. Ming is very involved physically. Without support from either proper positioning or handling, he would not be able to move or play. The most motor control that Ming has is with his head. When he is placed in his wheelchair with his head in a midline position, he is able to turn his head to the right. His head turning is slow but he has enough force to activate a pressure leaf switch. The leaf switch is mounted on the right side of his head rest for play.

Finding a suitable switch site can be difficult. A trial-and-error process might be needed to find the best placement. Don't worry if the first site does not work out over time. The child could have been so excited about the new switch that you did not realize how much energy was needed for activation. It is important to keep trying. Also, remember that a child who is limited now may have more functional movement patterns in the future. For example, a child who is quadriplegic and does not have an effective eye gaze or head control would not be suited to switch use. This child would need to start with basic skills in visual tracking and head control before effectively using a switch. Yet with such training, the child might eventually be able to reliably operate a switch to turn a tape recorder or TV off and on or control a motorized wheelchair.

Battery-Operated Toys

Just as there is a variety of switches to work with and choose from, there is also a variety of battery-operated toys. When purchasing battery-operated toys, consider the sensory input they provide: auditory, visual, or tactile. Table 3 (page 66) gives some examples of toys and their sensory inputs. The toys should also have a variety of movement patterns. Stationary toys stay in one place and do not move around the table or floor. The Drumming Bear is a stationary toy. Horizontal toys, such as the Walking Cow and Police Car, move around the table or floor. Vertical toys, such as the Fireman on the Ladder, move up and down. Finally, some toys combine movement patterns. For example, the Penguin Roller Coaster and a race track are toys that combine movement patterns. The toys chosen also need to be incorporated into the play routines in the child's environment (Gossens and Crain 1986; Musselwhite 1986). The interventionist needs to go beyond the concept of cause and effect. Once a child learns that the toy can be activated by hitting a switch, it is no longer a challenge. It is no wonder that children become bored quickly with switch toys if they are never asked to do anything more challenging than turn them off and on. A thematic or unit approach to play can be helpful for alleviating this boredom. Incorporating the toys into the themes allows you to expand on the toy. The following are some examples that work.

These brief examples show how to expand play schemes that involve battery-operated toys. Every battery-operated toy can fit into a theme. Using some creativity will help you make games with the toys. Children can learn much more than cause and effect when working with a switch toy. They can also learn turn taking, scanning, following directions, opposites, identification and classification, choice-making, and matching when playing with a switch toy.

Theme: Fire Trucks (May, Week 1)

Toy: Fireman on Ladder

Purpose: horizontal tracking, turn taking, pretend play, scanning, peer interaction, choice-making

Game: Create a building out of a cardboard box. Cut out windows and have small people made out of paper taped in the windows. Have children sit in a circle. Each child will take a turn saving a person from the burning building.

Expansion of Game: Save the person on the top of the building (opposites). Save your favorite person (choice-making). Save the person in blue (categories). Save the person that I am holding (matching).

Theme: Fire Trucks (May, Week 1)

Toy: fan

Purpose: tactile input, turn taking, pretend play, concepts, peer interaction

Game: Make a stick of fire out of red construction paper and a craft stick. Have children sit in a circle. One child will hold the "fire" and another child will operate the fan. The teacher can ask the question "Who is hot?" The child with the fan will need to find the fire and blow it out with the fan. Crackling red cellophane paper can be used if a child has a visual disorder.

Expansion of Game: Other children hold blue sticks for cold (categories). Have a child give "fire" to a friend (choice-making).

Theme: At the Farm (July, Week 3)

Toy: Walking and Mooing Cow

Purpose: identification and classification, environmental clues, pretend play, turn taking

Game: Create a barn out of a cardboard box and place the cow and other animals around the farm. Have the children sit in a circle. Each child will take a turn to make the cow walk inside the barn for milking.

Expansion of Game: A child can make the cow follow directions (stop and go), stop inside (opposites), walk to the chicken (identification and classification), or walk to a favorite animal (choice-making).

TABLE 3

Types of Battery-Operated Toys

Sensory Input	Battery-Operated Toy	Manufacturer
Visual	Big Red Locomotive (shining light)	Toys for Special Children
	Fancy Feet Caterpillar (blinking nose and antennae)	Handicapped Children's Technological Services
	Fireman's Hat	Radio Shack
	Space ship or police car with light	Radio Shack
Auditory	Barking Dog	Crestwood
	Drumming Bear	Steven Kanor
	Mooing Cow	Toys for Special Children
	Tape recorder	Toys for Special Children
	Whistle Locomotive	Handicapped Children's Technological Services
Tactile	Bumble Ball	Ertil Co.
	Fan	Steven Kanor
	Vibrating pillows	Steven Kanor
	Vibrating tube	Steven Kanor

Theme: Bugs (August, Week 3)

Toy: Fancy Feet Caterpillar

Purpose: letter and color identification, categories, concepts

Game: Make an apple tree out of construction paper. Create different colored apples from construction paper and label some of the apples with the letter A and the others with the letter B. The hungry caterpillar is going to eat the fallen green apple or the apple with the letter B.

Expansion of Game: Hold up an apple with the letter A and have the child move the caterpillar to find that apple (matching). Have the child move the caterpillar to his favorite colored apple (choice-making). Create some paper worms and have the child move the caterpillar to the worm, not the apple (discrimination).

Switches and battery-operated toys can bring a lot of fun to children and therapists during intervention. The proper selection of the switch and the switch site are crucial for effective interaction. Thematic units will help organize battery-operated switch toys into entertaining games that address many educational goals.

Augmentative Communication

The word *augment* means to enhance or support. Therefore, augmentative communication includes any aids, techniques, and approaches that support an individual's efforts to communicate. Aids are any objects that are used when communicating with others and can include items such as paper, pencils, phones, picture boards, and computers. Techniques are the methods that are used when communicating with others. These methods can include gestures, facial expressions, direct selection, and scanning. An approach is the way that aids and techniques work together to make the communication attempt meaningful. An example of an unsuccessful approach would be a person who could not read receiving a letter from a doctor. The communication attempt was not successful because the person receiving the letter was not able to understand it. In this example, it

was the communication aid that hindered the communication. If the person received a phone call from the doctor about the same information, the communication attempt would have been successful.

A child might need an augmentative communication system for any number of reasons:

- a child has a significant discrepancy between receptive and expressive language
- current speech and communication skills limit further development
- decreased opportunities exist for participation in daily activities in school, home, and community due to communication problems
- communication opportunities are restricted to specific partners, such as Mom or a teacher, or specific environments
- there is evidence of frustration from the child or the communication partners (Shane and Bashir 1980)

The team can address the issues surrounding the need for an augmentative communication system as part of the ongoing assessment of the child.

Team Members in the Assessment Process

Augmentative communication can mean the difference between communication and no communication. An augmentative communication system allows children to have more control over their lives and to have opportunities to interact with their peers and with adults. Finding an appropriate augmentative communication system for a child is a collaborative effort. The speech-language pathologist, occupational therapist, physical therapist, teacher, and the family all have valuable input to the process. The team also needs a member who is an expert in augmentative communication. This person might be the speech-language pathologist or a technology specialist. If there is no team expert, an outside referral must be made.

Each team member provides valuable information about the functioning level of a child. Table 4 gives some examples of the specific areas that each member may be able to address. All of this information needs to be collected before a specific system can be developed. This process cannot be jumped into quickly and without planning. An unplanned process will result in an inappropriate system. When all of the information has been gathered, the team can collaborate with the augmentative communication expert to choose an appropriate system.

There is a difference between an augmentative communication system and an augmentative communication device. The system is the "total" way that a child communicates. It includes the child's aids as well as the techniques used for communication. Children can communicate with a variety of techniques (for example, gestures, facial expressions, and direct selection) and a variety of aids (such as computers, picture boards, and voice output devices). So each child communicates with specific aids and specific techniques. A device is the specific aid that is used by a child; for instance, Whisper Wolf or Cannon Communicator. The device is not the only way that a child communicates. The child may also use nonverbal communication or gestures. For example, Ian, who is able to wave "hello" and shake his head for "no," would not need these symbols on his picture communication board. Ian is able to communicate these ideas through gestures. Keep in mind that a device is not the only way a child can communicate. The augmentative communication expert will address the child's complete communication needs and abilities to create a communication system that can include an augmentative communication device.

When an appropriate system is devised, it is imperative to have the system functioning in the early intervention environment. This includes the playground, snack time, field trips, and all other aspects of the program. The final part of this section provides examples of some augmentative communication systems and how they can be incorporated into the intervention program.

Incorporating Systems into the Intervention Program

Picture communication boards are fairly common in many early intervention programs. The pictures are symbolic representations of objects, people, places, feelings, and other abstract concepts. The user must be able to select a picture to communicate. Touching the picture, pointing, eye gazing, or using a head stick pointer are most of the ways in which a child can select a picture. Using picture communication boards has advantages and disadvantages. One advantage is that the boards are very durable. Contact paper and lamination have made these systems waterproof and resistant to daily wear and tear. A child can use these systems even during the messiest tactile activity. These systems are also very portable. The boards can be easily carried by the child or an adult. The boards are lightweight and can be constructed in a variety of shapes and sizes to meet various needs.

TABLE 4

Assessment Areas for Team Members

Team Members	Assessment Areas
Classroom Teacher	cause and effect object permanence identification classification discrimination understanding opposites means vs. end problem solving
Occupational Therapist	visual acuity horizontal and vertical scanning figure-to-ground contrast eye-hand coordination fine motor movements positioning oral-motor movements
Physical Therapist	consistent motor movements seating and positioning range of motion reflexes endurance
Speech-Language Pathologist	oral-motor movements expressive language nonverbal communication receptive language following directions hearing
Family Members	child's likes and dislikes other communication environments attention span endurance nonverbal communication

Finally, the cost of making boards is low. The picture symbols, paper, glue, scissors, and contact paper are the only materials needed.

These systems have disadvantages as well. The most significant disadvantage pertains to the vocabulary. The vocabulary on the picture board is fixed; therefore, it cannot be used in every activity or intervention session. The child may become bored using the same symbols over and over again. Also, the symbols cannot address all of the communication needs for each activity. A picture board would need to be constructed for each planned activity. For example, if the day includes circle time, sensory play, snack, quiet time, and gross motor, and finishes up with a game, the interventionist would need a picture board for each of these different activities. The result would be a lot of picture boards. The interventionist would have to take time away from other activities to create all of these boards. This problem also occurs with many preprogrammed devices. The Whisper Wolf and the Intro Talker, for example, contain preprogrammed symbols and are voice-output devices. The interventionist will need to preprogram the device for each activity. Again this process is time-consuming and requires additional training.

Sign language is another augmentative system that can be incorporated into the classroom. Instead of having only one child learn the signs, the whole class can learn them. If a cooking activity is planned, each child will learn the sign for "cookie." Circle time is another wonderful opportunity for the whole class to incorporate sign. Many songs, such as "Wheels on the Bus" or "If You're Happy and You Know It," have movement and signs associated with them. The class can learn the sign for "bus" when singing "Wheels on the Bus." Storybook time also lends itself to signing. When looking at a picture book, sign and name the pictures. Incorporate signs into simple fairy tales and nursery rhymes.

Summary

Remember that technology includes anything that makes life easier. Therefore, technology can be considered a tool for completing a task or a function within society. Without incorporating technology effectively, computers will collect dust because they are not being used and children will sit around bored with turning on and off the same battery-operated switch toy. Keep in mind that children will be excluded if they do not have an appropriate system to communicate. Technology is a tool that empowers children with disabilities to interact with their world.

9 Monitoring Individual Intervention Programs

As interventionists in activity-based programs, our goal is to help children achieve desired developmental outcomes as they engage in functional, meaningful, and enjoyable activities. How do we know if we have accomplished this goal? We do so by monitoring the intervention program that the team has designed for each child. Monitoring involves examining and evaluating the intervention endeavors to identify any adjustments that need to be made. Often, monitoring is considered onerous busywork. It is important to remember, however, that even the most carefully planned and skillfully executed programs may need fine-tuning. Program monitoring, therefore, is an opportunity to make a child's program more effective, functional, or enjoyable. It should enhance intervention efforts, not detract from them. This chapter presents an approach for developing a monitoring plan. It also describes some strategies for collecting and analyzing data.

Developing a Monitoring Plan

Informal program monitoring occurs constantly during intervention sessions as interventionists observe children and respond to their behavioral cues. Program monitoring also occurs as teams debrief after a session and during team meetings when they discuss what worked, what didn't work, and what to do differently next time. Most teams also need a more systematic monitoring strategy to make sure they consider all aspects of intervention. A plan ensures that monitoring is conducted in a thorough, yet efficient, manner. A monitoring plan should be simple and enable the team to gather sufficient information to make needed adjustments in a child's program. It should not be so complicated and elaborate that it

overwhelms the intervention efforts. To develop a monitoring plan, a team needs to make decisions about the following program aspects:

- target—what will be monitored?
- schedule—how often will monitoring take place?
- circumstances—when and where will monitoring take place?
- method—how will information be gathered and analyzed?

Targets

Children's goals and objectives are the most common targets for monitoring. This type of monitoring is called *outcome monitoring* because it examines the results of intervention. It answers the question, "Were the child's goals achieved?" Of course, that is a very broad question. As a result, single goals, learning objectives, or task-analyzed segments of objectives are individually monitored.

In addition to goals and objectives, let's also consider the intervention process itself, another aspect of the program that can be monitored. The goals stated at the beginning of this chapter contained references to process (engagement in functional, meaningful, and enjoyable activities) as well as results (desired developmental outcomes). A monitoring plan, therefore, might also address both of these aspects. *Process monitoring* examines the way that intervention was provided. It answers the question, "Did we do what we had planned?" The answer to this question is important for several reasons. It can sometimes explain why desired outcomes were not achieved. Think about a child who is not reaching a goal that involves choice-making. Process monitoring could indicate that the child was not provided with opportunities to make choices in the classroom.

It could also reveal that the child's attempts to indicate choices went largely unrecognized. This information can help the team make decisions about how the program should be modified. In this instance, the team could make changes to ensure that opportunities for choice-making exist and that attempts at choice-making are reinforced. If, however, process monitoring indicated that the program had been implemented as it was planned, different adjustments, such as use of peer models or verbal prompts, might be made.

Process monitoring can provide information about the qualitative aspects of intervention. Just as interventionists use task analysis to narrow the focus of outcome monitoring, teams can also target specific aspects of the intervention process. Depending on their needs, teams may address areas such as the pace of activities, transition between activities, children's enjoyment of activities, or classroom atmosphere. Finally, process monitoring is a valuable staff development tool. It can help interventionists focus on their own actions and responses during intervention to ensure that they are supporting and enhancing children's learning experiences.

The information about schedules, circumstances, and methods discussed in the next sections are presented from an outcome-monitoring perspective. The reader should remember, however, that the same principles apply to process monitoring. The only difference is that the target shifts from outcomes to processes.

Schedule

Some interventionists feel obligated to collect data on each of the children's goals every day. Some behaviorally based programs allow for daily data collection. In most settings, however, this is an unrealistic expectation. Often data is collected but never analyzed. If data is not used to evaluate or adjust the child's program, the data collection effort was nothing more than busywork for the interventionist. The frequency of data collection should be driven by the team's need and ability to make adjustments in the child's program. There is no simple formula to determine how frequently data should be gathered. The frequency of data collection will differ depending on the goal, the child, and the team. Once a month, or even quarterly, may be sufficient for

certain objectives. Conversely, high-priority goals require more frequent data collection and analysis, perhaps on a weekly basis. Each team must decide what is useful and manageable for them. Most teams attempt to stagger data collection so that it is spaced throughout the week, month, or quarter. This process allows them to analyze the data as it is collected and put it to immediate use. It also prevents the overload that can occur if all data collection and analysis efforts are compressed into a short period of time.

Circumstances

When planning activities, teams have already identified opportunities for children to develop and exhibit certain developmental behaviors in various environments. Planning makes it easy for the team to select an activity that has a high probability of eliciting the target behavior. When selecting the activity during which data will be collected, it is important to consider whether the target goal addresses skill acquisition or generalization. Acquisition goals are more easily monitored during planned activities because the environment has been designed to facilitate and support certain abilities. Generalization goals need to be monitored in a variety of routine and spontaneous activities as well as in different environments.

Methods

Data collection involves observing and recording behaviors. Many interventionists find it difficult to facilitate an intervention session and simultaneously record data. They feel it interferes with the flow of the activities and impairs their ability to interact effectively. In the case of process monitoring, it is very demanding to observe and record one's own behavior during a session. In this type of situation, a team approach is quite helpful. One member of the team acts as the facilitator of the session while another team member serves as the observer and recorder. Another option is to record the session on videotape for later analysis. Sometimes, however, when neither technology nor other team members are available, the interventionist must observe and record as well as participate in the session. Recording does not necessarily have to be done with pencil and paper. Some interventionists have developed creative approaches to observation such as moving rubber bands from one wrist to the other as behaviors occur. Although acting as a facilitator and recorder at the same time is not an optimal situation, brief (5 to 10 minutes) data collection periods allow most interventionists to collect sufficient data without serious detriment to either the session or data collection.

Methods for collecting and analyzing data fall into one of two broad categories. Quantitative methods deal with numerical measurement, whereas qualitative methods are concerned with descriptions and relationships. Either of these can be used to collect and analyze data in an activity-based program. The method chosen depends upon the way in which an outcome, goal, or objective is stated. A match must be made between the way the goal or objective is written and the data collection/analysis strategy that is used. Consider the following objective: Tikia will walk ten feet while an adult holds one hand. In order to determine if Tikia achieved the goal, we need to measure how far she walked. A quantitative approach is therefore needed. Another of Tikia's goals is: Tikia will explore and manipulate objects using a variety of play schemes. For this goal, a description of Tikia's play schemes and the situations in which she used them would be appropriate, thus indicating the need for a qualitative approach.

Quantitative Methods

Several quantitative strategies are frequently used to monitor outcomes. One quantitative technique involves simple measurement. To collect information on Tikia's walking goal, we would simply measure how far she walked. Another quantitative method is event recording in which a tally or count is made of specific events, actions, objects, or behaviors. Placing a mark on a chart when a child uses the toilet is an example of event recording. Other examples include counting the number of times a child imitates a physical movement, the number of rings placed on a stacking pole, or the number of syllables in a child's utterance.

Some objectives are written not in terms of number or distance, but in terms of time. For these goals, duration and latency recording are appropriate. Duration recording measures the extent of time during which a behavior occurs. This type of recording could be used to monitor the amount of time that a child engages in a specific activity or to measure a child's tolerance for a new orthotic. Latency recording measures the length of time that elapses between the onset of a stimulus and the occurrence of a behavior. Latency recording would be appropriate to determine the time between presentation of a switch toy and a child's activation of the toy. This method could also be used to measure the time between the presentation of a direction and a child's response to it.

A final quantitative strategy involves the use of permanent products. A permanent product is something tangible that can be measured after a behavior takes place. Permanent products include artwork, scribbles, or writing samples. A collection of permanent products is called a *portfolio* and can be used as a record of a child's abilities. For example, if a child's goal was to draw a face containing eyes, a nose, and a mouth, the drawing itself (a permanent product) would provide appropriate data for analysis.

Quantitative data is analyzed by comparing the collected data with previously established criteria. The criteria may be stated as part of the learning objective. Tikia's walking objective established a distance of ten feet as the criterion for achievement. Other times, a comparison is made between the collected data and a baseline that was established before intervention began. Consider the following goal: Tikia will increase her vocalizations 60% over baseline. In this instance, collected data would be compared with the abilities that Tikia displayed at the time the goal was written. Line graphs and bar charts are visual representations of data and can be useful tools not only for analyzing data but for communicating quantitative results to others.

Qualitative Methods

The qualitative methods most frequently used for monitoring individual programs are rating scales and anecdotal records. Rating scales provide descriptive information in an abbreviated form. Teams develop rating scales and determine the specificity of the coding categories based on the child's goals, abilities, and the aspect of the goal selected for monitoring. One example is an assistance scale that can be used to record the type of support needed to complete hand washing. An illustration of an assistance scale is provided in figure 2. Other rating scales might include those based on categories of social play (solitary, parallel, associative) or types of imitation (motor, facial, vocal, verbal).

Anecdotal records provide a description of what children do and how they do it. Because descriptive measures emphasize the quality of performance, this type of data collection is especially appropriate for goals involving social-emotional development and cognitive processes. The time elapsed between when the child was observed and when the information was recorded affects the accuracy of anecdotal notes. Some interventionists have found it useful to take notes on sticky labels that can be added to the child's folder at the end of the day. Although it is tempting to "observe now, record later," the caliber of the data will be significantly reduced. It is also important to remember that the quality of anecdotal data depends on the amount and type of detail provided in the record. Writing detailed anecdotal records can be very time-consuming and

teams should be aware of the time required when developing their monitoring plan.

The goal of a qualitative approach is to both describe and explain what was observed. Analysis involves reading, reviewing, and examining the data to identify patterns and relationships. Analysis also involves searching for factors that influence the child's ability to achieve the desired outcomes and evaluating the impact of these factors on the child's program.

Modifying the Program

Once data has been collected and analyzed, the resulting information should be used to make appropriate adjustments in the child's individual program. Program modification involves revising a team's plan for a child; therefore, the strategy for making these modifications involves repeating the strategic planning steps presented in chapters 2, 5, 6, and 7.

Name: Molly		
Activity: hand washing		
Day/Time	Code	Notes/Comments
		Coding Key: H—hand-over-hand assistance P—physical prompt G—gestural prompt V—verbal prompt I—independent completion O—other (specify)

Figure 2. Sample Assistance Scale

▤10 Sample Activities for Use Throughout the Year

How to Use This Chapter

This chapter contains a series of sample activities that are appropriate for activity-based intervention. As mentioned in the introduction, these fall into the category of planned activities. Any intervention program would also incorporate a certain number of routine and child-initiated activities. Examples of such activities are not included here, since the focus of this book is on planned activities. Nevertheless, it is expected that some activities from these other categories would be included in an ongoing intervention program.

Some generic goals accompany each activity. These goals are organized roughly in a hierarchy, beginning with basic sensory responses, moving through increasingly complex motor and cognitive objectives, and ending with the most complex tasks of social interaction. As with the goals, the activities within each weekly set are also roughly hierarchial. Thus, each suggested activity may have a sensory component, but the activities at the beginning of the set will stress more basic sensory and motor goals whereas the later activities will require more complex cognitive, language, and social objectives. This arrangement provides built-in sensorimotor preparation time so that children with sensory or motor difficulties will be given the maximum opportunity to be ready physically and neurologically to benefit from the more complex learning opportunities presented later in the set.

Although it is important to progress from easier activities to those that are more challenging, the sequence of activities should not be inflexible. Adapt the sequence to suit the needs of your group and situation. Another possible arrangement is a "stations" approach (described in chapter 2) in which several of the activities are set up at the same time in different parts of the room. The children then move from station to station. Adults usually need to provide some structure to this arrangement, such as limiting the number of children who can participate at each station and the amount of time children can play at a particular station. The goal, as always, is to achieve the appropriate balance between flexibility and structure.

Please remember, too, that generic goals are just that. They are not intended to take the place of individualized goals for each child. For example, trunk rotation may be listed as a possible goal associated with the Riding Toys activity (December, Week 1, Activity 1). Trunk rotation may be facilitated as the interventionist helps Tamika climb onto and off of the tricycle. Trunk rotation may not be a goal right now for Michael, who uses an adaptive tricycle that provides full back and side support. He may be working on developing reciprocal leg movements as he pushes his tricycle's adapted pedals. Not all goals listed for an activity will apply to all children, nor are all possible goals listed. Rather, general categories of goals are listed, leaving to the intervention team the task of selecting and modifying appropriate goals for each child.

One set of activities per week is presented, beginning with September and continuing through August. The activities are organized around weekly themes within a more general monthly theme. These themes tend to reflect the culture and seasonal patterns of the authors' mid-Atlantic U.S. background. Some of these themes are not applicable to all parts of the United States. For example, the winter theme features snow, which is not as relevant in southern states as it is in other areas of the country. We recognize these regional differences and encourage interventionists to modify and adapt activities so that they are more appropriate. Researching local traditions and incorporating them into intervention activities enhance children's learning and deepen the links they have with their community.

We have attempted to provide activities that are appropriate for children and families from a wide range of cultures. Since we are not equally familiar with all traditions, we may have made errors both of omission and of commission. If so, we apologize for any unintended insensitivity and would appreciate hearing your comments on the appropriateness of any of these activities for various populations. We also wish to emphasize that seasonal activities and themes are intended to represent cultural rather than religious expressions. We encourage interventionists to substitute or add activities that are appropriate to the cultures represented in their programs. We have found that such activities, when presented in an atmosphere of cultural exchange, have sometimes gone a long way toward promoting closer working relationships and establishing trust between families and interventionists, as well as among families of different backgrounds. We also urge interventionists to continue to explore and develop their cultural competence. This is an area in which one can never finish growing.

The activities presented in this chapter were developed for a once-a-week, center-based infant intervention group. Many of these activities were successfully used with infants between the ages of one and two years. Younger infants were also incorporated into the activities. We have tried to provide enough activities to fill a 2- to 3-hour session each week and, in some weeks, we have provided more than enough activities for that amount of time. We believe that the core of activities provided should be enough to spark additional ideas for intervention programs that run several days a week and maintain the weekly themes suggested.

It is not our intention to provide a "cookbook" for the intervention year, but instead to provide an outline to be adapted and filled in as appropriate for each individual program. Some activities may be too challenging for a group or may not provide enough challenge. We hope that the preceding chapters will help teams modify these activities to provide the appropriate amount of challenge for each group and, within each group, for each individual child. Some activities, as mentioned above, may not be regionally or culturally suitable. Please substitute, adapt, or modify as needed. We hope that the activities presented here will merely serve as springboards to the individual creativity of each interventionist and program. Have fun!

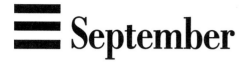# September

Week 1   Overall Theme: Who Am I?

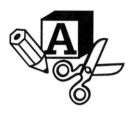

Activity 1: Mirror Exploration

Materials

mirrors, preferably full-length as well as hand-held

Goals

Sensory
- to improve body awareness
- to improve visual attending
- to increase attention span

Gross Motor
- to improve motor planning, balance, and coordination

Fine Motor
- to improve reach and grasp, grasp and release, hand manipulation, and midline skills

Cognitive
- to improve understanding of spatial relationships, imitation, and concept development
- to develop generalization skills

Language
- to improve following directions; taking turns; identifying/labeling body parts, actions, people, and relationships; requesting; initiating

Social
- to facilitate peer interaction

Directions

After introducing the session, provide small mirrors for the children to use to take turns looking at their reflections. Then move on to full-length mirrors (horizontal on the floor for infants who are not yet upright). Talk about body parts as the child looks at or moves different parts. Repeat each child's name frequently. Name body parts and see if children can identify them first on themselves, then on others. With more advanced children, encourage them to imitate each other—pick partners and be each other's "mirror." Adapt this activity for children who are not yet ready for more advanced activities by gently touching, rubbing, or patting hands, arms, and legs and naming the part touched while the child looks in the mirror.

Activity 2: Body Tracing

Materials

large roll of butcher paper

markers or crayons

Goals

Sensory
- to improve responses to sensory stimulation
- to increase attention span
- to increase body awareness

Gross Motor
- to improve motor planning

Cognitive
- to improve imitation, understanding of spatial relationships, and concept development
- to develop generalization skills

Language
- to improve following directions; taking turns; identifying/labeling body parts, actions, people, and relationships; requesting; and initiating

Directions

Unroll a section of paper on the floor and have a child lie on it while an adult traces the child's body. Name each body part as it is being traced. Repeat each child's name several times during the activity.

Activity 3: Rub-a-Dub-Dub

Materials

several items of various textures

Goals

Sensory
- to improve response to tactile stimulation
- to increase attention span
- to increase body awareness

Gross Motor
- to improve motor planning, balance, coordination, trunk rotation, and weight shifting

Fine Motor
- to improve reach and grasp, grasp and release, eye-hand coordination, and visual attending and tracking

Cognitive
- to improve imitation, concept development, and object permanence
- to develop generalization skills

Language
- to improve following directions; taking turns; identifying/labeling body parts, actions, people, and relationships; requesting; and initiating

Social
- to make choices
- to facilitate peer interaction

Directions

Show children a container full of different textured objects. Encourage them to choose different textured items to rub on themselves and each other. (Children should always ask before rubbing an item on someone else. Adults will probably have to facilitate this for the children. Adults should also ask before they rub an item on a child.) Talk about how the textures look and feel. Name the body parts being rubbed. Facilitate gross motor skills through positioning; for example, side-sitting while playing with the textures can facilitate balance and coordination. Positioning the materials so that the child has to reach to the sides can facilitate trunk rotation. Children who show signs of tactile defensiveness can benefit from deep pressure, brushing, or firm rubbing with hands or a washcloth before, during, and after this activity. Give them as much control as possible over their level of participation with the textures.

Activity 4: Paper-Plate Faces

Materials

paper plates	construction paper
yarn	tongue depressors
scissors	glue
paintbrushes (optional)	cotton swabs (optional)
table	chairs (adaptive seating as needed)
washcloths for cleanup	

Goals

Sensory
- to improve sensory awareness through tactile stimulation
- to increase visual attending
- to increase attention span

Fine Motor
- to improve hand/finger manipulation, eye-hand coordination, using both hands together, reach and grasp, grasp and release, and midline skills

Cognitive
- to improve understanding of spatial relationships, imitation, tool use, functional object use, and concept development
- to develop generalization skills
- to develop recall skills

Language
- to improve following directions; taking turns; increasing vocabulary; identifying/labeling objects, actions, characteristics, and relationships; initiating; and requesting

Social
- to make choices

Directions

Ahead of time, cut out eyes, noses, and mouths from the construction paper. Cut some yarn for hair. Position children seated around tables for fine motor activity. Give each child a paper plate. Show the children a sample of how the face will look when they are finished. Have them select the color eyes they want to use. Help children squeeze or spread glue onto their plates, encouraging them to stabilize the plates with one hand, if possible. Vary the activity by having them spread the glue with paintbrushes or cotton swabs. Help them put the eyes onto the glue. Repeat with noses, mouths, and hair. Provide as much assistance as needed. Use lots of language to describe what the children are doing, what features they are gluing, and who is gluing what. Let the pictures dry while completing another activity.

Snack

Materials

audio player	recording of "Aiken Drum"*
rice cakes	cups (adapted if necessary)
peanut butter	napkins
raisins	juice
olives	table
bananas	chairs (adaptive seating as needed)
table knives	washcloths for cleanup
plates	

Goals

Sensory
- to improve responses to sensory stimuli, especially tactile and olfactory
- to increase attention span

Fine Motor
- to improve using both hands together, reach and grasp, grasp and release, hand/finger manipulation, and eye-hand coordination

Self-Help
- to improve self-feeding skills
- to improve oral-motor skills

Cognitive
- to improve tool use, understanding of spatial relationships, functional use of objects, imitation, and concept development
- to develop generalization skills
- to develop recall skills

Language
- to improve following directions; taking turns; identifying/labeling objects, actions, people, and characteristics; initiating; and requesting

---

* This recording can be found in many children's/folk collections.

Social
- to make choices
- to facilitate peer interaction

Directions

Seat children appropriately for snack, using adaptive seating as needed. Play recording of "Aiken Drum" and assemble the snack as children watch. Tell them they are going to make "Aiken Drums." Give each child a table knife and a rice cake. Help them spread the peanut butter on the rice cake. Let them choose what they will use for eyes (olives suggested), nose (raisins), mouth (banana slice). Describe what they are doing, what the snack is made of, and what it looks like. Talk about how it looks like a face. Sing a version of "Aiken Drum" for each child's combination. Encourage communication, including ways to request more or indicate "all done." Offer juice as needed. Assist with self-feeding and drinking skills as needed.

Week 2

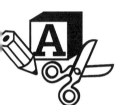

Overall Theme: Hands

Activity 1: Hands On

Materials

indoor climbing structure	toddler slide
inner tubes	indoor tunnel
ramp or other incline	rope
floor pillows/beanbag chairs	benches
bolsters	steps
indoor swing	

Goals

Sensory
- to improve responses to sensory stimulation
- to provide vestibular stimulation
- to provide proprioceptive stimulation
- to improve visual attending
- to increase attention span

Gross Motor
- to improve balance, coordination, motor planning, locomotion, trunk rotation, and weight shifting

Fine Motor
- to improve using both hands together, reach and grasp, and hand manipulation
- to increase upper body strength
- to improve shoulder girdle strength and stability

Cognitive
- to improve understanding of spatial relationships, imitation, problem solving, and concept development

Language
- to improve following directions; taking turns; identifying/labeling objects, actions, descriptions, and locations; requesting; and initiating

Social
- to make choices
- to facilitate peer interaction

Directions

Using the equipment available, set up an indoor obstacle course to facilitate gross motor and vestibular goals for individuals in the group. The materials listed above are just suggestions. Use the rope as a guide through the course. Assist the children through the obstacle course, having them hold onto the rope with their hands and follow it through the course activities. Encourage the children to use appropriate motor patterns throughout. Use lots of language to describe what is happening, who is doing what, and to indicate relationships; for example, "Tim is up on the slide; Maria is behind the beanbag."

Activity 2: Hands Down

Materials

Goals

Sensory
- to improve responses to sensory stimulation
- to provide proprioceptive input
- to improve body awareness
- to increase attention span

Gross Motor
- to improve coordination, motor planning, weight shifting, and reciprocal movement patterns

Fine Motor
- to improve shoulder girdle strength and stability
- to increase upper body strength

Cognitive
- to improve understanding of spatial relationships, imitation, and concept development

Language
- to improve following directions; taking turns; identifying/labeling actions, descriptions, and locations; requesting; and initiating

Directions

Have children take turns doing the wheelbarrow walk with adults supporting them at the legs or hips. You can introduce different textures for them to "walk" their hands over, but often a rug provides sufficient texture.

Activity 3: Hands Out

Materials

platform or hammock swing

variety of interesting small objects

Goals

Sensory
- to improve responses to vestibular stimulation
- to improve visual attending
- to increase attention span

Gross Motor
- to improve back extension against gravity and motor planning

Fine Motor
- to improve reach and grasp, grasp and release, hand manipulation, and eye-hand coordination
- to increase upper body strength

Cognitive
- to improve understanding of spatial relationships, imitation, and concept development

Language
- to improve following directions; taking turns; identifying/labeling people, actions, and relationships; requesting; and initiating

Directions

Position the hammock or platform swing so that the children are about 2 to 3 inches off the ground when on their tummies. Use the swing to support as much of their bodies as necessary. Encourage them to stretch out their arms. Gently move the swing back and forth, side to side, at diagonals, and even spinning in circles for those for whom this activity is appropriate. Scatter a variety of interesting small toys on the floor around the swing. Encourage the children to grab these objects as they swing by. Those who want to can try to grab objects with their eyes closed to heighten awareness of their hands even further.

Caution: Vestibular stimulation can have powerful effects. This activity should be planned in consultation with the physical or occupational therapist. Spinning, in particular, should be carried out only under the supervision of a trained occupational or physical therapist.

Activity 4: Hand Sounds

Materials

Goals

Sensory
- to increase attention span
- to improve auditory awareness

Gross Motor
- to improve balance and coordination

Fine Motor
- to improve using both hands together, hand manipulation, and midline skills

Cognitive
- to improve imitation and concept development

Language
- to improve following directions; taking turns; listening; identifying/labeling objects, actions, people, and concepts; initiating; and requesting

Directions

Explore hand sounds: clap, slap, tap, knock, snap, and drum fingers. How many different sounds can you make with your hands? Encourage children to imitate your sounds and actions. Talk about the sounds. How does it feel to make them? Can you make them louder? Softer? Incorporate concepts as appropriate to the level of the group.

Activity 5: Hands In

Materials

finger paint
spoons or tongue depressors for scooping paint
smocks
washcloths for cleanup
chairs (adaptive seating as needed)

finger-paint paper
container of water
soap for cleanup
table

Goals

Sensory
- to improve responses to sensory stimulation
- to increase attention span

Gross Motor
- to improve balance, coordination, and control of flexion/extension patterns

Fine Motor
- to improve visual attending and tracking, hand manipulation, midline skills, and finger isolation
- to increase upper body strength
- to improve shoulder girdle strength and stability

Cognitive
- to improve imitation, concept development, and sequencing
- to develop generalization skills

Language
- to improve following directions; taking turns; identifying/labeling objects, actions, descriptions, relationships, and people; initiating; and requesting

Social
- to make choices
- to facilitate peer interaction

Directions

Give each child a piece of finger-paint paper. Let each child select which color paint to use. Sprinkle each child's paper with water and put a dab of the selected paint on the paper. Provide physical assistance to children as needed. Encourage those children who are able to use individual fingers to make fingerprints and designs. Use lots of language to describe the motions and colors. This activity can facilitate even more peer interaction if the group works together on a single large sheet of paper.

Caution: Young children tend to eat the paint. If you think this will happen in your group, substitute colorful pudding for paint. Although you can't hang pudding paint pictures on the wall, remember that it is the process that is important here, not the final product.

Snack

Materials

thumbprint cookies (see Appendix C for recipe)	juice
	cups (adapted if necessary)
napkins	chairs (adaptive seating as needed)
table	washcloths for cleanup

Goals

Sensory
- to improve responses to sensory stimuli, especially tactile and olfactory
- to increase attention span

Fine Motor
- to improve reach and grasp, grasp and release, hand manipulation, and eye-hand coordination

Self-Help
- to improve self-feeding skills
- to improve oral-motor skills

Cognitive
- to improve functional object use, imitation, understanding of spatial relationships, and concept formation
- to develop generalization skills

Language
- to improve following directions; taking turns; identifying/labeling objects, actions, people, and characteristics; requesting; and initiating

Social
- to make choices
- to facilitate peer interaction

Directions

Seat children appropriately for snack, using adaptive seating as needed. Offer thumbprint cookies and talk about why they are called that. Encourage communication, including ways to request more or indicate "all done." Assist with self-feeding and oral-motor skills as needed. Offer juice and assistance with drinking skills as needed.

Week 3

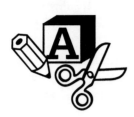

Overall Theme: Feet

Activity 1: Footpath

Materials

a variety of textured materials, such as:

cotton balls	styrofoam chips
sand	rice
cellophane grass	artificial grass (such as Astroturf®)
carpet squares	lamb's wool
cooked pasta (cooled)	
shallow containers	

Goals

Sensory
- to improve responses to tactile stimulation
- to improve body awareness

Gross Motor
- to improve motor planning, balance, coordination, locomotion, weight bearing, and weight shifting

Fine Motor
- to improve hand manipulation, finger isolation, and grasp and release

Cognitive
- to improve understanding of spatial relationships, imitation, concept development, and sequencing

Language
- to improve following directions; taking turns; identifying/labeling objects, people, and actions; initiating; and requesting

Social
- to facilitate peer interaction

Directions

Fill shallow containers with various textured materials. Construct a "path" with the containers. Help the children walk along the path, stepping in each container. Use lots of language to describe the activity. How does it feel? What does it feel like? How does sand feel after stepping in the spaghetti? Children could also be encouraged to explore the materials with their hands and compare how the different textures feel in their hands versus on their feet.

Activity 2: Kick Ball

Materials

several balls of various sizes

Goals

Sensory
- to provide proprioceptive stimulation
- to improve body awareness
- to increase attention span

Gross Motor
- to improve motor planning, trunk rotation, balance, coordination, weight shifting, and weight bearing

Cognitive
- to improve understanding of spatial relationships, imitation, and concept development

Language
- to improve following directions; taking turns; identifying/labeling objects, people, actions, locations, and relationships; initiating; and requesting

Social
- to facilitate peer interaction

Directions

Group the children in a circle and bring out the balls. Encourage children to kick them to one another. They can begin this activity in sitting and move to standing if they are ready. Name the child kicking the ball and the child catching it. Encourage children to name the child to whom they are kicking the ball. Describe the balls; for example, big yellow ball or little red ball.

Activity 3: Big Feet

Materials

several pairs of adult-sized shoes and slippers

Goals

Sensory
- to improve responses to sensory stimulation
- to increase attention span

Gross Motor
- to improve balance, coordination, visual attending and tracking, motor planning, and locomotion

Fine Motor
- to improve hand manipulation, midline skills, reaching and grasping, and using both hands together

Cognitive
- to improve classification, understanding of spatial relationships, functional object use, and concept development
- to develop generalization skills

Language
- to improve following directions; taking turns; identifying/labeling objects, actions, people, and characteristics; initiating; and requesting

Social
- to make choices
- to facilitate peer interaction

Directions

Have the children sit in a circle. Put the shoes in the center of the circle in a pile. Encourage the children to choose shoes to try on. Provide assistance as needed. Encourage those children who are walking to try walking while wearing the "big shoes." Use lots of language to describe these activities.

Activity 4: Foot Painting

Materials

finger paint
spoons or tongue depressors
  for scooping paint
soap for cleanup
table

finger-paint paper
container of water
washcloths for cleanup
chairs (adaptive seating
  as needed)

Goals

Sensory
- to improve responses to sensory stimulation
- to increase attention span

Gross Motor
- to improve balance, coordination, control of flexion/extension patterns, and motor planning

Fine Motor
- to improve visual attending and tracking

Cognitive
- to improve imitation, concept development, and sequencing
- to develop generalization skills

Language
- to improve following directions; taking turns; identifying/labeling objects, actions, descriptions, relationships, and people; initiating; and requesting

Social
- to make choices
- to facilitate peer interaction

Directions

Position children in sitting so their bare feet will reach the floor or a low table and so that their feet are free to move. Put a piece of finger-paint paper on the floor or table under their feet. Let each child select which color paint to use. Sprinkle each paper with water and put a dab of the selected color paint on the paper. Encourage children to paint with their feet. Provide physical assistance to children as needed. Use lots of language to describe the motions and colors. This activity can facilitate even more peer interaction if the group works together on a single large sheet of paper.

Caution: Young children tend to eat the paint. If you think this will happen in your group, substitute colorful pudding for paint. Although you can't hang pudding paint pictures on the wall, remember that it is the process that is important here, not the final product.

Snack

Materials

Bigfoot cookies*	juice
napkins	cups (adapted if necessary)
table	chairs (adaptive seating as needed)
washcloths for cleanup	

Goals

Sensory
- to improve responses to sensory stimuli, especially tactile and olfactory
- to increase attention span

Fine Motor
- to improve reach and grasp, grasp and release, hand/finger manipulation, and eye-hand coordination

Self-Help
- to improve self-feeding skills
- to improve oral-motor skills

Cognitive
- to improve functional object use, understanding of spatial relationships, imitation, and concept formation
- to develop generalization skills

Language
- to improve following directions; taking turns; identifying/labeling objects, actions, people, and characteristics; requesting; and initiating

Social
- to make choices
- to facilitate peer interaction

Directions

Seat children appropriately for snack, using adaptive seating as needed. Offer Bigfoot cookies and talk about why they are called that. Encourage communication, including ways to request more or indicate "all done." Assist with self-feeding and oral-motor skills as needed. Offer juice and assistance with drinking skills as needed.

---

* Bigfoot cookies are simply sugar cookies that have been cut in the shape of a foot. These can be made by tracing around a child's foot on a piece of cardboard and using the tracing as a pattern. Or they can simply be cut in the general shape of a foot.

Week 4

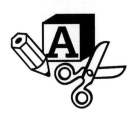

Overall Theme: Apples

Activity 1: Obstacle Course

Materials

indoor climbing structure	toddler slide
inner tubes	indoor tunnel
ramp or other incline	carpet squares
floor pillows/beanbag chairs	benches
bolsters	steps
indoor swing	a variety of apples (such as red, green,
containers for apples (baskets work best)	plastic, wooden)

Goals

Sensory
- to provide proprioceptive stimulation
- to improve visual attending
- to increase attention span

Gross Motor
- to improve balance, coordination, motor planning, locomotion, trunk rotation, weight bearing, and weight shifting

Fine Motor
- to improve using both hands together, reach and grasp, grasp and release, and hand manipulation
- to increase upper body strength
- to improve shoulder girdle strength and stability

Cognitive
- to improve object permanence, imitation, problem solving, classification, and concept development
- to develop generalization skills

Language
- to improve following directions; taking turns; identifying/labeling objects, actions, descriptions, and locations; requesting; and initiating

Social
- to make choices
- to facilitate peer interaction

Directions

Using the equipment available, set up an indoor obstacle course to facilitate the gross motor and vestibular goals for children in the group. The materials listed above are just suggestions. Place the apples at various points throughout the obstacle course. Make sure that some are hidden, some partially hidden, and some in plain sight. Assist the children through the obstacle course. A "path" of carpet squares can provide a structure to follow through the course. Encourage the children to use appropriate motor patterns throughout. Help them find the apples as they go through the course. Be sure to provide enough apples for each child to find at least two or three. Collect the apples in baskets or other containers. Depending on their abilities, children can be encouraged to carry their own baskets filled with apples.

Activity 2: Apple Roll

Materials

apples from previous activity

Goals

Sensory
- to increase attention span

Gross Motor
- to improve motor planning, trunk rotation, sitting balance, coordination, and weight shifting

Fine Motor
- to improve reach and grasp, grasp and release, eye-hand coordination, visual attending and tracking, and hand manipulation
- to increase upper body strength
- to improve shoulder girdle strength and stability

Cognitive
- to improve understanding of spatial relationships, imitation, and concept development
- to develop generalization skills
- to develop recall skills

Language
- to improve following directions; taking turns; identifying/labeling objects, people, actions, locations, and relationships; initiating; and requesting

Social
- to make choices
- to facilitate peer interaction

Directions

Seat the children in a circle on the floor and put the apples in the center of the circle. Encourage children to roll the apples to one another. Name the children who are rolling and catching the apples. Encourage the children to announce ahead of time to whom they are rolling an apple. Describe the apples; for example, big yellow apple or little red apple.

Activity 3: Sorting Apples

Materials

apples from previous activities

pictures of apples

Goals

Sensory
- to increase attention span

Gross Motor
- to improve balance, coordination, weight shifting, and trunk rotation

Fine Motor
- to improve reach and grasp, grasp and release, visual attending and tracking, eye-hand coordination, and hand manipulation

Cognitive
- to improve problem solving, picture-object association, imitation, classification, and concept development
- to develop generalization skills
- to develop recall skills

Language
- to improve following directions; taking turns; identifying/labeling objects, actions, locations, and relationships; initiating; and requesting

Social
- to make choices
- to facilitate peer interaction

Directions

Show the children the pictures of the apples and ask what they are. Ask which apples go with which pictures; for example, red with red, yellow with yellow. You may want to add some additional pictures to the collection to see how the children respond. Position children to facilitate gross motor goals during this activity.

Activity 4: Making Applesauce

Materials

apples	sharp knives
potato masher	cooking pot
water	stove
potholders	spoon
table	chairs (adaptive seating as needed)
washcloths for cleanup	

Goals

Sensory
- to improve responses to sensory stimuli, especially tactile and olfactory
- to increase attention span

Fine Motor
- to improve using both hands together, reach and grasp, grasp and release, and hand manipulation

Cognitive
- to improve functional object use, understanding of spatial relationships, classification, sequencing, imitation, and concept development
- to develop generalization skills

Language
- to improve following directions; taking turns; identifying/labeling objects, actions, characteristics, and relationships; initiating; and requesting

Social
- to make choices
- to facilitate peer interaction

Directions

Tell children that they are going to help make applesauce. Have them help peel and chop the apples. Give each child some apple pieces to put into the pot. Add water to the pot and put the pot on the stove to cook while continuing with the rest of the planned activities. As the apples cook, mash them from time to time with the potato masher for softer texture. If you use sweet apples, such as a mixture of golden delicious and some other slightly more tart apple, you will not need to add sugar. Use lots of language to discuss the process, including the changes happening to the ingredients as they cook. How do they look, taste, feel, smell before cooking? After cooking?

Activity 5: Apple Prints

Materials

apples	knife
tempera paint	construction paper
paper plates, pie tins, or saucers	smocks
table	chairs (adaptive seating as needed)
washcloths for cleanup	

Goals

Sensory
- to improve sensory awareness and responsiveness

Fine Motor
- to improve reach and grasp, grasp and release, eye-hand coordination, hand manipulation skills, using both hands together, and midline skills
- to increase upper body strength
- to improve shoulder girdle strength and stability

Cognitive
- to improve sequencing, imitation, and concept development
- to develop generalization skills
- to develop recall skills

Language
- to improve following directions; taking turns; increasing vocabulary; identifying/labeling objects, actions, people, places, characteristics, and relationships; requesting; and initiating

Social
- to make choices
- to facilitate peer interaction

Directions

Set up the activity on a small table. Seat the children or let them work in standing, according to the needs of the group. Have children identify the apples as an adult cuts them in halves. Cut some in half crosswise and some in half lengthwise. Compare the similarities and differences between the two types of pieces. Have children choose which color paper, apple half, and color paint they want to use. Demonstrate dipping the apple in the paint and pressing it onto the paper to make a print. Assist the children as needed with making their own prints. Talk about the feel of the paint and the apples, the colors being used, and the actions. Encourage children to trade apples and colors of paint with each other.

Snack

Materials

applesauce from Activity 4	bowls
spoons (adapted if necessary)	juice
cups (adapted if necessary)	napkins
table	chairs (adaptive seating as needed)
washcloths for cleanup	

Goals

Sensory
- to improve responses to sensory stimuli, especially tactile and olfactory
- to increase attention span

Fine Motor
- to improve using both hands together, reach and grasp, grasp and release, hand/finger manipulation, and eye-hand coordination

Self-Help
- to improve self-feeding skills
- to improve oral-motor skills

Cognitive
- to improve tool use, understanding of spatial relationships, functional object use, imitation, concept development, and sequencing
- to develop generalization skills
- to develop recall skills

Language
- to improve following directions; taking turns; identifying/labeling objects, actions, people, and characteristics; initiating; and requesting

Social
- to make choices
- to facilitate peer interaction

Directions

Seat children appropriately for snack. Have them pass out napkins and spoons, if appropriate. Serve small quantities of the applesauce. Talk about making the applesauce. How has it changed? How is it still the same? Provide assistance with self-feeding and oral motor skills as needed. Offer juice and provide assistance with drinking as needed.

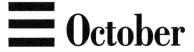 October

Week 1

Overall Theme: Autumn Leaves

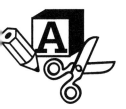

Activity 1: Leaf Walk

Materials

access to outdoors, if possible
bags or baskets for carrying leaves
strollers or other adaptive means of
  locomotion for children who are
  nonambulatory

a variety of leaves in various
  stages of color

Goals

Sensory
- to improve sensory awareness
- to increase attention span
- to improve auditory and visual attending skills

Gross Motor
- to improve walking, stooping/squatting, weight shifting, weight bearing, balance, coordination, and motor planning

Fine Motor
- to improve eye-hand coordination, reach and grasp, grasp and release, hand manipulation, and finger isolation (pointing)
- to increase upper body strength

Cognitive
- to improve classification, imitation, and concept development
- to develop generalization skills

Language
- to improve following directions; taking turns; increasing vocalization/ vocabulary; identifying and labeling objects, actions, characteristics, relationships, and locations; initiating; requesting; and questioning

Social
- to make choices
- to facilitate peer interaction

Directions

Have children hike along a path outdoors, if possible. Otherwise, set up a "path" indoors with leaves placed along the way. Let the children who are walking push the strollers for the children who are using them, thus helping the walking children to improve their upper body strength. Talk with the children about what they see, hear, and smell. Help them collect leaves in their bags or baskets. Ask questions about what they are doing and about the leaves they have found.

Activity 2: Leaf Piles

Materials

collection of fallen leaves

small slide (optional)

Goals

Sensory
- to improve responses to sensory stimulation
- to provide vestibular stimulation
- to provide proprioceptive stimulation
- to improve visual attending
- to increase attention span

Gross Motor
- to improve balance, coordination, motor planning, locomotion, trunk rotation, segmental rolling, and weight shifting

Fine Motor
- to improve using both hands together, reach and grasp, and grasp and release
- to increase upper body strength
- to improve shoulder girdle strength and stability

Cognitive
- to improve understanding of spatial relationships, object permanence, imitation, problem-solving, classification, and concept development
- to develop generalization skills

Language
- to improve following directions; taking turns; listening; auditory discrimination; identifying/labeling objects, actions, descriptions, and locations; requesting; and initiating

Social
- to facilitate peer interaction

Directions

This activity is best done outdoors, but leaves may be brought indoors if necessary. Assemble a pile of leaves. Encourage children to walk through the leaves, roll in the leaves, and jump in the leaves. A small slide may be set up so that the children land in the leaves when they slide down the slide. Throughout the activity, use lots of language to describe what is happening. How do the leaves look? Feel? Smell? Sound? Do they sound different when someone walks through them than they do when someone jumps in them?

Caution: Any child with a history of asthma or allergies may have difficulty with leaf molds and should not be covered with leaves.

Activity 3: Leaf Match

Materials

leaves collected in Activity 1

Goals

Sensory
- to improve visual attending
- to increase attention span

Gross Motor
- to improve balance, coordination, weight shifting, and trunk rotation

Fine Motor
- to improve reach and grasp, grasp and release, visual attending and tracking, eye-hand coordination, and hand/finger manipulation

Cognitive
- to improve problem solving, imitation, classification, and concept development
- to develop generalization skills
- to develop recall skills

Language
- to improve following directions; taking turns; identifying/labeling objects, actions, locations, and relationships; initiating; and requesting

Social
- to make choices
- to facilitate peer interaction

Directions

Gather the children together with the leaves they have collected. Have them spread out their leaves on the floor (or table) to see who has leaves that match. The children can match leaves by color, shape, or other features. Encourage children to talk about why the leaves they select match. Describe the features of all the leaves.

Activity 4: Leaf Prints

Materials

crayons	drawing paper
tape	leaves from previous activity
table	chairs (adaptive seating as needed)

Goals

Sensory
- to improve visual attending
- to increase attention span

Fine Motor
- to improve hand/finger manipulation, eye-hand coordination, using two hands together, reach and grasp, grasp and release, and midline skills
- to improve shoulder girdle strength and stability

Cognitive
- to improve tool use, concept development, and imitation
- to develop generalization skills

Language
- to improve following directions; taking turns; increasing vocabulary; identifying/labeling objects, actions, characteristics, and relationships; initiating; and requesting

Social
- to make choices
- to facilitate peer interaction

Directions

Seat children appropriately for fine motor activity. Have each child select one or more leaves (up to about five). Arrange the leaves under a sheet of drawing paper. Tape the edges of the paper to the table. Have children choose crayons to use. Show them how to rub the crayon across the paper to produce a leaf print. Talk about the process as you go through each step.

Leaf prints may be made in alternative ways, including dipping the leaves in paint and pressing a piece of paper over them, pressing leaves into clay, and finger-painting with leaves under the paper. Choose the activity that best meets the needs and abilities of the group.

Snack

Materials

gelatin jigglers prepared ahead of time in the shape of leaves (see recipe in Appendix C)
napkins
table
washcloths for cleanup

juice
paper plates
cups, adapted as needed
spoons (optional)
chairs (adaptive seating as needed)

Goals

Sensory
- to improve responses to sensory stimuli, especially tactile and olfactory
- to increase attention span

Fine Motor
- to improve reach and grasp, grasp and release, hand/finger manipulation, and eye-hand coordination

Self-Help
- to improve self-feeding skills
- to improve oral-motor skills

Cognitive
- to improve tool use, understanding of spatial relationships, imitation, sequencing, and concept development
- to develop generalization skills
- to develop recall skills

Language
- to improve following directions; taking turns; identifying/labeling objects, actions, people, and characteristics (color, texture, shape); requesting; and initiating

Social
- to make choices
- to facilitate peer interaction

Directions

Seat children at a table. Have them help pass out plates, if appropriate. Show children the jigglers. Encourage them to touch and describe the jigglers. Have children choose the shape and color they want. Facilitate appropriate feeding skills as necessary for each individual. Encourage communication, including ways to request more or indicate "all done." Offer juice and provide assistance as needed. Children may be offered spoons to use with the jigglers if appropriate and if spoon feeding is a goal.

Week 2

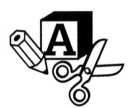

Overall Theme: Orange

Activity 1: Obstacle Course

Materials

indoor climbing structure
inner tubes
ramp or other incline
orange contact paper
benches
steps
orange beanbags

toddler slide
indoor tunnel
carpet squares
floor pillows/beanbag chairs
bolsters
indoor swing
containers for beanbags

Goals

Sensory
- to provide proprioceptive stimulation
- to provide vestibular stimulation
- to increase visual attending
- to increase attention span

Gross Motor
- to improve balance, coordination, motor planning, locomotion, trunk rotation, and weight shifting

Fine Motor
- to improve using both hands together, reach and grasp, and grasp and release
- to increase upper body strength
- to improve shoulder girdle strength and stability
- to improve object permanence, imitation, problem solving, understanding of spatial relationships, and concept development

Language
- to improve following directions; taking turns; identifying/labeling objects, actions, characteristics, and locations; requesting; and initiating

Social
- to make choices
- to facilitate peer interaction

Directions

Using the equipment available, set up an indoor obstacle course to facilitate the gross motor and vestibular goals of the individuals in the group. The materials listed above are just suggestions. Place the orange beanbags at various points throughout the obstacle course. Be sure that some are hidden, some partially hidden, and some in plain sight. Assist the children through the obstacle course. A "path" of carpet squares can provide a structure to follow through the course. Attach orange contact paper to carpet squares to enhance the color effect. Encourage the children to use appropriate motor patterns throughout. Help them find the beanbags as they go through the course. Be sure there are enough beanbags for each child to find at least two to three. Collect the beanbags in buckets or baskets, preferably orange ones. Depending on their abilities, children can be encouraged to carry their own buckets filled with beanbags.

Activity 2: Beanbags

Materials

several beanbags, preferably orange
basket or bin

Goals

Sensory
- to provide proprioceptive stimulation
- to increase attention span

Gross Motor
- to improve balance, weight shifting, and coordination

Fine Motor
- to improve eye-hand coordination, reach and grasp, grasp and release, and throwing
- to increase upper body strength
- to improve shoulder girdle strength and stability

Cognitive
- to improve understanding of spatial relationships, imitation, and concept development

Language
- to improve following directions; taking turns; identifying/labeling objects, actions, locations, and relationships; initiating; and requesting

Social
- to make choices
- to facilitate peer interaction

Directions

This activity usually works best if children are seated in a circle with the "target" (basket or bin) in the middle. Each child can take a beanbag from the bucket or adults can begin the activity by tossing beanbags to each child.

Encourage children to throw the beanbags into the target or to each other. They may need help to accomplish this task. Children who are not yet ready to throw can often begin by placing the beanbags into the container. Talk about the actions, who is throwing, and who is catching. Encourage children to name the person they would like to catch the beanbag. Emphasize the orange beanbags. An orange target (maybe a pumpkin) can be painted or glued onto the side of the container as a variation of this activity.

Activity 3: Orange Toys

Materials

a variety of toys, predominately orange; for example:

bristle blocks	blocks
pegs	beads
books	puzzles

Goals

Sensory
- to improve visual attending
- to increase attention span

Fine Motor
- to improve hand/finger manipulation, reach and grasp, grasp and release, and eye-hand coordination

Cognitive
- to improve understanding of spatial relationships, imitation, problem-solving, picture-object association, and concept development
- to develop generalization skills

Language
- to improve following directions; taking turns; increasing vocalizations/ vocabulary; identifying and labeling objects, actions, characteristics, and locations; requesting; and initiating

Social
- to make choices
- to facilitate peer interaction

Directions

Set up "stations" for the various toys. Allow children to wander to a station and begin playing. An adult can then assist with the play, expanding and guiding as appropriate. Depending on the child's needs, gross motor goals can be incorporated into these activities by positioning the stations so that the child stands or kneels to play, for example. Encourage children to take turns with an adult or peer to stack blocks and knock them down. Use lots of language to describe what is happening. Emphasize the orange color of all the toys.

Activity 4: Finger Painting

Materials

orange finger paint	finger-paint paper
spoons or tongue depressors for scooping paint	container of water
	smocks
soap for cleanup	table
chairs (adaptive seating as needed)	washcloths for cleanup

Goals

Sensory
- to improve responses to sensory stimulation
- to increase attention span

Gross Motor
- to improve balance, coordination, and control of flexion/extension patterns

Fine Motor
- to improve visual attending and tracking, hand/finger manipulation, finger isolation, midline skills, and using both hands together
- to increase upper body strength
- to improve shoulder girdle strength and stability

Cognitive
- to improve imitation and concept development
- to develop generalization skills

Language
- to improve following directions; taking turns; identifying/labeling objects, actions, descriptions, relationships, and people; initiating; and requesting

Social
- to facilitate peer interaction

Directions

Give each child a piece of finger-paint paper. Sprinkle each child's paper with water and put a dab of the orange finger paint on it. Provide physical assistance to children as needed. Use lots of language to describe the motions and colors. This activity can facilitate even more peer interaction if the group works together on a single large piece of paper.

Caution: Younger children tend to eat the paint. If you think this will happen in your group, substitute colored pudding for paint. Although you can't hang pudding paint pictures on the wall, remember that it is the process that is important here, not the final product.

Snack

Materials

oranges	knives	table
plates	napkins	washcloths for cleanup
cups (adapted as needed)	orange juice	chairs (adapted seating as needed)

Goals

Sensory
- to improve responses to sensory stimulation, especially tactile and olfactory
- to increase attention span

Fine Motor
- to improve reach and grasp, grasp and release, hand/finger manipulation, and eye-hand coordination

Self-Help
- to improve self-feeding skills
- to improve oral-motor skills

Cognitive
- to improve functional object use, understanding of spatial relationships, imitation, and concept development
- to develop generalization skills

Language
- to improve following directions; taking turns; identifying/labeling objects, actions, locations, and relationships; initiating; and requesting

Social
- to make choices
- to facilitate peer interaction

Directions

Have children help pass out plates and napkins, if appropriate. Cut the oranges into quarters. Encourage the children to identify the oranges before you cut them and again afterward. Give each child a section of an orange. Provide assistance with feeding and oral-motor skills as needed. Offer juice and provide assistance with drinking skills as needed. Also, encourage children to identify the juice.

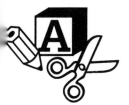

Week 3

Overall Theme: Pumpkins

Activity 1: Obstacle Course

Materials

indoor climbing structure	toddler slide
inner tubes	indoor tunnel
ramp or other incline	carpet squares
floor pillows/beanbag chairs	benches
bolsters	steps
indoor swing	a variety of mini-pumpkins (real, plastic,
containers for pumpkins	stuffed)

Goals

Sensory
- to provide proprioceptive stimulation
- to provide vestibular stimulation
- to improve visual attending
- to increase attention span

Gross Motor
- to improve balance, coordination, motor planning, locomotion, trunk rotation, weight bearing, and weight shifting

Fine Motor
- to improve using both hands together, reach and grasp, grasp and release, and hand manipulation
- to increase upper body strength
- to improve shoulder girdle strength and stability

Cognitive
- to improve object permanence, imitation, problem-solving, classification, understanding of spatial relationships, and concept development
- to develop generalization skills

Language
- to improve following directions; taking turns; identifying/labeling objects, actions, descriptions, and locations; requesting; and initiating

Social
- to make choices
- to facilitate peer interaction

Directions

Using the equipment available, set up an indoor obstacle course to facilitate the gross motor and vestibular goals for individuals in the group. The materials listed above are just suggestions. Place the pumpkins at various points throughout the obstacle course. Have some hidden, some partially hidden, and some in plain sight. Assist the children through the obstacle course. A "path" of carpet squares can provide a structure to follow through the course. Encourage the children to use appropriate motor patterns throughout. Help them find the pumpkins as they go through the course. Be sure there are enough pumpkins for each child to find at least two or three. Collect the pumpkins in baskets or other containers. Depending on their abilities, children can be encouraged to carry their own baskets filled with pumpkins.

Activity 2: Decorating Pumpkins

Materials

pumpkins from previous activity	stickers
markers	table
chairs (adaptive seating as needed)	standers (if needed)

Goals

Sensory
- to increase attention span
- to improve body awareness

Gross Motor
- to improve balance, coordination, motor planning, and weight bearing

Fine Motor
- to improve using both hands together, reach and grasp, grasp and release, visual attending and tracking, eye-hand coordination, and hand/finger manipulation
- to improve shoulder girdle strength and stability

Cognitive
- to improve understanding of object permanence, imitation, and concept development
- to develop generalization skills
- to develop recall skills

Language
- to improve following directions; taking turns; identifying/labeling objects, actions, characteristics, and locations; requesting; and initiating

Social
- to make choices
- to facilitate peer interaction

Directions

Have children stand or sit around the table. Help the children decorate the pumpkins using markers and stickers. Encourage them to hold the pumpkin with one hand while decorating with the other (most will need an adult's help to do this). Talk about how they are decorating the pumpkin. Does it have a face? Where are the eyes? Nose? Mouth? Where are your eyes? Nose? Mouth?

Activity 3: Carving a Pumpkin

Materials

pumpkin	knife
large spoon	candle
matches	newspapers
table	chairs (adaptive seating as needed)
washcloths for cleanup	

Goals

Sensory
- to improve responses to sensory stimulation
- to increase attention span

Gross Motor
- to improve trunk rotation

Fine Motor
- to improve visual attending and tracking, reach and grasp, grasp and release, hand/finger manipulation, finger isolation, using both hands together, and midline skills
- to increase upper body strength
- to improve shoulder girdle strength and stability

Cognitive
- to improve object permanence, understanding of spatial relationships, tool use, functional use of objects, imitation, and concept development
- to develop generalization skills
- to develop recall skills

Language
- to improve following directions; taking turns; identifying/labeling objects, actions, characteristics, relationships, emotions, and people; initiating; and requesting

Social
- to make choices
- to facilitate peer interaction

Directions

Seat children in a circle on the floor or around a small table, as appropriate. Show them the big pumpkin. Compare it to the little pumpkins they have been playing with and decorating. Decide together whether to carve a friendly face or a scary face on the big pumpkin. Where should the eyes go? Should they be round or square or triangles? Discuss the other features. Carve the pumpkin. Have the children reach in to pull out the seeds and flesh. Encourage them to play with the pumpkin's flesh. What do the insides look like? Smell like? Feel like? Taste like? Do the insides make sounds? When finished carving the pumpkin, you can place the candle inside, light it, and replace the pumpkin's top. (This activity can be vastly simplified for younger groups. Just omit most of the higher-level language and let them play with the pumpkin's flesh.)

Activity 4: Making Pumpkin Bread

Materials

cooked pumpkin	cooking oil	electric hand mixer (optional)
eggs	water	smocks
flour		potholders
sugar	measuring cups	table
baking powder	measuring spoons	oven
baking soda	mixing spoon	washcloths for cleanup
salt	mixing bowl	chairs (adaptive seating as needed)
cinnamon	loaf pan	
cloves		

Note: see Appendix C for a pumpkin bread recipe.

Goals

Sensory
- to improve responses to sensory stimulation, especially tactile and olfactory
- to increase attention span

Fine Motor
- to improve using both hands together, midline skills, hand/finger manipulation, visual attending and tracking, reach and grasp, grasp and release, and eye-hand coordination
- to increase upper body strength

Cognitive
- to improve understanding of spatial relationships, tool use, sequencing, conservation of volume, functional object use, imitation, and concept development
- to develop generalization skills
- to develop recall skills

Language
- to improve following directions; taking turns; identifying/labeling objects, actions, locations, and relationships; initiating; and requesting

Social
- to make choices
- to facilitate peer interaction

Directions

Pumpkin bread takes a long time to bake. Bake a loaf ahead of time so the group can eat while the loaf they have helped to make is baking.

Encourage children to name the objects and ingredients to be used as they are needed. Have children help combine ingredients for making pumpkin bread. They can take turns pouring ingredients into the bowl, holding the mixer, and stirring with a spoon. Be sure to let them taste and smell the different ingredients as they are added.

Snack

Materials

pumpkin bread
knife
paper napkins
chairs (adaptive seating as necessary)

milk or juice
cups (adapted, if necessary)
table
washcloths for cleanup

Goals

Sensory
- to improve responses to sensory stimuli, especially tactile and olfactory
- to increase attention span

Fine Motor
- to improve reach and grasp, grasp and release, hand/finger manipulation, and eye-hand coordination

Self-Help
- to improve self-feeding skills
- to improve oral-motor skills

Cognitive
- to improve understanding of spatial relationships, concept development, and imitation
- to develop generalization skills
- to develop recall skills

Language
- to improve following directions; taking turns; identifying/labeling objects, actions, people, and characteristics; requesting; and initiating

Social
- to make choices
- to facilitate peer interaction

Directions

Seat children appropriately for snack, using adaptive seating as needed. Have children help pass out napkins, if appropriate. Show children the pumpkin bread and talk about making it—how the batter looked, smelled, felt; what went into the batter; and where the pumpkin is. Talk about how the bread looks, smells, tastes, and feels now. What is the same? What is different? Encourage communication, including ways to request more or indicate "all done." Assist with self-feeding skills as needed. Offer milk or juice and provide assistance as needed

Week 4   Overall Theme: Multisensory Carnival

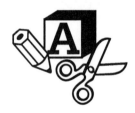

Activity 1: Touchy-Feely

Materials

a variety of unusual sensory materials, such as:

cold cooked spaghetti	latex gloves filled with sand, air, or ice
olives	pudding

bench or table
containers for items as needed

Goals

Sensory
- to improve responses to sensory stimulation, especially tactile and olfactory
- to increase attention span

Gross Motor
- to improve motor planning, balance, coordination, weight bearing, and weight shifting

Fine Motor
- to improve using both hands together, midline skills, reach and grasp, grasp and release, and hand/finger manipulation
- to increase upper body strength

Cognitive
- to improve understanding of spatial relationships, imitation, classification, and concept development

Language
- to improve following directions; taking turns; identifying/labeling objects, actions, locations, and relationships; initiating; and requesting

Social
- to make choices
- to facilitate pretend play
- to facilitate peer interaction

Directions

Set up items on a bench or table. Display "heavy hands" (gloves filled with sand), "light hands" (gloves filled with air), and "cold hands" (frozen gloves). For an added effect, add nail polish to the fingertips of the gloves. Fill shallow containers with pudding, cold cooked spaghetti, olives, and other edible items with unusual textures. Let the children explore these items. If appropriate to their motor goals, the children may stand for this activity. Otherwise, provide appropriate seating. Use lots of language to ask about and describe the children's experiences.

Activity 2: Pumpkin Patch

Materials

straw
mini-pumpkins

Goals

Sensory
- to improve responses to sensory stimulation
- to provide proprioceptive stimulation
- to increase attention span

Gross Motor
- to improve balance, coordination, motor planning, locomotion, trunk rotation, weight bearing, and weight shifting

Fine Motor
- to improve using both hands together, reach and grasp, grasp and release, and hand manipulation
- to increase upper body strength
- to improve shoulder girdle strength and stability

Cognitive
- to improve imitation, problem solving, classification, object permanence, and concept development
- to develop generalization skills
- to develop recall skills

Language
- to improve following directions; taking turns; identifying/labeling objects, actions, descriptions, and locations; requesting; and initiating

Social
- to make choices
- to facilitate peer interaction

Directions

This activity works best outdoors but can be set up indoors if necessary. Spread straw on the ground or floor to create a "pumpkin patch." Hide mini-pumpkins in the straw. (Don't hide them so well that the children can't find them.) Help the children find the pumpkins. Encourage them to walk, roll, and crawl through the straw. Facilitate movement as needed.

Caution: Children and adults with allergies may have difficulty with this activity. If you think the straw will present difficulties for some people in the group, choose an alternative way to hide the pumpkins, such as in a wading pool filled with small balls or a box of styrofoam chips.

Activity 3: Dress-Up

Materials

a variety of large clothing items and costume pieces, including:

hats	wigs	capes
wings	false noses	glasses
make-up for face painting		
washcloths for cleanup	mirrors	soap for cleanup

Goals

Sensory
- to improve responses to sensory stimulation
- to improve visual attending
- to improve body awareness
- to increase attention span

Gross Motor
- to improve motor planning, balance, coordination, trunk rotation, weight bearing, weight shifting, and walking

Fine Motor
- to improve reach and grasp, grasp and release, eye-hand coordination, hand/finger manipulation, and finger isolation
- to increase upper body strength

Self-Help
- to improve dressing/undressing skills

Cognitive
- to improve understanding of spatial relationships, functional object use, classification, imitation, sequencing, and concept development
- to develop generalization skills
- to develop recall skills

Language
- to improve following directions; taking turns; identifying/labeling objects, people, actions, and concepts; initiating; and requesting

Social
- to make choices
- to facilitate pretend play
- to facilitate peer interaction

Directions

Include a wide variety of textures and colors in the collections of clothing and costumes. Encourage children to choose the items they would like to try on. Use lots of language to describe the items and the children's activities. Provide assistance with dressing and undressing as needed. Encourage children to note the changes they see in the mirror as they try on different items. Use lots of language to describe these changes. Try some simple face painting with children's make-up.

Activity 4: Flashlights

Materials

flashlights
colored filters or cellophane for flashlights (optional)
glow-in-the-dark stickers or pictures
tent or table covered with a sheet

Goals

Sensory
- to increase attention span

Gross Motor
- to improve motor planning, balance, coordination, trunk rotation, weight bearing, and weight shifting

Fine Motor
- to improve visual attending and tracking, reach and grasp, eye-hand coordination, hand manipulation, finger isolation, and wrist rotation
- to increase upper body strength

Cognitive
- to improve understanding of spatial relationships, functional object use, classification, imitation, and concept development
- to develop recall skills

Language
- to improve following directions; taking turns; identifying/labeling objects, pictures, people, actions, and concepts; initiating; and requesting

Social
- to make choices
- to facilitate peer interaction

Directions

Set up a small tent or cover a table with one or more sheets to make an enclosed space. (This activity can also be done in an open room but the effects will be different.) Decorate the inside of the tent with glow-in-the-dark stickers or pictures. Place several different sizes of flashlights inside the tent. Cover some with filters or colored cellophane so that the beam of light is a different color, such as red, green, or blue. Bring the children into the tent in small groups, depending on the size of the space. Give them flashlights and let them explore. Then help them find specific pictures or trace patterns with their flashlights. Talk about what they are doing.

Snack

Materials

several small containers	chocolate or carob chips
raisins	crunchy cereal pieces
dried fruit bits	large cooking pot or bowl
wooden spoons	napkins
plates	cups (adapted as needed)
juice	chairs (adaptive seating as needed)
	table

Goals

Sensory
- to improve responses to sensory stimuli, especially tactile and olfactory

Self-Help
- to improve self-feeding skills
- to improve oral-motor skills

Fine Motor
- to improve eye-hand coordination, reach and grasp, grasp and release, hand manipulation, and visual attending and tracking

Cognitive
- to improve understanding of spatial relationships, sequencing, concept development, and imitation
- to develop generalization skills
- to develop recall skills

Language
- to improve following directions; taking turns; identifying/labeling objects, actions, people, and characteristics; initiating; and requesting

Social
- to make choices
- to facilitate peer interaction
- to facilitate pretend play

Directions

Place the ingredients in several small containers and put them on the table. The children may stand to do the mixing, if appropriate, and then sit to eat, or the entire activity can be done with the children seated if that is more appropriate. Tell the children they are going to make a "brew." Have each child choose an ingredient to add and throw a handful into the pot. (A large plastic cauldron from the garden shop or a large bowl is also effective since no actual cooking is required.) Ingredients are approximate. Combine whatever you like, in whatever proportions you and the children decide. When the children are finished adding ingredients, stir and stir the brew with the wooden spoons. Then eat the mixture. Offer assistance with feeding and oral-motor skills as needed. Offer juice and assistance with drinking skills as needed.

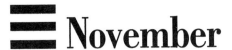
November

Week 1

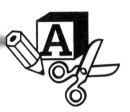

Overall Theme: Corn

Activity 1: Corn Field

Materials

corn stalks
tunnel
baskets or other containers

ears of dried corn (various kinds)
climbing gym

Goals

Sensory
- to improve responses to sensory stimulation
- to provide proprioceptive stimulation

Gross Motor
- to improve balance, coordination, motor planning, trunk rotation, weight bearing, weight shifting, and locomotion

Fine Motor
- to improve reach and grasp, grasp and release, eye-hand coordination, and hand manipulation
- to increase upper body strength
- to improve shoulder girdle strength and stability

Cognitive
- to improve problem solving, imitation, understanding of spatial relationships, object permanence, and concept development
- to develop generalization skills

Language
- to improve following directions; taking turns; identifying/labeling objects, actions, characteristics, locations, relationships, and people; initiating; and requesting

Social
- to make choices
- to facilitate representational/pretend play
- to facilitate peer interaction

Directions

Set up an area as a "corn field" by fastening stalks of corn to climbing equipment and concealing a tunnel between corn stalks. Place ears of dried corn (use different varieties) throughout the "corn field." Encourage children to explore. Facilitate a variety of appropriate movement patterns. Help children find the ears of corn. Provide baskets for the children so they can collect the corn.

Activity 2: Same and Different

Materials

ears of corn from previous activity

pictures of the different varieties of corn

Goals

Sensory
- to increase attention span

Gross Motor
- to improve balance, coordination, weight shifting, and trunk rotation

Fine Motor
- to improve reach and grasp, grasp and release, visual attending and tracking, eye-hand coordination, and hand manipulation

Cognitive
- to improve problem solving, picture-object association, imitation, classification, and concept development
- to develop generalization skills
- to develop recall skills

Language
- to improve following directions; taking turns; identifying/labeling objects, actions, locations, and relationships; initiating; and requesting

Social
- to make choices
- to facilitate peer interaction

Directions

Gather the children in a group. Share the different ears of corn with them. Talk about which ones are similar and why. Talk about which ones are different and why. Show the children pictures of the corn and encourage them to identify the pictures. Ask them which ears of corn go with which pictures. Position children to facilitate gross motor goals during this activity.

Activity 3: Grinding Corn

Materials

mortar and pestle	dried corn
table	chairs (adaptive seating as needed)

Goals

Sensory
- to improve responses to sensory stimulation
- to provide proprioceptive stimulation
- to improve visual attending
- to increase attention span

Gross Motor
- to improve weight bearing

Fine Motor
- to improve hand manipulation, eye-hand coordination, reach and grasp, grasp and release, using both hands together, and grading movements
- to increase upper body strength
- to improve shoulder girdle strength and stability

Cognitive
- to improve imitation, functional object use, understanding of spatial relationships, classification, and concept development
- to develop generalization skills
- to develop recall skills

Language
- to improve following directions; taking turns; increasing vocabulary; identifying/labeling objects, actions, characteristics, and relationships; initiating; and requesting

Social
- to make choices
- to facilitate pretend play
- to facilitate peer interaction

Directions

Display some dried corn cobs containing kernels, dried kernels, and a mortar and pestle. Explain to the children that corn used to be ground with a mortar and pestle. Assist children with trying to grind some of the dried kernels.

Activity 4: Corn Prints

Materials

dried corn cobs from previous activities   tempera paint
construction paper   paper plates, pie tins, or saucers
smocks   table
chairs (adaptive seating as needed)   washcloths for cleanup

Goals

Sensory
- to improve sensory awareness and responsiveness
- to improve visual attending
- to increase attention span

Gross Motor
- to improve weight bearing, weight shifting, balance, and coordination

Fine Motor
- to improve reach and grasp, grasp and release, eye-hand coordination, hand/finger manipulation skills, using both hands together, and midline skills
- to increase upper body strength
- to improve shoulder girdle strength and stability

Cognitive
- to improve sequencing, imitation, and concept development
- to develop generalization skills
- to develop recall skills

Language
- to improve following directions; taking turns; identifying/labeling objects, actions, people, places, characteristics, and relationships; requesting; initiating; and increasing vocabulary

Social
- to make choices
- to facilitate peer interaction

Directions

Set up the activity on a small table. Seat children or let them work in standing, according to the needs of the group. Have children identify the corncobs from the previous activities. Encourage children to choose which color paper and paint to use. Demonstrate rolling the corn cob in the paint and then rolling or pressing it on the paper to make a print. Assist the children as needed with making their own prints. Talk about the feel of the paint and the corn, the colors being used, and the actions required for the activity. Encourage children to trade paint and corn cobs with each other.

Activity 5: Corn Bread

Materials

yellow corn meal	eggs
flour	sugar
baking powder	salt
shortening	milk
measuring cups	measuring spoons
mixing bowl	mixing spoon
electric hand mixer (optional)	9" x 9" x 2" square baking pan
oven	potholders
smocks	table
chairs (adaptive seating as needed)	washcloths for cleanup

Note: see Appendix C for a corn bread recipe.

Goals

Sensory
- to improve responses to sensory stimulation, especially tactile and olfactory
- to increase attention span

Fine Motor
- to improve using both hands together, midline skills, hand/finger manipulation, visual attending and tracking, reach and grasp, grasp and release, and eye-hand coordination
- to increase upper body strength

Cognitive
- to improve understanding of spatial relationships, tool use, conservation of volume, functional object use, sequencing, imitation, and concept development
- to develop generalization skills
- to develop recall skills

Language
- to improve following directions; taking turns; identifying/labeling objects, actions, locations, and relationships; initiating; and requesting

Social
- to make choices
- to facilitate peer interaction

Directions

Corn bread takes a while to bake. Bake a pan of corn bread ahead of time, so the group can eat while the pan of corn bread they make is baking.

Encourage children to name the objects and ingredients to be used as they are needed. Have children help combine ingredients for making corn bread. They may take turns pouring ingredients into the bowl, holding the mixer, and stirring with a spoon. Be sure to let them taste and smell the different ingredients as they are added.

Snack

Materials

corn bread
knife
paper napkins
chairs (adaptive seating as necessary)

milk or juice
cups (adapted if necessary)
table
washcloths for cleanup

Goals

Sensory
- to improve responses to sensory stimuli, especially tactile and olfactory
- to increase attention span

Fine Motor
- to improve eye-hand coordination, reach and grasp, grasp and release, hand/finger manipulation, visual attending and tracking, midline skills, and using both hands together

Self-Help
- to improve self-feeding skills
- to improve oral-motor skills

Cognitive
- to improve understanding of spatial relationships, functional object use, concept development, and imitation
- to develop generalization skills
- to develop recall skills

Language
- to improve following directions; taking turns; identifying/labeling objects, actions, people, and characteristics; requesting; and initiating

Social
- to make choices
- to facilitate peer interaction

Directions

Seat children appropriately for snack, using adaptive seating as needed. Have children help pass out napkins, if appropriate. Show children the corn bread and talk about making it—how the batter looked, smelled, felt; what went into the batter; and where the corn meal is now. Talk about how the bread looks, smells, tastes, and feels now. What is the same? What is different? Encourage communication, including ways to request more or indicate "all done." Assist with self-feeding skills as needed. Offer milk or juice and provide assistance as needed.

Week 2

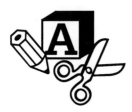

Overall Theme: Over the River and through the Woods

Activity 1: Over the River

Materials

scooter boards
tree branches
jingle bells
recording of "Over the River and
  through the Woods"

carpet squares or blankets
pictures of trees
audio player

Goals

Sensory
- to improve responses to vestibular stimulation
- to increase attention span

Gross Motor
- to improve motor planning, balance, and coordination

Fine Motor
- to improve reach and grasp and hand manipulation
- to increase upper body strength

Cognitive
- to improve imitation, understanding of spatial relationships, object-picture association, and concept development

Language
- to improve following directions; taking turns; identifying/labeling actions, people, locations, and relationships; increasing vocabulary; initiating; and requesting

Social
- to make choices
- to facilitate pretend play
- to facilitate peer interaction

Directions

Ahead of time, set up a space to represent "the woods." Use small tree branches, if possible, along with pictures of trees. Arrange carpet squares or blankets on the floor to represent the "river." Seat children on scooter board "sleighs." Encourage them to choose where they would like to sit. Play the song "Over the River and through the Woods" while pulling the "sleighs" along the path. Give the children jingle bells to shake. Use lots of language to describe what the children are doing and who is doing what.

Activity 2: Boats across the River

Materials

rocking boat
platform swing
mat

Goals

Sensory
- to improve responses to sensory stimulation
- to provide vestibular stimulation

Gross Motor
- to improve balance, coordination, motor planning, trunk rotation, and weight shifting

Fine Motor
- to improve reach and grasp and grasp and release
- to increase upper body strength

Cognitive
- to improve problem solving, imitation, and understanding of spatial relationships
- to develop generalization skills

Language
- to improve following directions; taking turns; identifying/labeling objects, actions, descriptions, locations, relationships, and people; initiating; and requesting

Social
- to make choices
- to facilitate representational/pretend play
- to facilitate peer interaction

Directions

Talk about other ways to get over the "river," including the use of a boat. Tell children they are going for a "boat" ride across the river. Let them choose whether they want to ride on the platform swing "boat" or the rocking "boat." Be sure to position a mat under the swing to protect children in case of accidental falls. Let half of the group use each piece of equipment, then switch. Encourage them to problem solve getting on and off the equipment, making it move, and making it stop. Use lots of language to describe these activities. Also, use language to set the scene for pretend play. Describe the boat, where they are going, and what they are doing. Impose some movements to facilitate sensorimotor goals as indicated for the group.

Activity 3: Riding Horses through the Woods

Materials

bolster swing
bolsters on floor
rocking horses
stick horses

Goals

Sensory
- to improve responses to vestibular stimulation

Gross Motor
- to improve balance, weight shifting, motor planning, and coordination

Cognitive
- to improve imitation, understanding of spatial relationships, and concept development

Language
- to improve following directions; taking turns; increasing vocalizations/vocabulary; identifying/labeling actions, objects, people, and characteristics (such as fast or slow); initiating; and requesting

Social
- to make choices
- to facilitate pretend play
- to facilitate peer interaction

Directions

Talk about other ways to get through the "woods." Riding horses might be one way. Help children, one at a time, onto the bolster swing. Make horse noises and/or sing horse songs while swinging the swing back and forth. Help children adjust to the movements. Children can "ride" the bolsters on the floor while waiting their turn for the swing. Help them practice weight shifting from side to side and balancing. With some help from an adult, one end of the bolster can rear up like a horse's head. Again, encourage children to make and imitate horse noises and sing horse songs during this activity. If appropriate, children can also use rocking horses or stick horses during this activity.

Activity 4: Grandma's House

Materials

toy kitchen set
child-sized table and chairs
doll clothes
toy dishes

dolls
accessories for dolls (such as bottles, brushes, and diapers)

Goals

Sensory
- to improve responses to sensory stimulation
- to increase attention span

Gross Motor
- to improve balance, coordination, weight shifting, and motor planning

Fine Motor
- to improve eye-hand coordination, reach and grasp, grasp and release, hand/finger manipulation, and using both hands together

Cognitive
- to improve functional object use, imitation, understanding of spatial relationships, and concept development
- to develop generalization skills
- to develop recall skills

Language
- to improve following directions; taking turns; identifying/labeling objects, actions, people, and characteristics; increasing vocabulary; initiating; and requesting

Social
- to make choices
- to facilitate representational/pretend play
- to facilitate peer interaction

Directions

Set up a corner, or use the regular housekeeping corner, to be "Grandma's House." (Avoid the stereotype of little old grey-haired ladies rocking in chairs and knitting.) Tell the children that they have arrived at Grandma's House as in the song "Over the River and through the Woods." Help them to set up Grandma's House. Encourage them to take turns playing Grandma, Grandpa, aunts, uncles, and cousins. Encourage them to "cook" dinner, including pudding and pumpkin pie, as in the song.

Activity 5: Making Pumpkin Pie

Materials

prepared pie crust
sugar
cinnamon
nutmeg
eggs

prepared pumpkin
salt
ginger
cloves
evaporated milk

Materials (continued)

mixing bowl	mixing spoon
electric mixer (optional)	measuring spoons
measuring cups	oven
potholders	smocks
table	chairs (adaptive seating as needed)
washcloths for cleanup	

Note: see Appendix C for a pumpkin pie recipe.

Goals

Sensory
- to improve responses to sensory stimulation, especially tactile and olfactory
- to increase attention span

Fine Motor
- to improve using both hands together, midline skills, hand/finger manipulation, visual attending and tracking, reach and grasp, grasp and release, eye-hand coordination
- to increase upper body strength

Cognitive
- to improve understanding of spatial relationships, tool use, conservation of volume, functional object use, sequencing, imitation, and concept development
- to develop generalization skills
- to develop recall skills

Language
- to improve following directions; taking turns; identifying/labeling objects, actions, locations, and relationships; initiating; and requesting

Social
- to make choices
- to facilitate peer interaction

Directions

Pumpkin pie takes a while to bake. Bake a pie ahead of time so the group can eat while the pie they make is baking.

Encourage children to name the objects and ingredients to be used as they are needed. Have children help combine ingredients for making the pie filling. They may take turns pouring ingredients into the bowl, holding the mixer, and stirring with a spoon. Be sure to let them taste and smell the different ingredients as they are added.

Snack

Materials

pumpkin pie	milk or juice
knife	cups (adapted if necessary)
paper napkins	paper plates
spoons and/or forks	table
chairs (adaptive seating as necessary)	washcloths for cleanup

Goals

Sensory
- to improve responses to sensory stimuli, especially tactile and olfactory
- to increase attention span

Fine Motor
- to improve eye-hand coordination, reach and grasp, grasp and release, hand/finger manipulation, visual attending and tracking, midline skills, and using both hands together

Self-Help
- to improve self-feeding skills
- to improve oral-motor skills

Cognitive
- to improve understanding of spatial relationships, functional object use, concept development, and imitation
- to develop generalization skills
- to develop recall skills

Language
- to improve following directions; taking turns; identifying/labeling objects, actions, people, and characteristics; requesting; and initiating

Social
- to make choices
- to facilitate peer interaction

Directions

Seat children appropriately for snack, using adaptive seating as needed. Have children help pass out napkins, if appropriate. Show children the pumpkin pie and talk about making it—how the filling looked, smelled, felt; what went into it; and where the pumpkin is. Talk about how the pie looks, smells, tastes, and feels now. What is the same? What is different? Encourage communication, including ways to request more or indicate "all done." Assist with self-feeding skills as needed. Offer milk or juice and provide assistance as required.

Week 3

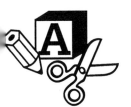

Overall Theme: Turkeys

Activity 1: Obstacle Course

Materials

indoor climbing structure	indoor tunnel
inner tubes	carpet squares
ramp or other incline	benches
floor pillows/beanbag chairs	steps
bolsters	assorted toy turkeys and pictures
indoor swing	of turkeys
toddler slide	

Goals

Sensory
- to provide proprioceptive stimulation
- to provide vestibular stimulation
- to increase attention span

Gross Motor
- to improve balance, coordination, motor planning, locomotion, trunk rotation, and weight shifting

Fine Motor
- to improve using both hands together, reach and grasp, and grasp and release
- to increase upper body strength
- to improve shoulder girdle strength and stability

Cognitive
- to improve imitation, problem solving, object permanence, understanding of spatial relationships, and concept development
- to develop generalization skills
- to develop recall skills

Language
- to improve following directions; taking turns; identifying/labeling objects, actions, descriptions, and locations; increasing vocabulary; requesting; and initiating

Social
- to make choices
- to facilitate pretend play
- to facilitate peer interaction

Directions

Using the equipment available, set up an indoor obstacle course to facilitate the gross motor and vestibular goals for the individuals in the group. The materials listed above are just suggestions. Place the toy turkeys at various points throughout the obstacle course. Have some hidden, some partially hidden, and some in plain sight. Assist the children through the obstacle course. A "path" of carpet squares can provide a structure to follow through the course. Encourage the children to use appropriate motor patterns throughout. Help them find the turkeys as they go through the course. Be sure there are enough turkeys for each child to find at least one. Encourage the children to help the turkeys through the obstacle course, too.

Activity 2: Turkey Gobble

Materials

toy turkeys   turkey puppets   dried corn

Goals

Sensory
- to increase sensory awareness and responsiveness, especially to tactile stimulation
- to provide vestibular stimulation

- to provide proprioceptive stimulation
- to improve visual attention
- to increase attention span

Gross Motor
- to improve motor planning, locomotion, balance, coordination, and weight shifting

Fine Motor
- to improve hand/finger manipulation, eye-hand coordination, reach and grasp, and grasp and release

Cognitive
- to improve cause and effect, imitation, and concept development
- to develop generalization skills
- to develop recall skills

Language
- to improve following directions; taking turns; identifying/labeling objects, actions, characteristics, and relationships; increasing vocalizations; initiating; and requesting

Social
- to make choices
- to facilitate peer interaction
- to facilitate pretend play

Directions

Have children imitate turkeys in a variety of ways. They can waddle like a turkey (provide assistance as needed). They can manipulate a toy turkey or pretend to feed one using the dried corn. (Remind them of their previous activities with corn.) Use lots of language to describe what the children and "turkeys" are doing, how they are moving, and who is moving. Be sure to encourage lots of gobbling.

Activity 3: Turkey Match

Materials

toy turkeys   photos or pictures matching the toy turkeys

Goals

Sensory
- to increase attention span

Gross Motor
- to improve balance, coordination, weight shifting, and trunk rotation

Fine Motor
- to improve reach and grasp, grasp and release, visual attending and tracking, eye-hand coordination, and hand/finger manipulation

Cognitive
- to improve problem solving, picture-object association, imitation, classification, and concept development
- to develop generalization skills
- to develop recall skills

Language
- to improve following directions; taking turns; identifying/labeling objects, actions, locations, and relationships; initiating; and requesting

Social
- to make choices
- to facilitate peer interaction

Directions

Gather the children together with the turkeys they have been using. Show them a picture corresponding to one of the turkeys and have the child who has that turkey put it with the picture. Continue the activity until all of the turkeys and pictures have been matched. Repeat the word *turkey* frequently and describe the turkeys. As before, encourage lots of gobbling.

Activity 4: Hand Print Turkeys

Materials

finger paint	finger-paint paper
paintbrushes (optional)	pie tins or paper plates
container of water	crayons or markers
soap for cleanup	smocks
chairs (adaptive seating as needed)	table
washcloths for cleanup	

Goals

Sensory
- to improve responses to sensory stimulation
- to provide proprioceptive stimulation
- to increase attention span

Gross Motor
- to improve balance, coordination, and control of flexion/extension patterns

Fine Motor
- to improve visual attending and tracking, hand/finger manipulation, using both hands together, midline skills, and finger isolation
- to increase upper body strength
- to improve shoulder girdle strength and stability

Cognitive
- to improve imitation and concept development
- to develop generalization skills

Language
- to improve following directions; taking turns; identifying/labeling objects, actions, descriptions, relationships, and people; initiating; and requesting

Social
- to make choices
- to facilitate peer interaction

Directions

Seat children appropriately for fine motor activity. Let children choose which color paint to use. Spread paint on their hands with a paintbrush or put some paint in a pie tin or paper plate and dip their hands in the paint. Press their hands on the papers to make hand prints. Allow the paint to dry and draw features (eyes, beak, wattles) on the turkeys, using the thumb prints for the heads. Add legs and feet at the wrist. Talk about this process with the children. Allow the children to finger-paint after they have made the turkey hand prints.

Alternatively, you can trace around the children's hands with a marker or crayon and then add legs and features as described above.

Activity 5: Paper-Bag Turkeys

Materials

construction paper	lunch bags
rubber bands or string	newspapers
scissors	feathers
glue	marking pens
table	chairs (adaptive seating as needed)
washcloths for cleanup	

Goals

Sensory
- to improve sensory awareness through tactile stimulation
- to improve visual attending
- to increase attention span

Fine Motor
- to improve hand/finger manipulation, eye-hand coordination, using both hands together, reach and grasp, and grasp and release

Cognitive
- to improve imitation and concept development
- to develop generalization skills
- to develop recall skills

Language
- to improve following directions; taking turns; increasing vocabulary/ vocalizations; identifying/labeling objects, actions, characteristics, and relationships; initiating; and requesting

Social
- to make choices

Directions

Ahead of time, cut out some turkey heads and necks from construction paper. Stuff a paper lunch bag lightly with crumpled-up newspaper. Close the end with a rubber band or tie it with string. Depending on the groups' abilities, you can do this ahead of time or let the children participate. Help the children spread glue on the bottom end of the stuffed bag and fasten the turkey's head on the bag. Glue some feathers on the opposite end to make the turkey's tail. Encourage children to choose which colors to use. Talk about turkeys. How are these turkeys like the other turkeys the children have played with and seen? How are they different? Encourage gobbling.

Snack

Materials

bread	turkey-shaped cookie cutters
mustard	napkins
cheese slices	cups (adapted if necessary)
milk or juice	chairs (adaptive seating as needed)
plates	table
table knives	

Goals

Sensory
- to improve responses to sensory stimuli, especially tactile and olfactory
- to increase attention span

Fine Motor
- to improve using both hands together, reach and grasp, grasp and release, hand/finger manipulation, and midline skills
- to improve shoulder girdle strength and stability

Self-Help
- to improve self-feeding skills
- to improve oral-motor skills

Cognitive
- to improve understanding of spatial relationships, imitation, functional object use, and concept development
- to develop generalization skills
- to develop recall skills

Language
- to improve following directions; taking turns; identifying/labeling objects, actions, people, and characteristics; imitating; and requesting

Social
- to make choices
- to facilitate peer interaction

Directions

Seat children appropriately for snack, using adaptive seating as needed. Tell them they are going to make sandwiches. As children watch, spread a slice of bread with mustard and add cheese. Give each child a table knife and a slice of bread. Help them spread the mustard and put the cheese slices on the bread. Top the cheese with a second slice of bread. Using the turkey cookie cutters, cut out turkey shapes from the sandwiches. Describe what they are doing, what the snack is made of, and what it looks like. Encourage communication, including ways to request more or indicate "all done." Offer milk or juice as needed. Assist with self-feeding/drinking skills as needed.

Week 4

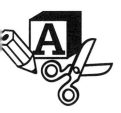

Overall Theme: Friends

Activity 1: Taking Turns

Materials

gross motor toys that facilitate turn taking, such as:

swings	see-saws
rocking horses	slides
riding toys	

Goals

Sensory
- to provide vestibular stimulation
- to provide proprioceptive stimulation
- to increase attention span

Gross Motor
- to improve balance, coordination, weight bearing, weight shifting, trunk rotation, reciprocal movement patterns, and motor planning

Fine Motor
- to improve reach and grasp and grasp and release
- to increase upper body strength
- to improve shoulder girdle strength and stability

Cognitive
- to improve imitation, understanding of spatial relationships, problem solving, and concept development
- to develop generalization skills

Language
- to improve following directions; taking turns; identifying/labeling objects, actions, people, and characteristics; initiating; and requesting

Social
- to make choices
- to facilitate peer interaction

Directions

Set up gross motor equipment that requires children to take turns or work together. As children play, facilitate their turn taking. With two-person equipment, such as a see-saw, emphasize the turn-taking aspect of the activity. Facilitate motor skills as appropriate.

Activity 2: Giving and Sharing

Materials

variety of small toys	large building blocks
assorted manipulatives	bell

Goals

Sensory
- to improve auditory attending
- to increase attention span

Gross Motor
- to improve motor planning, balance, coordination, weight bearing, and weight shifting

Fine Motor
- to improve hand/finger manipulation, eye-hand coordination, reach and grasp, and grasp and release
- to increase upper body strength

Cognitive
- to improve understanding of spatial relationships, imitation, problem solving, and concept development
- to improve generalization skills

Language
- to improve following directions; taking turns; increasing vocalizations/ vocabulary; requesting; initiating; and identifying/labeling objects, actions, characteristics, and locations

Social
- to make choices
- to facilitate peer interaction

Directions

Set up "stations" for the various toys. Allow children to wander to a station and begin playing. After a few minutes, ring the bell. Adults then help children choose another child to give their toy to or to share the toy with. This activity needs to be carried out in a sensitive manner so that children who are not developmentally ready for giving and sharing are not having toys wrenched from their hands despite their protests. Large cooperative toys, such as giant building blocks, that require two or more children for effective play can be used to facilitate "sharing." Children may trade toys or may simply be helped to invite another child to join them in a turn-taking activity.

Activity 3: Sharing Circle

Materials

games, songs, stories, and toys that each child enjoys at home

Goals

Sensory
- to increase attention span

Gross Motor
- to improve balance, coordination, weight shifting, and motor planning

Fine Motor
- to improve reach and grasp, grasp and release, hand/finger manipulation, and using both hands together

Cognitive
- to improve imitation and concept development
- to develop recall skills

Language
- to improve following directions; taking turns; identifying/labeling objects, actions, people, and characteristics; initiating; requesting; and listening

Social
- to facilitate peer interaction

Directions

Ask families ahead of time to bring a favorite short song, game, fingerplay, story, or toy for the child to share with the group. Emphasize *short*. Gather the children together (families should join the circle, too, if they are present). Help each child/ family to share their activity with the group.

Activity 4: Collages

Materials

pictures of friends (include pictures showing action, such as friends swinging together or eating together)	paper
	paintbrushes (optional)
	scissors
glue	cotton swabs (optional)
table	chairs (adaptive seating as needed)
washcloths for cleanup	

Goals

Sensory
- to improve responses to sensory stimulation
- to increase attention span

Fine Motor
- to improve hand/finger manipulation, eye-hand coordination, using two hands together, reach and grasp, grasp and release, and midline skills

Cognitive
- to improve classification, picture-object relationships, understanding spatial relationships, and concept development
- to develop generalization skills
- to develop recall skills

Language
- to improve following directions; taking turns; identifying/labeling objects, pictures, actions, and descriptions; initiating; and requesting

Social
- to make choices

Directions

Ahead of time, cut out a variety of pictures of friends. Include pictures representing friends interacting in a variety of ways. Choose pictures that portray people of a wide variety of ethnicities and ages. If you want to, you could include people interacting with their pets. Discuss whether animals and people can be friends. Position children appropriately for fine motor activity. Have children select which color paper to use. Show them the pictures and encourage them to identify or name the pictures. Let them choose several pictures to use in their collages. Help children squeeze or spread glue onto their papers, encouraging them to stabilize the paper with one hand, if possible. Vary the activity by encouraging them to spread the glue with paintbrushes or cotton swabs. Help them pat the pictures into place. Let the pictures dry while completing another activity. Talk about the pictures. What do friends do together?

Snack

Materials

favorite food from home to share	juice
paper plates	spoons and/or forks
napkins	cups (adapted as necessary)
table	chairs (adaptive seating as needed)
washcloths for cleanup	

Goals

Sensory
- to improve responses to sensory stimuli, especially tactile and olfactory
- to increase attention span

Fine Motor
- to improve using both hands together, reach and grasp, grasp and release, hand/finger manipulation, eye-hand coordination, and midline skills

Self-Help
- to improve self-feeding skills
- to improve oral-motor skills

Cognitive
- to improve tool use, understanding of spatial relationships, functional object use, imitation, concept development, and sequencing
- to develop generalization skills
- to develop recall skills

Language
- to improve following directions; taking turns; identifying/labeling objects, actions, people, and characteristics; initiating; and requesting

Social
- to make choices
- to facilitate peer interaction

Directions

Seat children appropriately for snack. Have them pass out napkins and spoons/forks, if appropriate. Serve small quantities of each dish brought from home. If families are present, they should join in the potluck feast. Identify who brought which food. Talk about how it tastes (positive stuff, please) and what is in each dish. Encourage communication, including asking for more and indicating "all done." Provide assistance with self-feeding and oral-motor skills as needed. Offer juice and provide assistance with drinking as needed.

December

Week 1

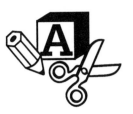

Overall Theme: Toys

Activity 1: Riding Toys

Materials

riding toys   tricycles (adapted if needed)   wagons

Goals

Sensory
- to provide vestibular stimulation
- to provide proprioceptive stimulation
- to increase attention span

Gross Motor
- to improve balance, coordination, motor planning, weight shifting, weight bearing, reciprocal movement, and trunk rotation

Cognitive
- to improve understanding of spatial relationships, imitation, problem solving, and concept development

Language
- to improve following directions; taking turns; identifying/labeling objects, actions, and people; initiating; and requesting

Social
- to make choices
- to facilitate peer interaction

Directions

Provide large wheeled toys at the appropriate developmental level for the group. Assist the children with choosing the toys they wish to use. Provide help as needed with moving the toys, steering, and getting on and off. Children who are more physically challenged can ride in wagons or in tandem with children who can operate the toys more independently. Use lots of language to describe what is happening and who is doing what.

Activity 2: Marching Toys

Materials

pictures of marching toys
marching toys (include switch-activated toys)
marching band instruments (such as a drum or cymbals)
audio player

marching music
construction paper marching band hats (optional)
alternative means of locomotion for children who are nonambulatory

Goals

Sensory
- to provide proprioceptive stimulation
- to provide vestibular stimulation
- to improve auditory attending
- to increase attention span

Gross Motor
- to improve walking, weight bearing, weight shifting, balance, coordination, and motor planning

Fine Motor
- to improve grasp and release, hand manipulation, eye-hand coordination, using two hands together, and midline skills

Cognitive
- to improve imitation, tool use, object-picture association, problem solving, and concept development
- to develop generalization skills
- to develop recall skills

Language
- to improve following directions; taking turns; identifying/labeling objects, actions, characteristics, relationships, and locations; initiating; and requesting

Social
- to make choices
- to facilitate pretend play
- to facilitate peer interaction

Directions

Show children the marching toys and the pictures. Include switch-activated toys as well as wind-up toys. Let them choose a toy to manipulate. Encourage them to activate the toys themselves or to ask for help when they need it. Talk about the toys—what they look like and what they do. Put on the marching music and show the children how to march like the toys. Let them choose hats to wear and instruments to use, if appropriate. Encourage them to march to the music. Children who are able may push children who are nonambulatory in strollers. As an alternative, children who are nonambulatory may activate one of the marching toys or play an instrument while the other children march.

Activity 3: Manipulative Toys

Materials

a variety of manipulative toys, for example:

interlocking blocks (such as Duplo™)	pop-up pals
	bristle blocks
square blocks	pegs
beads	books
puzzles	shape sorters

Goals

Sensory
- to improve visual attending
- to increase attention span

Fine Motor
- to improve hand/finger manipulation, eye-hand coordination, reach and grasp, grasp and release, and midline skills
- to improve shoulder girdle strength and stability

Cognitive
- to improve understanding of spatial relationships, imitation, problem solving, and concept development
- to improve generalization skills

Language
- to improve following directions; taking turns; increasing vocalizations/vocabulary; requesting and initiating; identifying/labeling objects, actions, characteristics, and locations

Social
- to make choices
- to facilitate peer interaction

Directions

Set up "stations" for the various toys. Allow children to wander to a station and begin playing. An adult can then assist with the play, expanding and guiding as appropriate. Depending on the child's needs, gross motor goals can be incorporated into these activities by positioning the stations so that the child stands or kneels to play, for example. Encourage children to take turns with an adult or peer in stacking blocks and knocking them down. Use lots of language to describe what is happening.

Activity 4: Toy Collage

Materials

pictures of toys (include those used in previous activities, if possible)
glue
cotton swabs (optional)
chairs (adaptive seating as needed)

scissors
paper
paintbrushes (optional)
table
washcloths for cleanup

Goals

Sensory
- to improve responses to sensory stimulation
- to increase attention span

Fine Motor
- to improve hand/finger manipulation, eye-hand coordination, using two hands together, reach and grasp, grasp and release, and midline skills

Cognitive
- to improve classification, picture-object relationships, and concept development
- to develop generalization skills
- to develop recall skills

Language
- to improve following directions; taking turns; identifying/labeling objects, pictures, actions, and descriptions; initiating; and requesting

Social
- to make choices

Directions

Ahead of time, cut out a variety of pictures of toys. Include those used in the previous activities if possible. Position children appropriately for fine motor activity. Have children select which color paper to use. Show them the pictures and encourage them to identify or name the pictures. Let them choose several pictures to use in their collages. Help children squeeze or spread glue onto their papers, encouraging them to stabilize the paper with one hand, if possible. Vary the activity by encouraging them to use paintbrushes or cotton swabs to spread the glue. Help them pat their pictures into place. Let the pictures dry while completing another activity.

Activity 5: Toy Cookies

Materials

sugar cookies baked in the shapes of various toys	frosting
	sprinkles
spoons	knives for spreading frosting
paper plates	table
chairs (adaptive seating as needed)	

Goals

Sensory
- to improve responses to sensory stimulation, especially tactile and olfactory
- to increase attention span

Fine Motor
- to improve using both hands together, midline skills, hand/finger manipulation, visual attending and tracking, reach and grasp, and grasp and release
- to increase upper body strength
- to improve shoulder girdle strength and stability

Cognitive
- to improve understanding of spatial relationships, tool use, functional use of objects, imitation, sequencing, and concept development
- to develop generalization skills
- to develop recall skills

Language
- to improve following directions; taking turns; identifying/labeling objects, actions, locations, and relationships; initiating; and requesting

Social
- to make choices
- to facilitate peer interaction

Directions

Be sure children are positioned for fine motor activity. Show children the cookies. Have them identify the shapes and relate them to the toys they have been playing with in the previous activities. Demonstrate spreading the frosting with a knife. Give each child a spoonful of frosting on a paper plate and have each one select a cookie to frost. Assist as needed. Demonstrate decorating the frosted cookie with the sprinkles. Have children choose the color sprinkles they wish to use. Assist as needed. Adjust the sequence to meet the needs of the group and repeat as needed. For example, some groups will need the activity broken into the steps suggested, while others will do better to see the entire sequence first. Some will be able to frost several cookies and then decorate them all with sprinkles, while others will need to complete each cookie separately. Remember to focus on the process.

Snack

Materials

cookies decorated in previous activity
cups (adapted as necessary)
chairs (adaptive seating as needed)
juice
napkins
washcloths for cleanup

Goals

Sensory
• to improve responses to sensory stimuli, especially tactile and olfactory
• to increase attention span

Fine Motor
• to improve using both hands together, reach and grasp, grasp and release, hand/finger manipulation, eye-hand coordination, and midline skills

Self-Help
• to improve self-feeding skills
• to improve oral-motor skills

Cognitive
• to improve tool use, understanding of spatial relationships, functional object use, concept development, sequencing, and imitation
• to develop generalization skills
• to develop recall skills

Language
• to improve following directions; taking turns; identifying/labeling objects, actions, people, and characteristics; initiating; and requesting

Social
• to make choices
• to facilitate peer interaction

Directions

Seat children appropriately for snack. Have them pass out napkins, if appropriate. Children may eat the cookies they have just decorated (if they have not already done so!). Encourage communication, including asking for more and indicating "all done." Provide assistance with self-feeding and oral-motor skills as needed. Offer juice and provide assistance with drinking as needed.

Week 2

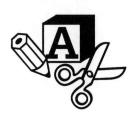

Overall Theme: Bird Feeders

Activity 1: Tree Walk

Materials

access to outdoors, if possible
bird feeder
strollers or other adaptive means of
  locomotion for children who are
  nonambulatory

a variety of evergreen
  (or other) branches

Goals

Sensory
- to increase sensory awareness and improve responses to sensory stimulation
- to increase attention span

Gross Motor
- to improve walking, weight shifting, balance, coordination, and motor planning

Fine Motor
- to improve eye-hand coordination, reach and grasp, grasp and release, hand manipulation, and finger isolation (pointing)
- to increase upper body strength
- to improve shoulder girdle strength and stability

Cognitive
- to improve classification skills, imitation, and concept development
- to develop generalization skills
- to develop recall skills

Language
- to improve following directions; taking turns; increasing vocalization/ vocabulary; identifying/labeling objects, actions, characteristics, relationships, and locations; initiating interactions; requesting; and questioning

Social
- to make choices
- to facilitate peer interaction

Directions

Have children hike along a path outdoors, if possible. Otherwise, set up a "path" indoors with evergreen or other branches placed along the way. Look for a good spot to hang the bird feeder. If appropriate, have the group help decide where to place the feeder. Make sure each child has a chance to examine the feeder before it is hung up. Let the children who are walking push the strollers for the children who are using them, thus helping the walking children to improve their upper body strength. Talk with the children about what they see, hear, and smell. Encourage them to describe the trees, branches, bird feeder, and seed, as well as any birds they happen to see. Talk about smells and textures as well as sights and sounds.

Activity 2: Paper Tree

Materials

large pieces of paper cut into the shape of trees
bird stickers
paper
tape
scissors
markers or crayons
easels (optional)

Goals

Sensory
- to increase attention span

Gross Motor
- to improve weight bearing, weight shifting, and balance

Fine Motor
- to improve hand/finger manipulation, eye-hand coordination, using both hands together, reach and grasp, and grasp and release
- to increase upper body strength
- to improve shoulder girdle strength and stability

Cognitive
- to improve understanding of spatial relationships, classification, imitation, and concept development
- to develop generalization skills
- to develop recall skills

Language
- to improve following directions; taking turns; increasing vocabulary; identifying/labeling objects, actions, characteristics, and relationships; initiating; and requesting

Social
- to make choices
- to facilitate peer interaction

Directions

Cut out large tree shapes ahead of time and fasten them to easels or to the wall. Have children choose bird stickers for their trees. Draw bird feeders or cut them from construction paper. Help the children "hang" the bird feeders in the trees with tape. Encourage them to reach up to put the birds and bird feeders in the trees. Use lots of language to talk about what they are doing.

This activity may also be done with children seated, if that is more appropriate. In that case, use smaller paper cutouts.

Activity 3: Pine Cone Bird Feeders

Materials

pine cones	scissors	yarn
peanut butter	bird seed	knives
chairs (adaptive seating as needed)	paper plates washcloths for cleanup	table

Goals

Sensory
- to improve sensory awareness through tactile stimulation
- to increase attention span

Fine Motor
- to improve hand/finger manipulation, eye-hand coordination, using both hands together, reach and grasp, grasp and release, and midline skills

Cognitive
- to improve imitation, understanding of spatial relationships, and concept development
- to develop generalization skills
- to develop recall skills

Language
- to improve following directions; taking turns; increasing vocabulary; identifying/labeling objects, actions, characteristics, and relationships; initiating; and requesting

Social
- to make choices

Directions

Position children for fine motor activity. Show them a sample of a completed feeder. Have children select the pine cones they want to use. Help children fasten the yarn to the pine cones so that they can be hung up. Secure the yarn with glue, if necessary. Show children how to spread peanut butter on their pine cones. Give each child a paper plate with a gob of peanut butter and a plastic knife for spreading. Provide assistance as needed. Finally, show them how to roll the peanut butter-covered pine cones in bird seed. Pour some bird seed on a paper plate and let children take turns rolling their pine cones in it. Encourage the children to name or describe the items they are using. Let children take their bird feeders home to hang up where they can watch the birds eat.

Activity 4: Talking Bird

Materials

battery-operated talking bird that records and plays back children's voices	bird seed blocks to use as pretend bird seed

Goals

Sensory
- to improve auditory attending

- to improve visual attending
- to increase attention span

Fine Motor
- to improve hand manipulation, reach and grasp, grasp and release, and eye-hand coordination

Cognitive
- to improve imitation, understanding of cause and effect, and concept development
- to develop generalization skills
- to develop recall skills

Language
- to improve following directions; taking turns; identifying/labeling objects, actions, people, and characteristics; listening skills; increasing vocalizations; requesting; and initiating

Social
- to make choices
- to facilitate representational/pretend play

Directions

Gather the children in a group. Introduce them to the talking bird by name. Demonstrate how the bird "talks" when you talk to it. Help the children take turns talking with the bird. Incorporate feeding the bird, if appropriate. Use real bird seed at first. Pretend to run out of seed, then help the children figure out that they can substitute the blocks as pretend food.

Snack

Materials

peanut butter	powdered milk
honey	candy sprinkles or chopped
raisins	nuts (optional)
mixing bowl	mixing spoon
measuring cups	paper plates
juice	napkins
cups (adapted if necessary)	table
chairs (adaptive seating as needed)	washcloths for cleanup

Note: see Appendix C for a peanut butter dough recipe.

Goals

Sensory
- to improve responses to sensory stimuli, especially tactile and olfactory
- to increase attention span

Fine Motor
- to improve reach and grasp, grasp and release, hand/finger manipulation, eye-hand coordination, midline skills, and using both hands together

Self-Help
- to improve self-feeding skills
- to improve oral-motor skills

Cognitive
- to improve functional object use, understanding of spatial relationships, imitation, and concept formation
- to develop generalization skills
- to develop recall skills

Language
- to improve following directions; taking turns; identifying/labeling objects, actions, people, characteristics; requesting; initiating

Social
- to make choices
- to facilitate peer interaction
- to facilitate representational/pretend play

Directions

Seat children appropriately for snack, using adaptive seating as needed. Have children help mix the peanut butter dough. Encourage them to identify each ingredient and action required. Give each child a small lump of the peanut butter mixture and let them shape it into balls, snakes, or logs. Let children choose what color candy sprinkles or decorations to use. Relate this activity to the earlier pine cone bird feeder activity. What is similar? What is different? Let children eat their creations. Encourage communication, including ways to request more or indicate "all done." Assist with self-feeding and oral-motor skills as needed. Offer juice and assistance with drinking skills as needed.

Week 3

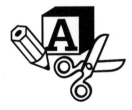

Overall Theme: Lights

Activity 1: Follow the Lights

Materials

indoor climbing structure	toddler slide
inner tubes	indoor tunnel
ramp or other incline	strings of colored mini-lights
floor pillows/beanbag chairs	benches
bolsters	steps
indoor swing	

Goals

Sensory
- to improve responses to sensory stimulation
- to provide vestibular stimulation
- to provide proprioceptive stimulation
- to increase attention span

Gross Motor
- to improve balance, coordination, motor planning, locomotion, trunk rotation, weight shifting, and weight bearing

Fine Motor
- to improve using both hands together, reach and grasp, grasp and release, visual attending and tracking, and hand manipulation
- to increase upper body strength
- to improve shoulder girdle strength and stability

Cognitive
- to improve understanding of spatial relationships, imitation, problem solving, and concept development
- to improve generalization skills

Language
- to improve following directions; taking turns; identifying/labeling objects, actions, descriptions, and locations; requesting; and initiating

Social
- to make choices
- to facilitate peer interaction

Directions

Using the equipment available, set up an indoor obstacle course to facilitate the gross motor and vestibular goals for the individuals in the group. The materials listed above are just suggestions. String the colored lights through the course and use them as a guide in sequencing activities. Assist the children through the obstacle course, having them follow the path marked by the lights. This activity can be even more effective if the room lights are dimmed, but this should be done only if the group can still negotiate the course safely. Encourage the children to use appropriate motor patterns throughout. Use lots of language to describe what is happening, who is doing what, and the relationships among objects; for example, "Tim is on the slide; Maria is behind the beanbag."

Activity 2: Flashlight Game

Materials

flashlights   colored filters for flashlights (optional)
seasonal pictures

Goals

Sensory
- to increase attention span

Gross Motor
- to improve motor planning, balance, coordination, trunk rotation, weight bearing, and weight shifting

Fine Motor
- to improve reach and grasp, grasp and release, visual attending and tracking, eye-hand coordination, hand manipulation, finger isolation, and wrist rotation
- to increase upper body strength
- to improve shoulder girdle strength and stability

Cognitive
- to improve understanding of spatial relationships, functional object use, classification, matching, imitation, and concept development
- to develop recall skills

Language
- to improve following directions; taking turns; identifying/labeling objects, pictures, people, actions, and concepts; initiating; and requesting

Social
- to make choices
- to facilitate peer interaction

Directions

Decorate the room with the seasonal pictures. Provide several flashlights of different sizes. Cover some with filters or colored cellophane to change the color of the beam of light, such as red, green, or blue. Give the children flashlights and let them explore. This activity is more effective if you can safely dim the room lights. Then help them find specific pictures or trace specific patterns with their flashlights. Adults can also "point" to various pictures with their flashlights and ask the children to name the picture, tell something about it, and find matching or related pictures. Talk about all aspects of the activity.

Activity 3: Candles

Materials

candleholders, such as Menorahs, yule logs, and candlesticks for Kwaanza	candles
	matches
	table
chairs (adaptive seating as needed)	construction paper
scissors	glue
washcloths for cleanup	

Goals

Sensory
- to improve responses to sensory stimulation
- to increase attention span

Fine Motor
- to improve hand/finger manipulation, visual attending and tracking, eye-hand coordination, using both hands together, reach and grasp, grasp and release, and midline skills

Cognitive
- to improve understanding of spatial relationships, functional object use, imitation, object-picture association, classification, and concept development
- to develop generalization skills
- to develop recall skills

Language
- to improve following directions; taking turns; increasing vocabulary; identifying/labeling objects, actions, characteristics, and relationships; initiating; and requesting

Social
- to make choices
- to facilitate peer interaction

Directions

If possible, have parents or staff members bring in candleholders. Light the candles for the class and explain some of the traditions associated with the holidays they celebrate. For the children, provide paper candleholders that have been prepared ahead of time. Let children choose the color paper they want to use to make candles. Help them cut or tear strips to make the candles. Help them tear small yellow paper strips for flames. Help them glue the candles to the candleholders and the flames to the candles. Use lots of language during the activity to relate the paper candleholders to the real ones and describe what the children see and do.

The candles may be prepared ahead of time if working with a very young class or if time is limited.

Activity 4: Big Sun

Materials

markers and/or crayons
scissors
easels (optional)

tape
large butcher paper or newsprint
washcloths for cleanup

Goals

Sensory
- to increase attention span
- to improve visual attending

Gross Motor
- to improve weight bearing, weight shifting, and balance

Fine Motor
- to improve hand/finger manipulation, eye-hand coordination, using both hands together, reach and grasp, and grasp and release
- to increase upper body strength
- to improve shoulder girdle strength and stability

Cognitive
- to improve imitation and concept development
- to develop generalization skills
- to develop recall skills

Language
- to improve following directions; taking turns; increasing vocabulary; identifying/labeling objects, actions, characteristics, and relationships; initiating; and requesting

Social
- to make choices
- to facilitate peer interaction

Is

ut large sun shapes ahead of time and fasten them to the easels or the wall.
activity can also be done with children seated, if more appropriate. In that case,
smaller paper cutouts. Have children color the suns with markers or crayons.
courage them to reach up to decorate the suns. Use lots of language to talk about
hat they are doing.

*Note: Some traditions celebrate winter solstice, the time when the days once again
begin to get longer, with the promise that the sun is returning to the land. This activity recognizes these traditions.*

Activity 5: Stained Glass

Materials

multicolored tissue paper	liquid laundry starch
heavy white paper	scissors
bowls	table
chairs (adaptive seating as needed)	washcloths for cleanup

Goals

Sensory
- to improve responses to sensory stimulation
- to increase attention span

Fine Motor
- to improve visual attending and tracking, hand/finger manipulation, reach and grasp, grasp and release, finger isolation, and eye-hand coordination
- to increase upper body strength
- to improve shoulder girdle strength and stability

Cognitive
- to improve understanding of spatial relationships, imitation, and concept development
- to develop generalization skills

Language
- to improve following directions; taking turns; identifying/labeling objects, actions, descriptions, relationships, and people; initiating; and requesting

Social
- to make choices
- to facilitate peer interaction

Directions

Ahead of time, cut out basic shapes from the heavy white paper. Position children appropriately for fine motor activity. Let them choose which colors of tissue paper to use. Help them tear the tissue paper into strips. Pour some liquid starch into shallow bowls and help the children dip the tissue strips into the starch. Then help them spread the starch-covered strips onto the white paper shapes. Use lots of language to talk about the process with the children; who is doing what; and how the tissue sounds, feels, and looks.

Snack

Materials

sugar cookie dough	hard candy or lollipops	flour
cutting board	cooking oil	cookie sheets
spatula	potholders	juice or milk
plates	napkins	chairs (adaptive
cups (adapted if necessary)	table	seating as needed)
washcloths for cleanup	oven	

Goals

Sensory
- to improve sensory awareness and responsiveness, especially tactile and olfactory
- to improve visual attending
- to increase attention span

Fine Motor
- to improve using both hands together, midline skills, hand/finger manipulation, eye-hand coordination, reach and grasp, and grasp and release
- to increase upper body strength
- to improve shoulder girdle strength and stability

Self-Help
- to improve self-feeding skills
- to improve oral-motor skills

Cognitive
- to improve tool use, understanding of spatial relationships, functional object use, imitation, sequencing, and concept development
- to develop generalization skills
- to develop recall skills

Language
- to improve following directions; taking turns; identifying/labeling objects, actions, characteristics, locations, and relationships; initiating; requesting; and increasing vocabulary

Social
- to make choices
- to facilitate peer interaction

Directions

Seat children appropriately at the table. Tell them they will be helping to make stained glass cookies. Place prepared cookie dough on a floured cutting board and demonstrate rolling pieces of dough into "snakes." Give each child a ball of dough and help to roll it into a snake. Then have the children make designs with their snakes. Place their snake designs on baking pans and put pieces of hard candy (or crushed lollipop) in the spaces of the designs. Let children choose which colors/flavors to use for their cookies. The heat will melt the candy to create a stained glass effect. If possible, let the children watch you put the cookies in the oven and take them out. Throughout the activity, use lots of language to talk about how the dough feels and smells, what the children are doing, the color and texture of the candy, and the shape of the cookies. Allow cookies to cool thoroughly before offering them to the children. Encourage them to choose which cookies they want. Talk about making the cookies and how the cookies are like the stained glass projects they just completed. Assist with self-feeding and drinking as needed.

Week 4

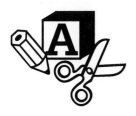

Overall Theme: Gingerbread House

Activity 1: Big Gingerbread House

Materials

large cardboard box, such as for
  a stove or washing machine
construction paper
tape
markers

low table
knife or other tools for cutting doors
  and windows in the box
scissors

Goals

Sensory
- to improve responses to sensory stimulation
- to increase attention span

Gross Motor
- to improve balance, coordination, motor planning, locomotion, trunk rotation, weight bearing, and weight shifting

Fine Motor
- to improve using both hands together, reach and grasp, grasp and release, visual attending and tracking, and hand/finger manipulation
- to increase upper body strength
- to improve shoulder girdle strength and stability

Cognitive
- to improve understanding of spatial relationships, object permanence, imitation, problem solving, sequencing, and concept development
- to develop generalization skills
- to develop recall skills

Language
- to improve following directions; taking turns; identifying/labeling objects, actions, descriptions, and locations; requesting; initiating; and increasing vocabulary

Social
- to make choices
- to facilitate pretend play
- to facilitate peer interaction

Directions

Prepare as much of this activity ahead of time as appropriate for the needs of your group. Make the box into a house by cutting out doors and windows. Cut out a few of the doors and windows on three sides only so that they open and close. Cut cookie and candy shapes from construction paper. Older preschoolers might enjoy participating in the preparation.

Have the pre-made house available for the group to look at. Talk about what it is and how it is made. The box is going to become a big gingerbread house. Let children choose which shapes they want to use for decorating the house. Assist them as needed with taping the decorations on the house. Encourage them to reach up and down as well as work at eye level.

Activity 2: Little Gingerbread House

Materials

cardboard gingerbread house from previous activity
variety of candies and cookies
knives
table
smocks
washcloths for cleanup

pre-made, undecorated gingerbread house
frosting
paper plates and/or bowls
chairs (adaptive seating or standers as needed)

Goals

Sensory
- to improve responses to sensory stimulation
- to increase attention span

Fine Motor
- to improve hand/finger manipulation, visual attending and tracking, eye-hand coordination, using two hands together, reach and grasp, and grasp and release

Cognitive
- to improve understanding of spatial relationships, problem solving, sequencing, classification, and concept development
- to develop generalization skills
- to develop recall skills

Language
- to improve following directions; taking turns; identifying/labeling objects, actions, and characteristics; initiating; and requesting

Social
- to make choices
- to facilitate peer interaction

Directions

This activity can be done with the children standing or seated at a table, depending on what is most appropriate for the group. Just as they made the big gingerbread house, they are now going to make a little gingerbread house. Give each child a bowl or plate with some frosting and a plastic knife. Candies and cookies should be sorted into bowls. Encourage children to choose which items they wish to use to decorate the house and to plan where to put each one. Have them identify the items and the parts of the house they are decorating. Demonstrate how to spread the frosting on the items and stick them on the house. They may also spread the frosting on the house and then stick on the items. Encourage requests to pass bowls or share items.

Activity 3: Gingerbread Doll House

Materials

cardboard gingerbread house
   from Activity 1
clothes for dolls
lotion, powder, diapers for dolls
doll houses, furniture, and
   other accessories
tape

dolls of various sizes, ethnicities,
   ages, and genders
brushes and combs for the dolls' hair
doll dishes, spoons, and bottles
construction paper
scissors

Goals

Sensory
- to improve responses to sensory stimulation
- to increase attention span

Gross Motor
- to improve motor planning, balance, and coordination

Fine Motor
- to improve hand/finger manipulation, using two hands together, midline skills, reach and grasp, and grasp and release

Cognitive
- to improve tool use, functional object use, imitation, understanding of spatial relationships, and concept development
- to develop generalization skills
- to develop recall skills

Language
- to improve turn taking; identifying/labeling objects, actions, descriptions, and relationships; increasing vocabulary; initiating; and requesting

Social
- to make choices
- to facilitate representational/pretend play
- to facilitate peer interaction

Directions

Decorate the doll houses with paper cutouts to resemble gingerbread houses. Set up the larger dolls and their accessories in or near the big gingerbread house from Activity 1. Ask the group to imagine what it would be like to live in a gingerbread house. Encourage them to act it out. Have the children choose to play at one house or the other. Observe and facilitate their play as needed. When facilitating play, try to model the next higher level of play. For example, if the child is hugging the doll, repeat that action and encourage brushing its hair or giving it a bottle. If a child is already doing those things, model sequencing behaviors such as heating the bottle and then giving it to the doll. Use lots of language to describe what the children are doing.

Activity 4: Story Time

Materials

illustrated story featuring gingerbread, such as "The Gingerbread Boy" or "Hansel and Gretel"

cushions or carpet squares (adapted seating as needed)

Goals

Sensory
- to improve auditory attending
- to increase attention span

Gross Motor
- to improve sitting balance and coordination

Fine Motor
- to improve hand/finger manipulation, eye-hand coordination, and using both hands together

Cognitive
- to improve object-picture association and concept development
- to develop generalization skills
- to develop recall skills

Language
- to improve following directions; taking turns; increasing vocabulary; and identifying/labeling objects, pictures, actions, characteristics, and relationships

Directions

Gather the children for story time. Each child should have a carpet square, cushion, or floor sitter. Share the selected story with the group. Encourage them to talk about the story, ask questions, and relate the story to the other activities of the day. At the same time, do not allow the group's conversation to wander too far from sharing the story together. It sometimes helps to tell the story in your own words while sharing the illustrations with the children. If appropriate, let the children take turns helping to flip the pages. Ask children to find various items in the illustrations or to describe what they see on the page.

Snack

Materials

gingerbread house from Activity 2   gingerbread people cookies
juice or milk   cups (adapted as needed)
napkins (optional)   table
chairs (adaptive seating as needed)   washcloths for cleanup

Goals

Sensory
- to improve responses to sensory stimuli, especially tactile and olfactory
- to increase attention span

Fine Motor
- to improve using both hands together, midline skills, hand/finger manipulation, eye-hand coordination, reach and grasp, and grasp and release

Self-Help
- to improve self-feeding skills
- to improve oral-motor skills

Cognitive
- to improve imitation, sequencing, functional object use, tool use, understanding of spatial relationships, and concept development
- to develop generalization skills
- to develop recall skills

Language
- to improve following directions; taking turns; identifying/labeling objects, actions, people, and characteristics; requesting; and initiating

Social
- to make choices
- to facilitate peer interaction
- to facilitate pretend play

Directions

Seat children appropriately for snack, using adaptive seating as needed. Have children help pass out napkins, if appropriate. Show children the gingerbread house and cookies. If they want to, help them break apart the gingerbread house and eat it. They may also eat the cookies. Review the preceding activities, including making the house and pretending to be gingerbread people. Encourage communication, including ways to request more or indicate "all done." Assist with self-feeding skills as needed. Offer milk or juice and provide assistance as needed.

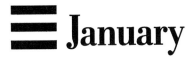

January

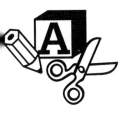

Overall Theme: Snow

Note: Most of these activities can be adapted for regions where snow is rare. For example, the Styrofoam Snow activity would be equally effective as Styrofoam Rain. Sledding could become Sliding or Scooter Boards.

Activity 1: Styrofoam Snow

Materials

large cardboard box or wading pool
cups or other containers for scooping chips
objects to hide in the chips

styrofoam packing chips to fill
  box or pool

Goals

Sensory
- to improve sensory awareness and responsiveness
- to facilitate increased body awareness

Gross Motor
- to improve motor planning, weight shifting, trunk rotation, sitting balance, and coordination

Fine Motor
- to improve grasp and release, visual tracking, and using both hands together
- to increase upper body strength

Cognitive
- to improve object permanence, understanding of spatial relationships, tool use, and concept development

Language
- to improve following directions; taking turns; imitation; identifying/labeling objects, people, and actions; initiating; and requesting

Social
- to facilitate peer interaction

Directions

Fill a box or wading pool with styrofoam chips so that the chips will be about waist high when the children are seated in them. Position children around the box or pool and allow them to play in the "snow" chips with their hands. This is a good opportunity to work on standing, side-sitting, or other therapeutic positioning. As they become comfortable with the chips, help them to climb into the box or pool or place them in it, preferably at least two at a time. A box big enough to contain at least four children is even better. If possible, remove most of the children's clothing before placing them in the chips. Some children may find the chips too uncomfortable on their bare skin. For these children, try just rolling up their shirt sleeves and pant legs to see if they can tolerate that degree of contact. Children with poor sitting balance can often be propped up in a corner and supported by the chips. Encourage children to move different body parts (Where are your feet?) and to identify parts being covered by the chips. Scoop up some of the chips and let them "snow" on the children. Pretend it is snowing and talk about snow. Encourage children to imitate scooping the chips and letting them create falling "snow." Hide objects in the chips and encourage the children to find and identify them. Place the objects all around the children so they have to reach to the front, sides, and behind them in order to retrieve the objects.

Caution: Many children will want to put the chips in their mouths. Watch carefully to prevent choking.

Activity 2: Sledding

Materials

scooter boards
saucer-shaped snow sleds
ramp or incline (optional)

Goals

Sensory
- to improve responses to vestibular stimulation

Gross Motor
- to improve motor planning, balance and coordination, reciprocal use of arms and legs, and acceptance of prone positioning
- to increase back strength

Fine Motor
- to improve weight bearing on open hands
- to increase upper body strength

Cognitive
- to improve imitation, understanding of spatial relationships, and concept development

Language
- to improve following directions; taking turns; identifying/labeling actions, people, locations, and relationships; initiating; and requesting

Social
- to facilitate peer interaction

Directions

Position children on appropriately sized scooter boards. Encourage the children to move themselves forward or backward. Gently pull or push them if they do not propel themselves. Some may be ready to go down a gentle incline, if available. During the activity, talk about going sledding through imaginary snow. Use lots of language to describe what the children are doing and who is doing it. You can also position the children in the saucers and rock, tilt, or gently spin them through the "snow."

Caution: Vestibular stimulation can have powerful effects. This activity should be planned in consultation with the physical or occupational therapist. Spinning, in particular, should be carried out only under the supervision of a trained occupational or physical therapist.

Activity 3: Big Snowballs

Materials

large therapy balls of several sizes
playground balls of various sizes
ramp or incline (optional)
stickers for snowpeople's faces (optional)

Goals

Sensory
- to improve responses to proprioceptive and vestibular stimulation
- to facilitate increased body awareness

Gross Motor
- to improve motor planning, trunk rotation, balance and coordination, sitting balance, and weight shifting

Fine Motor
- to improve using both hands together
- to increase upper body strength

Cognitive
- to improve concept development and understanding of spatial relationships

Language
- to improve following directions; taking turns; imitation; identifying/labeling objects, people, actions, locations, and relationships; initiating; and requesting

Social
- to facilitate peer interaction
- to develop representational play

Directions

Bring out therapy balls and allow the children to explore them. Patting the balls provides proprioceptive stimulation. Pushing the balls while walking provides practice with weight shifting, standing balance, and walking skills, as well as proprioceptive stimulation and strengthening of the upper body. Interventionists can support the children and bounce them on the balls to stimulate muscle tone or use gentle rocking to relax muscle tone. Trunk rotation, balance reactions, and improved use of abdominal muscles can also be facilitated. After these initial activities, model rolling the balls as if they were big snowballs. Rolling the balls over the children provides lots of proprioceptive stimulation. The children can also roll the balls down the incline. Model putting a smaller ball on top of a larger one to make a "snowperson." Represent the face with stickers, if desired. Many of the same activities can be repeated using the smaller balls.

Activity 4: Snow Scene Grab Bag

Materials

several snow scenes (plastic containers with winter scenes inside. "Snow" falls when the container is inverted and then turned right side up again.)
box or bag

Goals

Sensory
- to facilitate visual focusing and attending
- to increase attention span

Gross Motor
- to improve balance, coordination, and weight shifting

Fine Motor
- to improve using two hands together, midline skills, reaching and grasping, wrist rotation, and hand manipulation

Cognitive
- to improve understanding of spatial relationships, object permanence, and concept development
- to develop generalization skills

Language
- to improve following directions; taking turns; identifying/labeling objects and actions; requesting; and initiating

Social
- to make choices
- to facilitate peer interaction

Directions

Show children one or more of the snow scenes then place them all in a bag or box. Encourage children to reach into the container and take out one of the scenes. Help them play appropriately with it. Describe what they are doing and what happens in the snow scene as it is manipulated. Encourage children to trade scenes as they begin to tire of the particular one they have selected. Alternatively, all children could put the scenes back into the container and then each select another.

Activity 5: Gluing Snowpeople

Materials

dark-colored construction paper	styrofoam chips
white chalk or crayon	glue
paintbrushes (optional)	cotton swabs (optional)
table	chairs (adaptive seating as needed)
washcloths for cleanup	

Goals

Sensory
- to improve sensory awareness through tactile stimulation
- to increase attention span

Fine Motor
- to improve hand manipulation, eye-hand coordination, and using both hands together

Cognitive
- to improve imitation and concept development
- to develop generalization skills
- to develop recall skills

Language
- to improve following directions; taking turns; increasing vocabulary; and identifying/labeling objects, actions, characteristics, and relationships

Social
- to make choices

Directions

Prepare papers ahead of time by drawing the outline of a snowperson on each with white chalk or crayon. Position children for fine motor activity. Have children select which color paper to use. Help children squeeze or spread glue onto their papers, encouraging them to stabilize the paper with one hand, if possible. You can vary the activity by having the children spread the glue with paintbrushes or cotton swabs, as well as with their fingers. Help them put styrofoam chips onto the glue. Breaking the chips apart provides additional fine motor and sensory stimulation. Help them pat the styrofoam pieces into place. Use lots of language and encourage the children to describe what they are doing and using. Remind them that these are the chips they were playing with earlier in the box. Mention that the pictures look like snowpeople. Let the pictures dry while completing another activity.

Snack

Materials

vanilla ice cream	ice cream scoop
coconut	wax paper
spoons (adapted as needed)	juice
cups (adapted as needed)	table
chairs (adaptive seating as needed)	napkins
washcloths for cleanup	

Goals

Sensory
- to improve responses to sensory stimuli, especially tactile, temperature, and olfactory

Self-Help
- to improve self-feeding skills
- to improve oral-motor skills

Language
- to improve identifying/labeling objects, actions, people, and characteristics; taking turns; requesting; and concept development
- to develop generalization skills

Social
• to facilitate peer interaction

Directions

Seat children appropriately for snack, using adaptive seating as needed. Place wax paper on the table in front of each child. Sprinkle some flaked coconut "snow" on the wax paper. Give each child a round ball of ice cream scooped with the ice cream scoop. Allow the children to help scoop, if appropriate. Help children roll the ice cream in coconut with their hands. Comment on how cold the ice cream is, like snow. Talk about other ways this activity is like some of the previous activities. Encourage the children to describe what they are doing. Have children help pass out napkins and spoons, if appropriate. Facilitate appropriate feeding skills as necessary for each individual. Encourage communication, including ways to request more or indicate "all done." Offer juice and provide assistance as needed.

Week 2

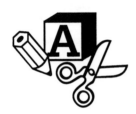

Overall Theme: More Snow

Note: As with the previous week's activities, these activities may be adapted to climates without snow. The theme for this set of activities might be Ball Play, for example.

Activity 1: Human Snowballs

Materials

wedge, ramp, or incline

Goals

Sensory
• to provide proprioceptive input
• to improve responses to vestibular stimulation
• to facilitate increased body awareness

Gross Motor
• to improve motor planning, trunk rotation, and rolling

Cognitive
• to improve imitation, understanding of spatial relationships; and concept formation
• to develop generalization skills

Language
• to improve following directions; taking turns; identifying/labeling people, actions, locations, and relationships; initiating; and requesting

Social
• to facilitate peer interaction
• to facilitate pretend play

Directions

Have children pretend to be snowballs and roll down the incline, like the big "snowballs" that they rolled the previous week. Provide the necessary facilitation for children who are physically challenged and be sure to use an incline that is appropriately steep for each individual. Children who are very insecure may need to roll on the flat floor or on a mat boosted up a tiny bit at one end with a towel. Older children may need a much steeper incline to maintain their interest in the activity. Use lots of language to talk about what the children are doing and what sensations they are experiencing.

Activity 2: Snowball Fight

Materials

white scrap paper
large boxes to store the "snowballs"

Goals

Sensory
- to improve sensory awareness and responsiveness

Gross Motor
- to improve balance and throwing skills

Fine Motor
- to improve hand manipulation, reach and grasp, controlled grasp and release, and midline skills
- to increase upper body strength

Cognitive
- to improve imitation, understanding of spatial relationships, cause and effect, and concept development
- to develop generalization skills

Language
- to improve following directions; taking turns; identifying/labeling objects, people, actions, descriptions, and locations; requesting; and initiating

Social
- to facilitate representational play
- to facilitate peer interaction

Directions

Help children make "snowballs" by crumpling white scrap paper into balls. Have them put the "snowballs" into a large box or basket. When the container is full, help them throw the balls at a target on the wall, into another container, or at each other.

Activity 3: Play Dough

Materials

homemade play dough   child-sized rolling pins
Plastic knives   cookie cutters
child-sized table   wooden hammers
washcloths for cleanup   chairs (adaptive seating as needed)

Note: see Appendix C for a play dough recipe

Goals

Sensory
- to improve responses to sensory stimulation, especially tactile
- to increase attention span

Fine Motor
- to improve using both hands together, midline skills, hand and finger manipulation, and visual attending
- to increase upper body strength

Cognitive
- to improve tool use, understanding of spatial relationships, functional use of objects, and imitation

Language
- to improve following directions; taking turns; sequencing; identifying/labeling objects, actions, locations, and relationships; initiating; and requesting

Social
- to make choices
- to facilitate peer interaction

Directions

Prepare the dough ahead of time. Don't use food coloring so that the white dough will resemble snow. Start with a large ball of dough on the table. Encourage children to explore it, including asking for some or trying to break some off. Give each child a chunk and help them roll it into balls. They can make one large ball or several small balls. Show them how to model snowpeople with the dough. Other ways of exploring with the dough include patting it into a flat pancake shape, poking it with isolated fingers, pinching it to make mountains, rolling it into a snake shape, rolling it with rolling pins, cutting it with the knives or cookie cutters, or hammering it with the hammers. Throughout the activity, use lots of language to describe what is happening. Compare the dough balls—big, little, lumpy, smooth. Describe the feel of the dough. Compare the dough snowballs with the paper snowballs. How are they the same? How are they different?

Activity 4: Gluing Snowpeople

Materials

dark-colored construction paper	uncooked rice
white chalk or crayon	glue
paintbrushes (optional)	cotton swabs (optional)
table	chairs (adaptive seating as needed)
washcloths for cleanup	

Goals

Sensory
- to improve sensory awareness through tactile stimulation
- to increase attention span

Fine Motor
- to improve hand and finger manipulation, eye-hand coordination, and using both hands together

Cognitive
- to improve imitation skills
- to develop generalization skills
- to develop recall skills

Language
- to improve following directions; taking turns; increasing vocabulary; and identifying/labeling objects, actions, characteristics, and relationships

Social
- to make choices

Directions

Prepare papers ahead of time by drawing the outline of a snowperson on each piece with white chalk or crayon. Position children for fine motor activity. Have children select which color paper to use. Help them squeeze or spread glue onto their papers, encouraging them to stabilize the paper with one hand, if possible. You can vary the activity by having the children spread the glue with paintbrushes or cotton swabs, as well as with their fingers. Help them sprinkle rice onto the glue and pat it into place. Use lots of language and encourage the children to describe what they are doing and using. Mention that the pictures look like snowpeople. Compare the feel of the rice with the feel of the play dough. Let the pictures dry while completing another activity.

Snack

Materials

round crackers	cream cheese	raisins
juice	table knives	paper plates
napkins, if needed	cups (adapted as needed)	table
chairs (adaptive seating as needed)	washcloths for cleanup	

Goals

Sensory
- to improve responses to sensory stimuli, especially tactile and olfactory
- to increase attention span

Fine Motor
- to improve using both hands together, grasp and release, and hand manipulation

Self-Help
- to improve self-feeding skills
- to improve oral-motor skills

Cognitive
- to develop generalization skills
- to develop recall skills

Language
- to improve following directions; imitation; identifying/labeling objects, actions, people, and characteristics; taking turns; and requesting

Social
- to make choices
- to facilitate peer interaction

Directions

Seat children appropriately for snack, using adaptive seating as needed. As children watch, spread two or three crackers with cream cheese to make a "snowperson." Tell them they are going to make snowpeople, too. Give each child a table knife and two to three crackers. Help them spread the cream cheese on the crackers. Use the raisins to make the eyes, nose, and mouth. Describe what the children are doing, what the snack is made of, and what it looks like. Talk about how it looks like a snowperson. Encourage communication, including ways to request more or indicate "all done." Offer juice as needed. Assist with self-feeding and drinking skills as needed.

Week 3

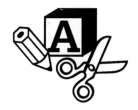

Overall Theme: Winter

Note: These activities can be modified as appropriate to your climate. For example, Winter Walk could become The Walk, and Winter Clothes could become Dress-Up. You could also substitute a unifying theme appropriate to your climate.

Activity 1: Winter Walk

Materials

indoor climbing structure
inner tubes
ramp or other incline
floor pillows/beanbag chairs
bolsters
indoor swing

toddler slide
indoor tunnel/barrel
carpet squares
benches
steps

Goals

Sensory
- to provide proprioceptive stimulation
- to provide vestibular stimulation
- to increase attention span

Gross Motor
- to improve balance, coordination, motor planning, locomotion, trunk rotation, and weight shifting

Fine Motor
- to improve using both hands together, reach and grasp, and visual attending
- to increase upper body strength
- to improve shoulder girdle strength and stability

Cognitive
- to improve imitation, problem solving, understanding of spatial relationships, and concept formation

Language
• to improve following directions; taking turns; identifying/labeling objects, actions, characteristics, and locations; requesting; and initiation

Social
• to make choices
• to facilitate peer interaction
• to facilitate pretend play

Directions

Using the equipment available, set up an indoor obstacle course to facilitate the gross motor and vestibular goals for the individuals in the group. The materials listed on the previous page are just suggestions. Assist the children through the obstacle course. A "path" of carpet squares can provide a structure to follow through the course. Encourage them to use appropriate motor patterns throughout. Talk about winter weather and winter weather activities. Also talk about the cold and how animals find warm homes for the winter. As the children go through the course, help them act out winter weather activities or pretend finding warm homes as if they were bunnies, squirrels, or birds.

Activity 2: Winter Clothes

Materials

hats	coats	mittens
scarves	boots	sweaters
dolls or stuffed animals	large mirror	

Note: All clothes should be a little too big for the children to facilitate dressing and undressing.

Goals

Sensory
• to increase sensory awareness and improve sensory responsiveness
• to improve body awareness

Gross Motor
• to improve motor planning, balance, coordination, and imitation

Fine Motor
• to improve midline skills and hand and finger manipulation
• to increase upper body strength

Self-Help
• to improve dressing, undressing, and fastening skills (buttoning and zipping)

Cognitive
• to improve understanding of spatial relationships, association, classification, imitation, and concept formation
• to develop generalization skills

Language
• to develop taking turns; sequencing; identifying/labeling objects, actions, people, characteristics, relationships, and body parts; following directions; initiating; and requesting

Social
- to make choices
- to facilitate peer interaction
- to facilitate representational and pretend play

Directions

Direct children to the pile of clothing. Encourage them to select items, identify them, try them on, and look at themselves in the mirror. Encourage lots of language to describe the articles of clothing, including what they look like and feel like. Listen to the sounds the boots make. Do the clothes smell different than usual? Use lots of language to describe what the children are doing; for example, "You're putting the sleeve over your arm," or "You're putting your foot in the boot." Talk about for what kinds of weather you would wear the different items: boots in the rain or snow and a sweater when it's cool but a coat when it's cold. Assist children with dressing and fastening skills as appropriate. Encourage them to try the clothing on the dolls. How does it fit? How do they look? How is this the same as when the children tried on the clothing? How is it different?

Activity 3: Fine Motor Free Play

Materials

a variety of manipulative toys, preferably with a winter theme; for example:

puzzles	books	sewing cards
blocks	pegs	bristle blocks
interlocking blocks (such as Duplo™)	beads/laces	

Goals

Sensory
- to increase attention span

Fine Motor
- to improve hand/finger manipulation and eye-hand coordination

Cognitive
- to improve understanding of spatial relationships, imitation, problem solving, and picture-object association
- to improve generalization skills

Language
- to improve concept formation; taking turns; increasing vocalizations/vocabulary; requesting and initiating; following directions; and identifying and labeling objects, actions, characteristics, and locations

Social
- to make choices
- to facilitate peer interaction

Directions

Set up "stations" for the various toys. Allow children to wander to a station and begin playing. An adult can then assist with the play, expanding and guiding as appropriate. Depending on the child's needs, gross motor goals can be incorporated into these activities by positioning the stations so that the child stands or kneels to play, for example. Encourage children to take turns with an adult or peer in stacking blocks and knocking them down. Use lots of language to describe what is happening. Emphasize the winter theme where appropriate.

Activity 4: Winter Scene

Materials

dark construction paper
white chalk
table
chairs (adaptive seating as needed)
washcloths for cleanup

Goals

Sensory
- to increase sensory awareness and improve sensory responsiveness
- to increase attention span

Fine Motor
- to improve hand manipulation, eye-hand coordination, visual focusing and tracking, and using two hands together
- to increase shoulder girdle strength and stability

Cognitive
- to improve tool use, imitation, and concept development
- to develop generalization skills

Language
- to improve following directions; taking turns; and identifying/labeling objects, actions, characteristics, and relationships

Social
- to make choices
- to facilitate peer interaction

Directions

Position children appropriately for fine motor activity. Encourage them to choose which color paper to use. Give each child a piece of white chalk and encourage scribbling or whatever marks the children choose to make on their papers.

Snack

Materials

fruit	vanilla	milk
ice cream	sugar (optional)	ice cubes
blender	knives	spoons
cups (adapted as needed)	straws (optional)	washcloths for cleanup
table	chairs (adaptive seating as needed)	

Goals

Sensory
- to improve responses to sensory stimuli, especially tactile, temperature, and olfactory
- to increase attention span

Fine Motor
- to improve using both hands together, grasp and release, hand manipulation, and imitation

Self-Help
- to improve self-feeding skills
- to improve oral-motor skills

Language
- to improve following directions; identifying/labeling objects, actions, and characteristics, and relationships; taking turns; initiating; and requesting

Social
- to make choices
- to facilitate peer interaction

Directions

Tell children they are going to help make milk shakes. Show them the fruit and encourage them to name each piece. Have them help slice the fruit. Give each child some fruit pieces to put into the blender. Show them the milk and have them name it. Have the children help pour some milk into the blender. Repeat with the ice cream, having them help scoop some into the blender. Add a little vanilla. Let the children each have a chance to smell the vanilla. Add one or two ice cubes, if needed. Count "1-2-3, On" before turning the blender on, since the noise may frighten some children. If possible, set up a capability switch so that the children can turn the blender off and on themselves. Use lots of language to discuss the process, including the changes happening to the ingredients in the blender. Let the children help pour milk shakes into cups and drink with straws, if appropriate. Describe the milk shakes with the children. Provide assistance with oral-motor skills as needed.

Week 4

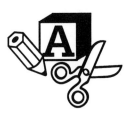

Overall Theme: Winter

Note: These activities should be modified as appropriate for your climate. For example, Sleigh Rides could become Buggy Rides or Wagon Rides in areas where the idea of sleigh riding is not a part of the history and culture; local vegetation could be substituted for evergreens in the Evergreen Walk.

Activity 1: Sleigh Rides

Materials

scooter boards
sleigh ride music (optional)
sleigh bells/jingle bells (optional)

hula hoops
pictures of sleigh riding

Goals

Sensory
- to improve responses to vestibular stimulation
- to provide proprioceptive stimulation

Gross Motor
- to improve motor planning, balance and coordination, reciprocal use of arms and legs, and acceptance of prone position

Fine Motor
- to improve grasp and release and understanding of spatial relationships
- to increase upper body strength

Cognitive
- to improve concept development
- to develop generalization skills

Language
- to improve following directions; taking turns; imitation; identifying/labeling actions, people, locations, and relationships; initiating; requesting

Social
- to facilitate representational/pretend play skills
- to facilitate peer interaction

Directions

Have some children lie prone on scooter boards. Have them hold onto hula hoops while other children or adults hold the other side of the hoops and pull the children on the scooter boards. Talk about what is happening; compare the activity with real sleigh rides. If possible, play sleigh ride music. Have the children carry, wear, or shake bells while riding and while pulling. This activity can be adapted by using wagons for those children for whom scooter boards are not appropriate.

Activity 2: Teddy Bear Sledding

Materials

scooter boards   saucer-shaped snow sleds
ramp or incline (optional)   teddy bears, dolls, or other stuffed animals

Goals

Sensory
- to improve responses to vestibular stimulation

Gross Motor
- to improve motor planning, balance and coordination, reciprocal use of arms and legs, and acceptance of prone position

Fine Motor
- to improve weight bearing on open hands
- to increase upper body strength

Cognitive
- to improve understanding of spatial relationships, concept development, and imitation
- to develop generalization skills

Language
- to improve following directions; taking turns; identifying/labeling actions, people, locations, and relationships; initiating; and requesting

Social
- to facilitate representational and pretend play
- to facilitate peer interaction

Directions

Position children on appropriate-sized scooter boards. Encourage them to move themselves forward or backward. Gently pull or push them if they do not propel themselves. Some may be ready to go down a gentle incline, if available. During the activity, talk about going sledding through the snow. Use lots of language to describe what the children are doing and who is doing what. You can also position the children in the saucers and rock, tilt, or gently spin them through the pretend snow. Have the children repeat these activities using the teddy bears on the scooter boards and saucers.

Caution: Vestibular stimulation can have powerful effects. This activity should be planned in consultation with the physical or occupational therapist. Spinning, in particular, should be carried out only under the supervision of a trained occupational or physical therapist.

Activity 3: Rice Table

Materials

sand table (can be filled with sand, rice, beans, or other dry textured material)
containers for scooping and hiding
small objects for hiding and finding
adaptive standers to allow children access to sand table, if needed

Goals

Sensory
- to improve sensory awareness/body awareness through tactile stimulation

Gross Motor
- to improve motor planning, standing balance, and weight shifting

Fine Motor
- to improve eye-hand coordination, wrist rotation, finger isolation (poking in rice), and hand manipulation skills
- to increase upper body strength

Cognitive
- to improve understanding of spatial relationships, object permanence, tool use, and imitation

Language
- to improve taking turns; identifying/labeling objects, actions, people, places, characteristics, and relationships; requesting; initiating; and following directions

Social
- to facilitate peer interaction

Directions

Remove the cover from the sand table and put containers and other objects into the rice or other material. Encourage children to play in the rice with their hands and fill the containers then pour out the rice. Hide objects in the rice and encourage children to find them. Encourage children to find specific objects and to name them before picking them up. Some children may want to hide objects for the adults to find. Ask children what they are doing. Encourage them to trade objects frequently with other children.

Activity 4: Evergreen Walk

Materials

access to outdoors, if possible
a variety of evergreen branches
strollers or other adaptive means of locomotion for children who are nonambulatory

Goals

Sensory
- to increase sensory awareness and improve responses to sensory stimulation
- to increase attention span
- to improve auditory and visual attending skills

Gross Motor
- to improve walking, stooping/squatting, weight shifting, balance, coordination, and motor planning

Fine Motor
- to improve eye-hand coordination, reach and grasp, hand manipulation, and finger isolation (pointing)
- to increase upper body strength

Cognitive
- to improve classification, imitation, and concept development
- to develop generalization skills

Language
- to improve following directions; taking turns; increasing vocalization/ vocabulary; identifying/labeling objects, actions, characteristics, relationships, and locations; initiating, requesting; and questioning

Social
- to facilitate peer interaction

Directions

Have children hike along a path outdoors, if possible. Otherwise, set up a "path" indoors with evergreen branches placed along the way. Encouraging them to march or hike with big, heavy steps will provide proprioceptive input and help them develop a variety of gross motor skills. Let the children who are walking push the strollers for the children who are using them, thus helping the walking children to improve their upper body strength. Talk with the children about what they see, hear, and smell. Help them collect evergreen branches. Ask questions about what they are doing and what they have found. Encourage describing the branches—what they feel like, look like, and smell like.

Activity 5: Snow Pictures

Materials

evergreen branches from previous activity	white paint
trays to contain paint for dipping	dark-colored paper
easels (optional)	table
chairs (adaptive seating as needed)	washcloths for cleanup

Goals

Sensory
- to improve responses to sensory stimulation
- to increase attention span

Gross Motor
- to improve hand manipulation and eye-hand coordination

Fine Motor
- to improve shoulder girdle strength and stability

Cognitive
- to improve tool use, imitation, and concept development
- to develop generalization skills

Language
- to improve following directions; taking turns; increasing vocabulary; and identifying/labeling objects, actions, characteristics, and relationships

Social
- to make choices
- to facilitate peer interaction

Directions

This activity can be done with children seated at a table, standing at a table, or standing at easels, depending on the children's motor goals. If the children will be seated, use small evergreen branches. You can use larger branches if the children will be standing at easels. Pour the paint into trays for easy dipping. The children can dip their branches into the paint and paint a snow scene on the paper using their branches as brushes. Encourage the children to choose which branch and which color paper to use. They may also want to trade branches during the activity. Use lots of language to describe what they are doing and creating.

Snack

Materials

whipped cream	graham crackers
table knives	plates (optional)
napkins (optional)	juice
cups (adapted as needed)	table
chairs (adaptive seating as needed)	washcloths for cleanup

Goals

Sensory
- to improve responses to sensory stimuli, especially tactile and olfactory
- to increase attention span

Fine Motor
- to improve using both hands together, grasp, and hand manipulation

Self-Help
- to improve self-feeding skills
- to improve oral-motor skills

Cognitive
- to improve imitation
- to develop generalization skills

Language
- to improve following directions; identifying/labeling objects, actions, people, and characteristics; taking turns; and requesting

Social
- to facilitate peer interaction

Directions

Seat children appropriately for snack, using adaptive seating as needed. As children watch, spread two or three graham crackers with whipped cream "snow." Tell them they are going to make snow crackers. Give each child a table knife and some graham crackers. Help them spread the whipped cream on the crackers. Describe what the children are doing, what the snack is made of, and what it looks like. Talk about how the whipped cream looks like snow. Encourage communication, including ways to request more or indicate "all done." Offer juice as needed. Assist with self-feeding/drinking skills as needed.

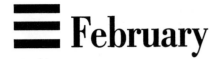

February

Week 1

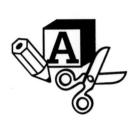

Overall Theme: Red

Note: To extend color themes, children can be asked to dress in the target color. They can also be given stickers in the target color to wear during the activities and to take home.

Activity 1: Obstacle Course

Materials

indoor climbing structure	toddler slide	inner tubes
indoor tunnel	ramp or other incline	carpet squares
red contact paper	floor pillows/beanbag chairs	benches
bolsters	steps	indoor swing
red beanbags	containers for beanbags	

Goals

Sensory
- to provide proprioceptive stimulation
- to increase attention span

Gross Motor
- to improve balance, coordination, motor planning, locomotion, trunk rotation, and weight shifting
- to strengthen the upper body

Fine Motor
- to improve using both hands together, reach and grasp, and visual attention
- to increase shoulder girdle strength and stability

Cognitive
- to improve object permanence, imitation, problem solving, and concept development

Language
- to improve following directions; taking turns; identifying/labeling objects, actions, descriptions, and locations; requesting; and initiating

Social
- to make choices
- to facilitate peer interaction

Directions

Using the equipment available, set up an indoor obstacle course to facilitate the gross motor and vestibular goals for individuals in the group,. The materials listed above are just suggestions. Place the red beanbags at various points throughout the obstacle course. Have some hidden, some partially hidden, and some in plain sight. Assist the children through the obstacle course. A "path" of carpet squares (preferably red) can provide a structure to follow through the course. Red contact paper can be attached to the carpet squares to enhance the color effect. Encourage the children to use appropriate motor patterns throughout. Help them find the beanbags as they go through the course. Be sure there are enough beanbags for each child to find at least two or three. Collect the beanbags in buckets or baskets, preferably red. Depending on their abilities, children can be encouraged to carry their own buckets filled with beanbags.

Activity 2: Beanbags

Materials

beanbags, preferably red   basket or bin to toss them in

Goals

Sensory
- to provide proprioceptive stimulation
- to increase attention span

Gross Motor
- to improve balance, weight shifting, throwing, and coordination

Fine Motor
- to improve eye-hand coordination, reach and grasp, and grasp and release
- to increase upper body strength

Cognitive
- to improve understanding of spatial relationships and imitation

Language
- to improve following directions; taking turns; identifying/labeling objects, actions, locations, and relationships; initiating; and requesting

Social
- to make choices
- to facilitate peer interaction

Directions

This activity usually works best if children are seated in a circle, with the target in the middle. Each child can take a beanbag from the bucket or adults can begin the activity by tossing beanbags to each child. Encourage children to throw the beanbags into the bucket or to each other. They may need help to accomplish this task. Children who are not yet ready to throw can participate by placing the beanbags in the container. Talk about the actions, who is throwing, and who is catching. Encourage children to name who they want to catch the beanbags. Emphasize the red beanbags. A red target (maybe heart-shaped) can be painted or glued onto the side of the container as a variation of this activity.

Activity 3: Red Toys

Materials

a variety of manipulative toys, predominately red in color; for example:
    interlocking blocks (such as Duplo™)   bristle blocks   wooden blocks
    pegs   beads   books

Goals

Sensory
- to increase attention span

Fine Motor
- to improve hand/finger manipulation and eye-hand coordination

Cognitive
- to improve understanding of spatial relationships, imitation, problem solving, picture-object association, and concept development
- to improve generalization skills

Language
- to improve taking turns; increasing vocalizations/vocabulary; requesting; initiating; following directions; and identifying/labeling objects, actions, characteristics, and locations

Social
- to make choices
- to facilitate peer interaction

Directions

Set up "stations" for the various toys. Allow children to wander to a station and begin playing. An adult can then assist with the play, expanding and guiding as appropriate. Depending on the child's needs, gross motor goals can be incorporated into these activities by positioning the stations so that the child stands or kneels to play, for example. Encourage children to take turns with an adult or peer in stacking blocks and knocking them down. Use lots of language to describe what is happening. Emphasize the red color of the toys.

Activity 4: Sponge Painting

Materials

sponges cut into heart shapes (or other shapes as desired)	red and white water-based paint
	red, white, and pink construction paper
trays to hold paint	table
chairs (adaptive seating as needed)	washcloths for cleanup

Goals

Sensory
- to improve responses to sensory stimulation
- to increase attention span

Fine Motor
- to improve hand manipulation, eye-hand coordination, using two hands together, and midline skills
- to increase shoulder girdle strength and stability

Cognitive
- to improve tool use, imitation, and concept development
- to develop generalization skills

Language
- to improve following directions; taking turns; increasing vocabulary; and identifying/labeling objects, actions, characteristics, and relationships

Social
- to make choices
- to facilitate peer interaction

Directions

Position children appropriately for fine motor activity. Have each child choose which color paper to use. Demonstrate dipping the sponges in the paint and pressing them on the paper to make prints. Let each child choose which sponge and color paint to use. Provide help with the activity as needed. Use lots of language to describe what they are doing. Emphasize the colors of the paint and paper. Some children may want to finger-paint instead or use the sponges in the same way as paintbrushes. This is fine. Remember that it is the process of exploration and learning that is important here, not the final product.

Activity 5: Making Cookie Dough

Materials

butter or shortening	sugar	eggs
flour	salt	cream of tartar
baking soda	vanilla	
mixing bowl	spoons	
electric hand mixer (optional)	measuring cups	
measuring spoons	airtight container for storage	
table	chairs (adaptive seating as needed)	
washcloths for cleanup		

Note: see Appendix C for a sugar cookie recipe.

Goals

Sensory
- to improve responses to sensory stimulation, especially tactile and olfactory
- to increase attention span

Fine Motor
- to improve using both hands together, midline skills, and hand/finger manipulation
- to increase upper body strength

Cognitive
- to improve understanding of spatial relationships, conservation of volume, functional use of objects, imitation, and concept development

Language
- to improve following directions; taking turns; sequencing; identifying/labeling objects, actions, locations, and relationships; initiating; and requesting

Social
- to make choices
- to facilitate peer interaction

Directions

Encourage children to name the objects and ingredients to be used as they are needed. Have children help combine ingredients for making sugar cookie dough. They can take turns pouring ingredients into the bowl, holding the mixer, and stirring with a spoon. Be sure to let them taste and smell the different ingredients as they are added. Refrigerate the dough for next week's activity.

Snack

Materials

a variety of red foods, such as:

cherries	strawberries	tomatoes
red cabbage	beets	red cookies
red apples	red gelatin	

napkins	spoons (adapted as needed)	cups (adapted as needed)
red juice	table	chairs (adaptive seating as
washcloths for cleanup	plates	needed)

Goals

Sensory
• to improve responses to sensory stimulation, especially tactile and olfactory

Fine Motor
• to improve eye-hand coordination, reach and grasp, grasp and release, hand/finger manipulation, finger isolation, using both hands together, and midline skills

Self-Help
• to improve self-feeding skills
• to improve oral-motor skills

Cognitive
• to develop classification and concept development
• to improve generalization skills

Language
• to improve taking turns; identifying/labeling objects, actions, locations, and relationships; initiating; and requesting

Social
• to make choices
• to facilitate peer interaction

Directions

Have children help pass out plates and napkins, if appropriate. Encourage them to identify the different foods and to request the one they want to try first. Encourage each child to try each food. Describe the appearance, taste, smell, feel of the foods with the children. Which ones do they like? Which ones do they dislike? What kinds of foods can be grouped together (fruits, vegetables, foods you eat with a spoon, foods you eat with your fingers)? Offer juice and provide assistance as needed.

Week 2

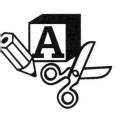

Overall Theme: More Red/Shapes

Activity 1: Blanket Swing/Pull

Materials

large blanket or sheet (with optional red fabric shapes sewn inside or drawn on the sheet with a marker)

Goals

Sensory
- to improve responses to sensory stimulation
- to provide vestibular stimulation
- to increase body awareness

Gross Motor
- to improve trunk rotation, rolling, and balance

Cognitive
- to improve imitation

Language
- to improve taking turns; identifying/labeling actions and relationships; initiating; and requesting

Social
- to facilitate peer interaction

Directions

One at a time, have each child lie on the blanket. Two adults lift the blanket gently off the ground a little bit and swing it. How vigorously to swing depends on the needs and tolerance of each child, which will vary widely from child to child. Be sure to stop from time to time and change directions—back and forth, side to side, up and down. To initiate rolling, gently pull up the blanket on one side, then the other. As the child becomes comfortable with this sensation, you can build the rolling into the side-to-side swinging. After everyone has had a turn, several (or even all, if the group is small enough) children at a time can sit on the blanket while an adult pulls it around the room. Children who are physically challenged can be supported by other children or by special positioning (for example, a beanbag chair), or they can lie on the blanket. Use lots of language to describe what is happening, who is on the blanket, how it is moving, and who is pulling or lifting it.

Activity 2: Balloons on a Blanket

Materials

several red balloons   blanket or sheet used in previous activity

Goals

Sensory
- to increase attention span

Gross Motor
- to improve balance, coordination, and motor planning

Fine Motor
- to improve visual attending and tracking, eye-hand coordination, and reach and grasp
- to increase upper body strength

Cognitive
- to improve concept development

Language
- to improve following directions; taking turns; identifying/labeling objects, actions, and descriptions; and requesting

Social
- to facilitate peer interaction

Directions

Seat children around the edge of the blanket and put the inflated balloons in the middle. Help them grasp the edges of the blanket and wave it up and down so that the balloons stay afloat. The activity can be expanded by having children (one at a time or several together) go under or on top of the blanket. Emphasize the up and down motion of the balloons as the blanket moves. Provide children with whatever adaptive seating or physical assistance they may need.

Activity 3: Collages

Materials

small pieces of various textured items, all red, white, or pink (cloth, sponge, styrofoam, pipe cleaners, feathers, ribbon, cellophane grass, wrapping paper, tissue paper, yarn, rice, macaroni)

glue	red markers or crayons
cotton swabs (optional)	paintbrushes (optional)
red, white, and pink construction paper	scissors
chairs (adaptive seating as needed)	table
washcloths for cleanup	

Goals

Sensory
- to improve sensory awareness through tactile stimulation
- to increase attention span

Fine Motor
- to improve hand manipulation, eye-hand coordination, and using two hands together

Cognitive
- to improve imitation and concept development

Language
- to improve following directions; taking turns; increasing vocabulary; and identifying/labeling objects, actions, characteristics, and relationships

Social
* to make choices

Directions

Position children for fine motor activity. Have children select which color paper to use. To emphasize the shape aspect of the activity, both the background papers and some of the textured materials can be cut into various shapes ahead of time. Help children squeeze or spread glue onto their papers, encouraging them to stabilize the paper with one hand if possible. This activity can be varied by having the children spread the glue with paintbrushes or cotton swabs, depending on their individual needs. Help each child choose the materials they want to use in their collage. Help them put the materials they have chosen onto the glue. Help them pat the materials into place. Use lots of language and encourage the children to describe what they are doing, the materials they are using, and how the materials feel. Let the pictures dry while completing another activity. Paper-folding can also be introduced into this activity, if appropriate.

Activity 4: Cookies

Materials

cookie dough (prepared the previous week)	flour
rolling pins	cutting board
cookie cutters (various basic shapes)	cookie sheets
spatulas	candy sprinkles and other decorations
potholders	oven
large plate for cooling cookies	table
chairs (adaptive seating as needed)	washcloths for cleanup

Goals

Sensory
* to improve responses to sensory stimulation, especially tactile and olfactory
* to increase attention span

Fine Motor
* to improve using both hands together, developing midline skills, and hand/finger manipulation
* to increase upper body strength

Cognitive
* to improve understanding of spatial relationships, functional use of objects, tool use, and imitation
* to develop recall skills

Language
* to improve following directions; taking turns; sequencing; identifying/labeling objects, actions, locations, and relationships; initiating; and requesting

Social
* to make choices
* to facilitate peer interaction

Directions

Seat children appropriately at the table. Tell the children they will be helping to make cookies with the dough they made last week. Place prepared cookie dough on a floured cutting board and demonstrate rolling out the dough with a rolling pin. Give each child a ball of dough and help them to roll it out. Use small, child-sized rolling pins, if possible, to facilitate midline goals. Children can also use their hands to pat the dough flat, if preferred. Show children how to press the cookie cutters into the dough to make shapes. Let each child choose a cookie cutter. Help them to press the cutters into their dough and place the cookies onto cookie sheets. Let children choose which sprinkles they wish to use to decorate their cookies. Help them to shake the sprinkles onto the cookies. If possible, let the children watch you put the cookies in the oven and take them out. Throughout the activity, use lots of language to talk about how the dough feels and smells, what the children are doing, the color and texture of the sprinkles, and the shapes of the cookies.

Snack

Materials

cookies made in the previous activity
cups (adapted if necessary)
table
washcloths for cleanup

milk or juice
napkins
chairs (adaptive seating as necessary)

Goals

Sensory
• to improve responses to sensory stimuli, especially tactile and olfactory

Fine Motor
• to improve eye-hand coordination, reach and grasp, grasp and release, hand/finger manipulation, finger isolation, using both hands together, and midline skills

Self-Help
• to improve self-feeding skills
• to improve oral-motor skills

Cognitive
• to improve concept development and sequencing skills
• to improve generalization skills
• to develop recall skills

Language
• to improve taking turns; identifying/labeling objects, actions, people, and characteristics

Social
• to make choices
• to facilitate peer interaction

Directions

Seat children appropriately for snack, using adaptive seating as needed. Have children help pass out napkins, if appropriate. Show children cookies and have them choose which one they want. Talk about making the cookies and how the dough looked, smelled, and felt. Talk about how the cookies look, smell, and feel now. What is the same? What is different? Talk about how the cookies are shaped like valentines (hearts). How are they like other valentines (hearts) the children have seen? Encourage communication, including ways to request more or indicate "all done." Assist with self-feeding skills as needed. Offer milk or juice and provide assistance as needed.

Week 3

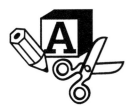

Overall Theme: Families

Note: This might be an appropriate time to invite extended family members to visit the program.

Activity 1: Ball Family

Materials

large, medium, and small therapy balls

Goals

Sensory
- to improve responses to proprioceptive and vestibular stimulation
- to facilitate increased body awareness

Gross Motor
- to improve motor planning, trunk rotation, sitting balance and coordination, and weight shifting

Fine Motor
- to improve using both hands together
- to increase upper body strength

Cognitive
- to improve understanding of spatial relationships and concepts
- to develop generalization skills

Language
- to improve following directions; taking turns; imitation; identifying/labeling objects, people, actions, locations, and relationships; initiating; and requesting

Social
- to develop representational play
- to facilitate peer interaction

Directions

Bring out the therapy balls. Introduce the ball "family"—mama ball, papa ball, sister ball, grandma ball. Try to represent the different relationships you are aware of in the children's families. Allow children to explore the balls. Patting them provides proprioceptive stimulation. Pushing them while walking provides practice with weight shifting, standing balance, and improving walking skills, as well as proprioceptive stimulation and strengthening the upper body. Interventionists can support the children and bounce them on the balls to stimulate muscle tone or use gentle rocking to relax muscle tone. Trunk rotation, balance reactions, and improved use of abdominal muscles can also be facilitated. Having the children pass a ball around a circle encourages coordinated use of both hands as well as trunk rotation. Encourage children to roll balls back and forth to each other. Name the child rolling the ball and the child catching it. Encourage children to call out to whom they are rolling the ball.

Activity 2: Class Portrait

Materials

large roll of butcher or other heavy paper
markers (possibly scented)

Goals

Sensory
- to improve responses to sensory stimulation
- to increase body awareness

Gross Motor
- to improve motor planning and imitating

Cognitive
- to improve imitation and concept development
- to develop generalization skills

Language
- to improve following directions; identifying/labeling body parts, actions, people, and relationships; taking turns; requesting; and initiating

Directions

Unroll a section of paper on the floor and have a child lie on it while an adult draws around the child's body. Name each body part as it is being traced. Talk about making a "portrait" of the group this way.

Activity 3: Doll Families

Materials

dolls of various sizes, ethnicities, ages, and genders
clothes for dolls
brushes and combs for the dolls' hair
lotion, powder, and diapers for dolls
doll dishes, spoons, and bottles
doll houses, furniture, and other accessories

Goals

Sensory
- to improve responses to sensory stimulation

Gross Motor
- to improve motor planning, balance, and coordination

Fine Motor
- to improve hand manipulation, using two hands together, and midline skills

Cognitive
- to improve tool use, functional object use, imitation, and concept development
- to develop generalization skills

Language
- to improve turn taking; identifying/labeling objects, actions, descriptions, and relationships; initiating; and requesting

Social
- to make choices
- to facilitate representational/pretend play
- to facilitate peer interaction

Directions

Set up at least two activity stations—one with the doll houses and the other with the larger dolls and their accessories. Encourage the children to choose a station. Observe and facilitate their play as needed. Use lots of language to describe the doll "families" and what the children are doing. When facilitating play, try to model the next higher level of play. For example, if the child is hugging a doll, repeat that action and encourage brushing its hair or giving it a bottle. If a child is already doing those things, model sequencing behaviors, such as heating the bottle and then giving it to the doll.

Activity 4: Family Portraits

Materials

cutout pictures representing people of various ages, genders, and ethnicities	glue
table	construction paper
washcloths for cleanup	chairs (adapted seating as needed)

Goals

Sensory
- to improve sensory awareness through tactile stimulation
- to increase attention span

Fine Motor
- to improve hand manipulation, eye-hand coordination, and using both hands together

Cognitive
- to improve imitation, sequencing skills, and concept development

Language
- to improve following directions; taking turns; increasing vocabulary; identifying/labeling objects, actions, characteristics, and relationships

Social
- to make choices

Directions

Position children for fine motor activity. Have children select which color paper to use. Help children squeeze or spread glue onto their papers, encouraging them to stabilize the paper with one hand, if possible. Help each child choose the pictures to use in the collage. Ask for assistance from their families as to which relationships to represent, such as uncles, aunts, cousins, grandparents, brothers, and sisters. Help them pat the pictures into place. Use lots of language and encourage the children to describe what they are doing, the materials they are using, and who the pictures represent. Let the pictures dry while completing another activity.

Activity 5: Family Books

Materials

photos of each child's family members, pets, house, car, toys, whatever is special to the child (brought from home or previously taken for this activity)

cardboard sheets that have been   notebook rings
  3-hole punched   clear contact paper
scissors   table
chairs (adaptive seating as needed)

Goals

Sensory
- to improve responses to sensory stimulation
- to increase attention span

Fine Motor
- to improve visual attending, focusing, and hand manipulation

Cognitive
- to improve object-picture association and classification
- to develop generalization skills

Language
- to improve following directions; identifying/labeling objects, pictures, actions, and people; taking turns; initiating; requesting
- to develop an interest in reading

Directions

Have family members assist in this activity, if possible. Attach one photo to each cardboard "page" with clear contact paper. Place rings through the pre-punched holes so that the pages turn freely. Talk with the children about the pictures while working on this activity. When each child's book is finished, "read" it to the child. Each child will have his or her own book to take home and enjoy.

Snack

Materials

gingerbread people cookies   juice or milk
cups (adapted as needed)   napkins (optional)
table   chairs (adaptive seating as needed)
washcloths for cleanup

Goals

Sensory
- to improve responses to sensory stimuli, especially tactile and olfactory
- to increase attention span

Fine Motor
- to improve reach and grasp, grasp and release, eye-hand coordination, hand/finger manipulation, midline skills, and using both hands together

Self-Help
- to improve self-feeding skills
- to improve oral-motor skills

Cognitive
- to improve imitation, understanding of spatial relationships, functional object use, tool use, and concept development
- to develop generalization skills
- to develop recall skills

Language
- to improve taking turns; identifying/labeling objects, actions, people, and characteristics; requesting; and initiating

Social
- to make choices
- to facilitate peer interaction

Directions

Seat children appropriately for snack, using adaptive seating as needed. Have children help pass out napkins, if appropriate. Show children cookies and have them choose which one they want. Talk about cookie "families"; for example, which cookies are the mom cookies, the dad cookies, and the brother and sister cookies. Encourage communication, including ways to request more or indicate "all done." Assist with self-feeding skills as needed. Offer milk or juice and provide assistance as needed.

Week 4   Overall Theme: Mittens

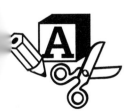

Activity 1: Obstacle Course

Materials

indoor climbing structure
inner tubes
ramp or other incline
floor pillows/beanbag chairs
bolsters
indoor swing
containers for mittens

toddler slide
indoor tunnel
carpet squares
benches
steps
several sets of mittens

Goals

Sensory
- to provide proprioceptive input
- to increase attention span

Gross Motor
- to improve balance, coordination, motor planning, locomotion, trunk rotation, and weight shifting

Fine Motor
- to improve using both hands together, reach and grasp, and visual attention
- to increase upper body strength
- to improve shoulder girdle strength and stability

Cognitive
- to improve object permanence, imitation, and problem solving

Language
- to improve following directions; taking turns; identifying/labeling objects, actions, descriptions, and locations; requesting; and initiating

Social
- to make choices
- to facilitate peer interaction

Directions

Using the equipment available, set up an indoor obstacle course to facilitate the gross motor and vestibular goals for individuals in the group. The materials listed above are just suggestions. Place the mittens at various points throughout the obstacle course. Have some hidden, some partially hidden, and some in plain sight. Assist the children through the obstacle course. A "path" of carpet squares can provide a structure to follow through the course. Encourage the children to use appropriate motor patterns throughout. Help them find the mittens as they go through the course. Be sure there are enough mittens for each child to find at least two or three. Collect the mittens in buckets, baskets, or bags. Depending on their abilities, children can be encouraged to carry their own bags filled with mittens.

Activity 2: Mitten Mash

Materials

sleeping bag, folding mat, or cloth tunnel (made by sewing a folded sheet down one side leaving both ends open) with large mitten shape fastened to the outside

Goals

Sensory
- to improve responses to sensory stimulation
- to provide proprioceptive stimulation
- to increase body awareness

Gross Motor
- to improve motor planning, crawling, and rolling

Fine Motor
• to increase shoulder girdle strength and stability

Cognitive
• to improve problem solving, object permanence, classification, imitation, understanding of spatial relationships, and concept development
• to develop generalization skills

Language
• to improve following directions; taking turns; identifying/labeling objects, actions, relationships, descriptions, and people; initiating; and requesting

Social
• to facilitate pretend play
• to facilitate peer interaction

Directions

Spread the sleeping bag, cloth tunnel, or folding mat on the floor like a giant mitten. Have the children crawl or scoot inside and roll across the floor. Adults can roll the children who cannot roll themselves. For many children, simply pressing down gently on their bodies while they are inside the "mitten" will provide the needed proprioceptive stimulation. Use lots of language to facilitate the pretend aspects of the activity for the children.

Activity 3: Mitten Match

Materials

several pairs of mittens

Goals

Sensory
• to improve responses to sensory stimulation
• to increase attention span

Gross Motor
• to improve balance and coordination, visual focusing, and tracking

Fine Motor
• to improve hand manipulation, reach and grasp, and midline skills

Cognitive
• to improve classification, functional object use, and concept development
• to develop generalization skills

Language
• to improve following directions; taking turns; identifying/labeling objects, actions, people, and characteristics; initiating; and requesting

Social
• to make choices
• to facilitate peer interaction

Directions

Put the mittens collected during the first activity in a pile in the center of the circle. Have the children sit around the circle. Help them to match the mittens. There are several ways to try this. An adult can give each child a mitten and provide help with finding a match. As an alternative, each child can select a mitten and then look for its match. To encourage more interaction, each child can be given two mismatched mittens and they can then trade with each other to get matched pairs. Initially, the mittens should be very dissimilar. As the children develop more skill, the mittens used could be more and more alike. You can also use this activity to review the colors previously introduced—red, for example.

Activity 4: Mitten Manipulatives

Materials

mittens for each child
a variety of toys enjoyed by the group, such as:

blocks	talking toys (for example, See N Say™)	cash register
puzzles	interlocking blocks	stacking cubes

Goals

Sensory
- to improve responses to sensory stimulation
- to increase body awareness

Gross Motor
- to improve motor planning, balance and coordination, and locomotion

Fine Motor
- to improve hand/finger manipulation, using two hands together, and midline skills

Cognitive
- to improve understanding of cause-and-effect and means-end concepts

Language
- to improve following directions; taking turns; identifying/labeling objects, actions, people, descriptions, locations, and relationships; initiating; and requesting

Social
- to facilitate peer interaction

Directions

Set up a variety of toys the children enjoy. Put a pair of mittens on each child and let them have free play time. Encourage communication skills if they need help either operating the toys or getting the mittens off. After a few minutes, remove one mitten from each child and allow the activity to continue. After another few minutes, remove each child's other mitten, if the children have not already done so. Use lots of language to talk about the activity. What was different with the mittens on?

Caution: This activity may be too frustrating for some children, especially those who may already be physically challenged. If so, simply substitute fine motor free play or some other more appropriate activity.

Activity 5: Mitten Rub

Materials

several pairs of mittens
soft bristle nonscratching brushes, such as hospital scrub brushes

Goals

Sensory
- to improve responses to sensory stimulation, especially tactile
- to increase body awareness

Fine Motor
- to improve visual attending and tracking, midline skills, and hand manipulation and control

Cognitive
- to improve concept development

Language
- to improve following directions; taking turns; identifying/labeling objects, actions, characteristics, relationships, and people; initiating; and requesting

Social
- to make choices
- to facilitate peer interaction

Directions

Have children choose mittens again. Help them put on the mittens and rub hands and arms firmly. Adults should provide help and may need to do the rubbing to be sure it is firm. Include hands, forearms, and palms, if possible. Brushes may also be used. Be sure to use firm strokes.

Note: This activity helps to normalize sensitivity to tactile stimulation. It can be used at any time a child is having difficulty with tactile activities. At the same time, rubbing and brushing should not be forced on a child if the child shows strong resistance. Sometimes rubbing or pressing with the bare hand is acceptable to a child even when using a mitten or brush is not. Children showing normal reactions to touch will also benefit from this activity by increasing their awareness of their bodies.

Activity 6: Mitten Paint

Materials

finger paint
spoons or tongue depressors for
    scooping paint
smocks
washcloths for cleanup
chairs (adaptive seating as needed)

finger-paint paper cut in large
    mitten shapes
container of water
soap for cleanup
table

Goals

Sensory
- to improve responses to sensory stimulation
- to increase attention span

Gross Motor
- to improve balance and coordination and control of flexion/extension patterns

Fine Motor
- to improve visual attending and tracking, hand manipulation and control
- to increase upper body strength
- to increase shoulder girdle strength and stability

Cognitive
- to improve concept development
- to develop generalization skills

Language
- to improve following directions; taking turns; identifying/labeling objects, actions, descriptions, relationships, and people; initiating; and requesting

Social
- to make choices
- to facilitate peer interaction

Directions

Give each child a large mitten shape. Let each select which color paint to use. Sprinkle each child's paper with water and put a dab of the selected color paint on it. Let the children finger-paint. Provide physical assistance to children as needed. Use lots of language to describe the motions and colors. This activity can facilitate even more peer interaction if the group works together to paint a giant mitten.

Caution: Younger children tend to eat the paint. If you think this will happen in your group, substitute colorful pudding for paint. Although you can't hang pudding paint pictures on the wall, remember that it is the process that is important here, not the final product.

Snack

Materials

pita or "pocket" bread
table knives
plates
juice
table
washcloths for cleanup

fillings (peanut butter, cream cheese, egg salad)
napkins (optional)
cups (adapted as needed)
chairs (adaptive seating as needed)

Goals

Sensory
- to improve responses to sensory stimuli, especially tactile and olfactory
- to increase attention span

Fine Motor
- to improve using both hands together, grasp and release, and hand manipulation

Self-Help
- to improve self-feeding skills
- to improve oral-motor skills

Cognitive
- to improve imitation
- to develop generalization skills
- to develop recall skills

Language
- to improve following directions; taking turns; identifying/labeling objects, actions, people, and characteristics; initiating; and requesting

Social
- to make choices
- to facilitate peer interaction

Directions

Seat children appropriately for snack, using adaptive seating as needed. As children watch, show them how to open their pocket bread and put filling into it, just like they put their hands into the mittens. Give each child a table knife and a piece of pocket bread. Help them choose a filling and spread it in the pocket. Describe what the children are doing, what the snack is made of, and what it looks like. Talk about how it looks like a mitten and also how it is not like a mitten. Encourage communication, including ways to request more or indicate "all done." Offer juice as needed. Assist with self-feeding/drinking skills as needed.

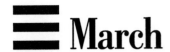

March

Week 1

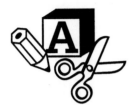

Overall Theme: Air/Wind

Activity 1: Poppin' Paper Bags

Materials

several brown paper lunch bags
stickers to decorate bags
markers or crayons to decorate bags

Goals

Sensory
- to provide proprioceptive stimulation
- to increase attention span

Gross Motor
- to improve coordination, motor planning, and locomotion

Fine Motor
- to improve using both hands together, reach and grasp, visual attention, and tracking
- to increase shoulder girdle strength and stability

Cognitive
- to improve understanding of means-ends and cause-and-effect relationships, object permanence, imitation, and concept development

Language
- to improve following directions; taking turns; identifying/labeling objects, actions, descriptions, and locations; requesting; and initiating

Social
- to make choices
- to facilitate peer interaction

Directions

Show the children the paper bags. Help them to decorate the bags if they wish. Adults can demonstrate blowing air into the bags and popping them with their hands and/or feet. Encourage children to imitate these actions.

Activity 2: Balloons

Materials

helium balloons (at least one per child)
string for balloons
stickers to decorate balloons (optional)

ordinary balloons, some blown up and some not
markers to decorate balloons (optional)

Goals

Sensory
- to increase attention span

Gross Motor
- to improve balance, coordination, motor planning, and locomotion

Fine Motor
- to improve using both hands together, reach and grasp, visual attention, and tracking
- to increase shoulder girdle strength and stability

Cognitive
- to improve understanding of means-end and cause-and-effect relationships, object permanence, imitation, and concept development

Language
- to improve following directions; taking turns; identifying/labeling objects, actions, descriptions, and locations; requesting; and initiating

Social
- to make choices
- to facilitate peer interaction

Directions

Encourage children to reach up for helium balloons and to use hand-over-hand action to pull them down from the ceiling using the attached strings. Children not yet ready for that activity can be encouraged to bat at the helium balloons while an adult holds them within range. Helium balloons, especially the shiny mylar kind, also make excellent targets for visual tracking. Regular balloons can be placed on the floor, partially hidden by furniture or equipment. Encourage children to find the balloons. They can bat them, throw them, kick them, and catch them. Children can also be encouraged to pull the balloons behind them on strings as they walk either forward or backward, encouraging more advanced and coordinated motor movements. Help the children decorate the balloons using markers and stickers. Encourage them to hold the balloons with one hand while decorating with the other. Most children will need an adult's help to do this. Adults may also want to blow up some balloons and release them without tying the ends. Encourage the children to follow the balloons visually and to talk about what happens.

Caution: Small pieces of broken balloons present a choking hazard. This activity must be carefully monitored.

Activity 3: Fan

Materials

large box fan	streamers	ribbons
balloons	tape	scissors
on/off capability switch set		

Goals

Sensory
- to improve sensory awareness and responsiveness
- to increase attention span

Fine Motor
- to improve visual attention and tracking

Cognitive
- to improve understanding of cause-and-effect, means-ends relationships, and imitation

Language
- to improve following directions; taking turns; identifying/labeling objects, actions, characteristics, locations, and relationships; initiating; and requesting

Directions

Plug the fan into a capability switch so that it can be turned off and on with the switch rather than with its regular control. Attach streamers and ribbons to the fan's grill so that the air will blow them when it is turned on. Balloons may also be tied to the fan's grill. Turn the fan on. Encourage the children to talk about what happens. Label the actions as well as the objects. Encourage the children to touch the streamers as they blow. Position the switch so that the children can discover how to activate it. The switch is particularly useful for children who are more physically challenged because it gives them a way to participate actively with the other children.

Caution: Children should be closely monitored to ensure that they do not attempt to stick their fingers into the fan.

Activity 4: Streamers

Materials

paper streamers   cloth streamers (optional)
pinwheels (optional)

Goals

Gross Motor
- to improve balance, coordination, and motor planning

Fine Motor
- to improve eye-hand coordination, visual tracking, and grasp and release
- to increase upper body strength

Cognitive
- to improve understanding of spatial relationships and imitation
- to develop generalization skills

Language
- to improve following directions; taking turns; identifying/labeling objects, actions, locations, and relationships; initiating; and requesting

Social
- to make choices
- to facilitate peer interaction

Directions

When children begin to tire of the fan activities (Activity 3), an adult should initiate activities with the streamers and pinwheels. Encourage children to make the streamers move in the way that they did when the fan blew them. They can run with the streamers and reach up high and wave streamers, for example. Use lots of language, showing and telling where the streamers are going and who is doing what type of action. Assist the children who are more physically challenged with the movements they need to make the streamers move. Streamers may also be attached to body parts other than the arms or hands for variety. Notice if any children show signs of visual or tactile defensiveness during this activity. If so, provide these children with more space and fewer materials to explore. Allow these children as much control as possible of their participation in the activity.

Activity 5: Collage

Materials

pieces of streamers	ribbon
fabric cut in balloon shapes	scissors
construction paper	glue
paintbrushes (optional)	cotton swabs (optional)
table	chairs (adaptive seating as necessary)
washcloths for cleanup	

Goals

Sensory
• to improve sensory awareness through tactile stimulation

• to increase attention span

Fine Motor
• to improve hand manipulation, eye-hand coordination, and using both hands together

Cognitive
• to improve imitation and concept development

• to develop generalization skills

• to develop recall skills

Language
• to improve following directions; taking turns; increasing vocabulary; and identifying/labeling objects, actions, characteristics, and relationships

Social
• to make choices

Directions

Position children for fine motor activity. Have children select the color paper they want to use. Help children squeeze or spread glue onto their papers, encouraging them to stabilize the paper with one hand, if possible. Vary the activity by allowing them to spread the glue with paintbrushes or cotton swabs. Help each child choose the materials to use for the collage. Help the children put the materials they have chosen onto the glue and pat them into place. Use lots of language and encourage the children to describe what they are doing and the materials they are using. Remind them that these materials look like the ones they were using earlier. Let the pictures dry while completing another activity.

Snack

Materials

rice cakes	cups (adapted if necessary)	plates
cream cheese	table	washcloths for cleanup
peanut butter	table knives for spreading	
jelly or fruit spread	napkins	
juice	chairs (adaptive seating as needed)	

Goals

Sensory
- to improve responses to sensory stimuli, especially tactile and olfactory
- to increase attention span

Fine Motor
- to improve using both hands together, grasp and release, and hand manipulation

Self-Help
- to improve self-feeding skills
- to improve oral-motor skills

Cognitive
- to improve imitation
- to develop generalization skills
- to develop recall skills

Language
- to improve following directions; taking turns; identifying/labeling objects, actions, people, and characteristics; requesting; and initiating

Social
- to make choices
- to facilitate peer interaction

Directions

Seat children appropriately for snack, using adaptive seating as needed. As children watch, spread a rice cake with jelly or other topping. Tell them they are going to make balloon snacks. Give each child a table knife and a rice cake. Help them spread the topping of their choice on the rice cake. Describe what they are doing, what the snack is made of, and what it looks like. Talk about how the snack looks like a balloon. Encourage communication, including ways to request more or indicate "all done." Offer juice as needed. Assist with self-feeding/drinking skills as needed.

Week 2

Overall Theme: Bubbles and Balls

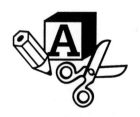

Activity 1: Ball Pool

Materials

commercial ball pool or other large container (such as a wading pool) filled with lightweight plastic balls about 3 inches in diameter
toddler slide ending in the ball pool (optional)

Goals

Sensory
- to improve responses to tactile and proprioceptive stimulation
- to improve responses to vestibular stimulation
- to facilitate increased body awareness

Gross Motor
- to improve motor planning, trunk rotation, sitting, balance, and coordination

Fine Motor
- to improve grasp, throwing/releasing
- to increase upper body strength

Cognitive
- to improve understanding of spatial relationships, imitation, and concept development

Language
- to improve following directions; taking turns; identifying/labeling objects, people, actions, locations, and relationships; initiating; and requesting

Social
- to facilitate peer interaction

Directions

Allow children to explore the ball pool. Encourage them to climb in and out independently, assisting them as necessary with using appropriate motor patterns. Use lots of language to describe the actions and who is doing what; for example, "John threw the red ball." Encourage children to name objects, actions, and people. "Bury" body parts under the balls and have the children "find" them again; for instance, "Where's Geoff's leg? There it is!" Help children climb up the stairs of the slide and slide down into the balls. Encourage them to use a variety of sliding positions, such as sitting, or feet first, or backward. Do not insist on a particular position if the child expresses apprehension or fear. Children who cannot climb the slide may be placed on it and helped to slide down. Children with tactile defensiveness may benefit from brushing, rubbing with a washcloth, or bear hugging before and after playing in the ball pool. Watch children's reactions to help you know who might need this additional attention.

Activity 2: Big Balls

Materials

large therapy balls in appropriate sizes for the children in the group
smaller balls, preferably in the same colors as the therapy balls
dolls or stuffed animals

Goals

Sensory
- to improve responses to proprioceptive and vestibular stimulation
- to facilitate increased body awareness

Gross Motor
- to improve motor planning, trunk rotation, sitting, balance, coordination, and weight shifting

Fine Motor
- to improve using both hands together
- to increase upper body strength

Cognitive
- to improve concept development, understanding of spatial relationships, and imitation

Language
- to improve following directions; taking turns; identifying/labeling objects, people, actions, locations, and relationships; initiating; and requesting

Social
- to facilitate peer interaction
- to facilitate representational play

Directions

Bring out the therapy balls and encourage children to explore them. Patting them provides proprioceptive stimulation. Pushing them while walking provides practice with weight shifting, standing balance, and improving walking skills, as well as proprioceptive stimulation and strengthening the upper body. Interventionists can support the children and bounce them on the balls to stimulate muscle tone or use gentle rocking to relax muscle tone. Trunk rotation, balance reactions, and improved use of abdominal muscles can also be facilitated. Having the children pass the ball around a circle encourages coordinated use of both hands as well as trunk rotation. Encourage children to roll balls back and forth to each other. Name the child rolling the ball and the child catching it. Encourage children to call out ahead of time to whom they are rolling the ball. Smaller balls can also be introduced and compared to the larger ones. Many of the same activities can be repeated using the smaller balls. Have dolls or stuffed animals available for children to act out bouncing on the balls, if appropriate.

Activity 3: Big Bubbles, Little Bubbles

Materials

hoop for making super big bubbles   smaller bubble hoops of various kinds
bubble soap   containers for bubble soap

Goals

Gross Motor
- to improve balance, weight shifting, motor planning, and coordination

Fine Motor
- to improve eye-hand coordination, visual tracking, reach and grasp, and hand/finger manipulation
- to increase upper body strength

Self-Help
- to improve oral-motor skills

Cognitive
- to improve tool use, imitation, and understanding of spatial relationships
- to develop generalization skills

Language
- to improve following directions; taking turns; identifying/labeling objects, actions, locations, and relationships; initiating; and requesting

Social
- to facilitate peer interaction

Directions

This activity is a good one to do outside if the weather permits. Introduce the bubbles using the small, familiar wands. Encourage the children to reach up to pop or catch the bubbles and to follow the bubbles with their eyes. Encourage the children to try to blow bubbles themselves. Introduce the big bubble wand and make big bubbles. Alternate big bubbles with little bubbles and talk about "big" and "little." Encourage children to chase and pop the big bubbles, too. Stepping or jumping on the bubbles provides proprioceptive stimulation and helps to improve one-leg balance and co-ordination for walking and running. Children who are more physically challenged can be assisted to reach and pop the bubbles. Have children help each other to pop, chase, and catch the bubbles.

Activity 4: Bubble Cups

Materials

empty tubs from soft margarine
  (or similar containers)
rubber bands

plastic straws
paper towels
dishwashing liquid

Goals

Fine Motor
- to improve eye-hand coordination, hand and finger manipulation, and finger isolation

Self-Help
- to improve oral-motor skills

Cognitive
- to improve imitation
- to develop generalization skills

Language
- to improve following directions; taking turns; identifying/labeling objects, actions, locations, and relationships; initiating; and requesting

Directions

Prepare several bubble cups ahead of time. To make a bubble cup, place a paper towel soaked in dishwashing liquid in an empty margarine tub. You may need to stretch it over the top and secure it with a rubber band. Punch two holes in the lid; one just big enough for a plastic straw to fit through and the other slightly bigger than the first. Put the lid on the margarine tub. Insert a plastic straw in the smaller hole. If necessary, cut the straw to make it shorter. When you are ready to introduce the activity, blow through the straw and bubbles should come out the other hole. Encourage children to poke the bubbles with their fingers. Some children may want to blow through the straws to make the bubbles. Use lots of language to describe what is happening, who is doing what, and where the bubbles are. Be careful that children just learning to use straws don't suck in and drink the liquid soap.

Activity 5: Soap Painting

Materials

soap flakes	water
eggbeater or hand mixer	construction paper
food coloring (optional)	sand, oatmeal, or other textured
table	material (optional)
chairs (adaptive seating as needed)	washcloths for cleanup

Goals

Sensory
- to improve responses to sensory stimulation, especially tactile and olfactory
- to increase attention span

Fine Motor
- to improve using both hands together, midline skills, hand/finger manipulation, and visual attending and tracking
- to increase upper body strength

Cognitive
- to improve imitation

Language
- to improve following directions; taking turns; identifying/labeling objects, actions, locations, and relationships; initiating; and requesting

Social
- to make choices
- to facilitate peer interaction

Directions

Mix the soap flakes with water to the desired consistency using the eggbeater or mixer. You can do this ahead of time or have the children assist you. Using an eggbeater is an excellent activity for promoting the use of both hands together at the midline. Food coloring and/or textured materials such as sand or dry oatmeal can be added, if desired. Let children choose the color paper they want to use. Help them to finger-paint with the soap mixture on the construction paper. Talk about what they are doing and encourage them to label their actions, describe the materials, and indicate that they are finished. To further facilitate peer interaction, let several children use a single large sheet of paper together. Let the paintings dry while completing another activity. Children who show signs of tactile defensiveness may benefit from brushing, firm pressure, or "squeezing" on their hands before and even during this activity to decrease their discomfort and increase their willingness to try the activity.

Snack

Materials

peanut butter	measuring cups	spoons
powdered milk	paper plates	napkins
raisins (optional)	cups (adapted if needed)	table
milk	chairs (adapted seating	
mixing bowl	washcloths for cleanup as needed)	

Goals

Sensory
- to improve responses to sensory stimulation, especially tactile and olfactory
- to increase attention span

Fine Motor
- to improve using both hands together, midline skills, hand and finger manipulation, and visual attending
- to increase upper body strength

Self-Help
- to improve self-feeding skills
- to improve oral-motor skills

Cognitive
- to improve tool use, understanding of spatial relationships, functional use of objects, and imitation
- to develop recall skills

Language
- to improve following directions; taking turns; sequencing; identifying/labeling objects, actions, locations, and relationships; initiating; and requesting

Social
- to make choices
- to facilitate peer interaction

Directions

Use ½ cup peanut butter for a group of 4 to 8 toddlers. Add enough powdered milk to the peanut butter to make a dough-like consistency. Raisins may be added if desired (they may present a choking hazard to younger children or to children whose feeding patterns are immature). The children may be encouraged to help with the mixing, as this promotes use of both hands together at midline, development of sequencing skills, turn taking, and a variety of other objectives. When the peanut butter dough has been mixed thoroughly, give each child a chunk and help them roll it into balls. They can make one large ball or several small balls. They could also pat it into a flat shape, poke it with isolated fingers, or roll it into a snake shape. Throughout the activity, use lots of language to describe what is happening. Have children identify the ingredients and tools as they are used in mixing the dough. Compare the children's dough balls—big, little, lumpy, smooth. Describe the feel of the dough. When children have finished shaping the dough, give them paper plates to put their shapes on. Encourage them to eat their shapes. Offer milk or other beverages as appropriate. Provide help with self-feeding and drinking skills as needed.

Week 3

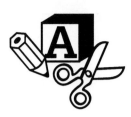

Overall Theme: Green

Activity 1: Obstacle Course

Materials

indoor climbing structure	toddler slide	inner tubes
indoor tunnel	ramp or other incline	carpet squares
green contact paper	floor pillows/beanbag chairs	benches
bolsters	steps	indoor swing
green beanbags	containers for beanbags	

Goals

Sensory
- to provide vestibular stimulation
- to provide proprioceptive stimulation
- to increase attention span

Gross Motor
- to improve balance, coordination, motor planning, locomotion, trunk rotation, and weight shifting

Fine Motor
- to improve using both hands together, reach and grasp, and visual attention
- to increase upper body strength
- to improve shoulder girdle strength and stability

Cognitive
- to improve object permanence, imitation, problem solving, and concept development

Language
- to improve following directions; taking turns; identifying/labeling objects, actions, descriptions, and locations; requesting; and initiating

Social
- to make choices
- to facilitate peer interaction

Directions

Using the equipment available, set up an indoor obstacle course to facilitate the gross motor and vestibular goals for individuals in the group. The materials listed above are just suggestions. Place the green beanbags at various points throughout the obstacle course. Have some hidden, some partially hidden, and some in plain sight. Assist the children through the obstacle course. A "path" of carpet squares can provide a structure to follow through the course. Green contact paper can be attached to the carpet squares to enhance the color effect. Encourage children to use appropriate motor patterns throughout. Help them find the beanbags as they go through the course. Be sure there are enough beanbags for each child to find at least two or three. Collect the beanbags in buckets or baskets, preferably green. Depending on their abilities, children can be encouraged to carry their own buckets filled with beanbags.

Activity 2: Beanbags

Materials

several beanbags, preferably green
basket or bin to toss them into

Goals

Sensory
• to provide proprioceptive stimulation
• to increase attention span

Gross Motor
• to improve balance, weight shifting, and coordination

Fine Motor
• to improve eye-hand coordination, reach and grasp, grasp and release, and throwing
• to increase upper body strength

Cognitive
• to improve understanding of spatial relationships and imitation

Language
• to improve following directions; taking turns; identifying/labeling objects, actions, locations, and relationships; initiating; and requesting

Social
• to make choices
• to facilitate peer interaction

Directions

This activity usually works best if children are seated in a circle with the "target" in the middle. Each child can take a beanbag from the bucket or the adults can begin the activity by tossing beanbags to each child. Encourage children to throw the bean-bags into the bucket or to each other. They may need help to accomplish this. Children who are not yet ready to throw may begin by placing the beanbags into the container. Talk about the actions, who is throwing, and who is catching. Encourage children to name who they want to catch the beanbag. Emphasize the green color of the beanbags.

Activity 3: Green Toys

Materials

a variety of manipulative toys, predominately green in color, for example:

| interlocking blocks (such as Duplo™) | bristle blocks | cubes |
| pegs | beads | books |

Goals

Sensory
• to increase attention span

Fine Motor
• to improve hand/finger manipulation and eye-hand coordination

Cognitive
- to improve understanding of spatial relationships, imitation, problem solving, picture-object association, and concept development
- to develop generalization skills

Language
- to improve taking turns; increasing vocalizations/vocabulary; requesting; initiating; following directions; and identifying/labeling objects, actions, characteristics, and locations

Social
- to make choices
- to facilitate peer interaction

Directions

Set up "stations" for the various toys. Allow children to wander to a station and begin playing. An adult can then assist with the play, expanding and guiding as appropriate. Depending on the child's needs, gross motor goals can be incorporated into these activities by positioning the stations so that the child stands or kneels to play, for example. Encourage children to take turns with an adult or peer to stack blocks and knock them down. Use lots of language to describe what is happening. Emphasize the green color of all the toys.

Activity 4: Collage

Materials

small pieces of various textured items, all green (cloth, sponge, styrofoam, pipe cleaner, feathers, ribbon, cellophane grass, wrapping paper, tissue paper, yarn, rice, macaroni)

green stickers	green markers or crayons
glue	paintbrushes (optional)
cotton swabs (optional)	scissors
construction paper	table
chairs (adaptive seating as needed)	washcloths for cleanup

Goals

Sensory
- to improve sensory awareness through tactile stimulation
- to increase attention span

Fine Motor
- to improve hand manipulation, eye-hand coordination, and using both hands together

Cognitive
- to improve imitation and concept development

Language
- to improve following directions; taking turns; increasing vocabulary; and identifying/labeling objects, actions, characteristics, and relationships

Social
- to make choices

Directions

Position children for fine motor activity. Have children select which color paper to use. Help children squeeze or spread glue onto their papers, encouraging them to stabilize the paper with one hand, if possible. Vary the activity by encouraging them to spread the glue with paintbrushes or cotton swabs. Help each child choose the materials to use in the collage. Help the children put the materials they have chosen onto the glue and pat them into place. Use lots of language and encourage the children to describe what they are doing, the materials they are using, and how the materials feel. Let the pictures dry while completing another activity.

Snack

Materials

green instant pudding (pistachio is green or
  green food coloring can be added to vanilla)
milk
cookies, such as vanilla wafers
juice
eggbeater or hand mixer
napkins
chairs (adaptive seating as needed)

mixing bowl
measuring cups
bowls
cups (adapted if needed)
mixing spoons
child-sized spoons
table
washcloths for cleanup

Goals

Sensory
- to improve responses to sensory stimulation, especially tactile and olfactory
- to increase attention span

Fine Motor
- to improve using both hands together, midline skills, and hand/finger manipulation
- to increase upper body strength

Self-Help
- to improve self-feeding skills
- to improve oral-motor skills

Cognitive
- to improve understanding of spatial relationships, conservation of volume, functional use of objects, imitation, and sequencing

Language
- to improve following directions; taking turns; sequencing; identifying/labeling objects, actions, locations, and relationships; initiating; and requesting

Social
- to make choices
- to facilitate peer interaction

Directions

Encourage children to name the objects to be used (bowl, spoons, pudding mix). Have children help open the pudding box and pour the contents into a mixing bowl. Have children identify the milk, pour it into a measuring cup, and then into the pudding. Mix the milk and pudding mix together using the eggbeater or mixer. This is an excellent activity for promoting the use of both hands together at the midline. Spoon individual servings into bowls and have children help hand them out, if appropriate. Give each child a spoon. Offer juice and cookies. Encourage children to initiate requests for more. Use lots of language to talk about what they are doing and encourage them to label objects, describe their actions, and indicate that they are finished. Provide assistance with feeding and drinking skills as needed.

Week 4

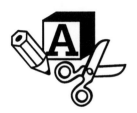

Overall Theme: Kites

Activity 1: Flying Kites

Materials

several kites in different sizes, shapes, colors

Goals

Sensory
- to improve sensory awareness and responsiveness

Gross Motor
- to improve balance, coordination, motor planning, and locomotion

Fine Motor
- to improve using both hands together, reach and grasp, visual attention, and tracking
- to improve shoulder girdle strength and stability

Cognitive
- to improve tool use, understanding of cause-and-effect and means-end relationships, understanding of spatial relationships, imitation, and concept development

Language
- to improve following directions; taking turns; identifying/labeling objects, actions, locations, and relationships; initiating; and requesting

Social
- to make choices
- to facilitate peer interaction

Directions

Introduce the kites at the end of opening circle time. Let the children explore them (gently). Encourage touching the different materials and talking about the sizes, shapes, and colors. Adults should repeat the word *kite* often in their comments. Eventually, help the children discover the kite strings. Encourage them to pull and drag the kites by the strings. Then show them how to run or walk quickly with the kites. Children who are more physically challenged may hold the kite strings while an adult pushes them in a wagon or stroller. Alternatively, the string may be tied to the child's arm or to the wagon. If the weather permits, this activity can be held outdoors.

Activity 2: Kite Grab Bag

Materials

several small paper kites with strings attached
a variety of manipulative toys or other materials, for example:

play dough	blocks
pegs	busy boxes

simple pictures or photos of the above manipulatives and materials

Goals

Sensory
- to improve sensory awareness and responsiveness
- to increase attention span

Gross Motor
- to improve balance, coordination, motor planning, and locomotion

Fine Motor
- to improve using both hands together, reach and grasp, visual attention and tracking, eye-hand coordination, and hand/finger manipulation
- to improve shoulder girdle strength and stability

Cognitive
- to improve tool use, understanding of cause-and-effect and means-end relationships, problem solving, picture-object association, understanding of spatial relationships, imitation, and concept development
- to develop generalization skills

Language
- to improve following directions; taking turns; identifying/labeling objects, actions, locations, and relationships; initiating; and requesting

Social
- to make choices
- to facilitate peer interaction

Directions

Attach pictures of the manipulatives and materials to be included to the backs of the small kites. Set up the toys in a nearby part of the room. Position the kites so that the children have to reach up to grab the strings. Help the children each select one kite. Then help them find the activity pictured on their kite. Follow up by exploring the activity with the child and expanding play as appropriate. When children tire of the first activity they selected, help them exchange kites and find a new activity. At every point, use lots of language to describe what is happening and what the children are doing.

Activity 3: Painting Kites

Materials

large pieces of paper cut into kite shapes

tempera or water-color paints (washable markers can be used as an alternative)

towels for cleanup

chubby paintbrushes

tape

smocks

Goals

Sensory
- to increase attention span

Fine Motor
- to improve hand manipulation and eye-hand coordination
- to improve shoulder girdle strength and stability

Cognitive
- to improve tool use, concept development, and imitation
- to develop generalization skills

Language
- to improve following directions; taking turns; increasing vocabulary; identifying/labeling objects, actions, characteristics, and relationships

Social
- to make choices
- to facilitate peer interaction

Directions

Tape kite-shaped papers to a wall or other surface so that children will need to reach up to paint. Have the children choose which kite to paint and which colors to use. Help the children paint the kites. Describe their actions and the colors used. Additional peer interactions can be encouraged by making the kite-painting a group project, with all children painting one large kite.

Activity 4: Kite Tails

Materials

yarn or string for each kite made in Activity 3

tissue paper

various pieces of textured fabrics

tape

Goals

Sensory
- to improve responses to tactile stimulation
- to increase attention span

Fine Motor
- to improve hand manipulation, eye-hand coordination, and using two hands together
- to improve shoulder girdle strength and stability

Cognitive
- to improve imitation and concept development
- to develop generalization skills

Language
- to improve following directions; taking turns; increasing vocabulary; identifying/labeling objects, actions, characteristics, and relationships

Social
- to make choices
- to facilitate peer interaction

Directions

Give each child a piece of string. Help the children select pieces of fabric to tie to their kite tails. They can also tear tissue paper to make pieces for their kite tails. Have each child choose which piece to tie onto the string and have an adult do the actual tying. Tape each kite tail to the child's kite (completed in the preceding activity) when finished.

Snack

Materials

bread	plates
fillings for bread (such as peanut butter or cream cheese)	table
	table knives for spreading
juice	diamond-shaped cookie cutters
napkins	cups (adapted if necessary)
chairs (adaptive seating as needed)	

Goals

Sensory
- to improve responses to sensory stimuli, especially tactile and olfactory
- to increase attention span

Fine Motor
- to improve using both hands together, grasp, and hand manipulation
- to improve shoulder girdle strength and stability

Self-Help
- to improve self-feeding skills
- to improve oral-motor skills

Cognitive
- to improve imitation and concept development
- to develop generalization skills
- to develop recall skills

Language
- to improve following directions; taking turns; identifying/labeling objects, actions, people, and characteristics; requesting; and initiating

Social
- to make choices
- to facilitate peer interaction

Directions

Seat children appropriately for snack, using adaptive seating as needed. As children watch, spread peanut butter or another topping on the bread. Tell them they are going to make "kite sandwiches." Give each child a table knife and slice of bread. Help them spread the topping of their choice on the bread. Top with a second slice of bread. Help children cut kite-shaped sandwiches using the diamond-shaped cookie cutters. Describe what they are doing, what the snack is made of, and what it looks like. Talk about how it looks like a kite. Encourage communication, including ways to request more or indicate "all done." Offer juice as needed. Assist with self-feeding and drinking skills as needed.

Week 5

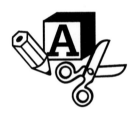

Overall Theme: Flying

Activity 1: Flying Kids

Materials

hammock swing

Goals

Sensory
- to improve responses to vestibular stimulation

Gross Motor
- to improve back extension against gravity and motor planning

Fine Motor
- to increase upper body strength

Cognitive
- to improve understanding of spatial relationships, imitation, and concept development

Language
- to improve following directions; taking turns; identifying/labeling people, actions, and relationships; requesting; and initiating

Social
- to facilitate pretend play

Directions

Begin this activity by elevating smaller children on their tummies in your arms so that they are "flying." Encourage them to stretch out their arms like wings. Two adults can sometimes "fly" larger children. This activity can also incorporate a variety of other gross motor goals, depending on the needs of the individual children. For example, "flying" on the tummy can also be used to stretch the upper back and shoulder muscles and break up a shoulder block. After the children have had a chance to observe and participate in this activity, introduce the hammock swing. Position it so that the children are just about 2 to 3 inches off the ground when on their tummies. Use the hammock to support as much of their bodies as necessary. Encourage them to stretch out their arms. Gently move the swing back and forth, side to side, diagonally, and even spinning in circles for those for whom this activity is appropriate.

Caution: Vestibular stimulation can have powerful effects. This activity should be planned in consultation with the physical or occupational therapist. Spinning, in particular, should be carried out only under the supervision of a trained physical or occupational therapist.

Activity 2: Flying Animals

Materials

a variety of puppets, stuffed toys, and pictures that represent flying animals, such as:

birds	grasshoppers	bees
butterflies	bats	flying squirrels

Goals

Sensory
- to improve responses to sensory stimulation
- to increase attention span

Gross Motor
- to improve motor planning and coordination

Fine Motor
- to improve reach and grasp, eye-hand coordination, visual attending, visual tracking, and hand manipulation
- to increase upper body strength

Cognitive
- to improve imitation, classification, functional object use, and concept development
- to develop generalization skills

Language
- to improve following directions; taking turns; identifying/labeling objects, people, actions, and relationships; requesting; and initiating

Social
- to make choices
- to facilitate pretend play
- to facilitate peer interaction

Directions

Show children the objects/pictures and encourage them to identify those they know. Help them to imitate the actions of the animals with which they are familiar. Demonstrate the actions using the puppets, stuffed toys, or adult's body in combination with the animal's picture. Encourage the children to choose a puppet or stuffed toy and imitate the actions of that particular animal. Provide physical assistance as needed.

Activity 3: Airplanes

Materials

a variety of toy airplanes and airport sets, including those that provide for toy people to be placed in the planes

Goals

Sensory
• to increase attention span

Fine Motor
• to improve hand/finger manipulation, reach and grasp, grasp and release, eye-hand coordination, and finger isolation

Cognitive
• to improve imitation, problem solving, understanding of spatial relationships, classification, and concept development
• to develop generalization skills

Language
• to improve taking turns; increasing vocalizations/vocabulary; requesting; initiating; following directions; and identifying/labeling objects, actions, characteristics, and locations

Social
• to make choices
• to facilitate pretend play
• to facilitate peer interaction

Directions

Set up the airplane/airport sets. Encourage the children to choose which one to play with. Demonstrate how the toys work, as necessary. Facilitate the exploration of the airport sets through motor skills as well as expanding the pretend play. Use lots of language to describe what is going on; for example, "The people are going in the plane," "Close the door," "The plane is flying."

Activity 4: Paper Airplanes

Materials

paper	crayons or markers
table	chairs (adaptive seating as needed)

Goals

Sensory
• to increase attention span

Fine Motor
• to improve hand manipulation, eye-hand coordination, visual focusing and tracking, and using two hands together
• to improve shoulder girdle strength and stability

Cognitive
- to improve tool use, imitation, and concept development
- to develop generalization skills
- to develop recall skills

Language
- to improve following directions; taking turns; and identifying/labeling objects, actions, and descriptions

Social
- to make choices
- to facilitate pretend play
- to facilitate peer interaction

Directions

Position children appropriately for fine motor activity. Give them paper and let them choose the crayons or markers they want to use. Encourage them to color all over their papers. When they have finished, fold their papers into colorful paper airplanes and help them to fly the planes.

Activity 5: Collages

Materials

pictures of things that fly— animals as well as airplanes	scissors	construction paper
	glue	paintbrushes (optional)
cotton swabs (optional)	table	chairs (adaptive seating as needed)
washcloths for cleanup		

Goals

Sensory
- to improve responses to sensory stimulation
- to increase attention span

Fine Motor
- to improve hand manipulation, eye-hand coordination, and using two hands together

Cognitive
- to improve classification, picture-object relationships, and concept development
- to develop generalization skills
- to develop recall skills

Language
- to improve following directions; taking turns; identifying/labeling objects, pictures, actions, and descriptions; initiating; and requesting

Social
- to make choices

Directions

Ahead of time, cut out a variety of pictures of things that fly, including those that have been presented in previous activities. Position children appropriately for fine motor activity. Have children select which color paper to use. Show them the pictures and encourage them to identify or name the pictures and to say anything else they remember about the object pictured. Let them choose several pictures to use in their collage. Help children squeeze or spread glue onto their papers, encouraging them to stabilize paper with one hand, if possible. Help them pat the pictures into place. Let the pictures dry while completing another activity.

Snack

Materials

celery sticks (bread sticks or even fruit leather can be substituted if celery is too challenging for the group's oral-motor skills)

peanut butter	table knives	napkins
paper plates	juice	cups (adapted as needed)
table	chairs (adaptive	
washcloths for cleanup	seating as needed)	

Goals

Sensory
- to improve responses to sensory stimuli, especially tactile and olfactory
- to increase attention span

Fine Motor
- to improve using both hands together, grasp and release, and hand manipulation
- to improve shoulder girdle strength and stability

Self-Help
- to improve self-feeding skills
- to improve oral-motor skills

Cognitive
- to improve imitation and taking turns
- to develop generalization skills
- to develop recall skills

Language
- to improve following directions; identifying/labeling objects, actions, people, and characteristics; requesting; and initiating

Social
- to make choices
- to facilitate peer interaction

Directions

Seat children appropriately for snack, using adaptive seating as needed. Have children hand out napkins and/or plates, if appropriate. Help children spread peanut butter on a celery stick, mounding it in the middle. Place another celery stick across the mound of peanut butter at a 90-degree angle to the bottom celery stick. Eat the celery "airplanes." Provide help with feeding and oral-motor skills as needed. Offer juice and provide assistance as needed.

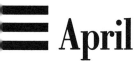

April

Week 1

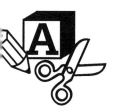

Overall Theme: Baby Animals

Note: You may want to modify this theme by concentrating on only a single animal each session; for example, puppies in one session, kittens in another, and bunnies in the next.

Activity 1: Obstacle Course

Materials

indoor climbing structure
inner tubes
ramp or other incline
floor pillows/beanbag chairs
bolsters
indoor swing

toddler slide
indoor tunnel
carpet squares
benches
steps

assorted toy animals (for example, stuffed, plastic, wooden) representing common baby animals (such as kittens, puppies, lambs, bunnies)

Goals

Sensory
- to provide vestibular stimulation
- to provide proprioceptive stimulation
- to increase attention span

Gross Motor
- to improve balance, coordination, motor planning, locomotion, trunk rotation, and weight shifting

Fine Motor
- to improve using both hands together, reach and grasp, and visual attention
- to increase upper body strength
- to improve shoulder girdle strength and stability

Cognitive
- to improve object permanence, imitation, problem solving, and concept development

Language
- to improve following directions; taking turns; identifying/labeling objects, actions, descriptions, and locations; requesting; and initiating

Social
- to make choices
- to facilitate pretend play
- to facilitate peer interaction

Directions

Using the equipment available, set up an indoor obstacle course to facilitate the gross motor and vestibular goals for the individuals in the group. The materials listed above are just suggestions. Place the toy animals at various points throughout the obstacle course. Have some hidden, some partially hidden, and some in plain sight. Assist the children through the obstacle course. A "path" of carpet squares can provide a structure to follow through the course. Encourage them to use appropriate motor patterns throughout. Help them find the baby animals as they go through the course. Be sure there are enough baby animals for each child to find at least one. Encourage the children to help their animals through the obstacle course, too. If appropriate, encourage them to move as their animals would move.

Activity 2: Pat the Bunny

Note: Other animals may be substituted in this activity. Older puppies or kittens might be more readily available. One of the authors has a pet rabbit who regularly visited the infant program for many years, thus this particular choice. Be cautious about exposing very young animals to very young children who can harm them without meaning to simply by patting or poking roughly.

Materials

pet rabbit
carrots or apple pieces

Goals

Sensory
- to improve responses to sensory stimulation, especially tactile
- to increase attention span

Fine Motor
- to improve reach and touch, grading movements, eye-hand coordination, and visual attending

Cognitive
- to improve concept development
- to develop generalization skills

Language
- to improve taking turns; identifying/labeling objects, actions, characteristics, and body parts; increasing vocalizations/vocabulary; initiating; and requesting

Directions

Introduce the rabbit in its cage or held in an adult's arms. Encourage children to touch the rabbit gently, and identify its eyes, nose, ears, and tail. Encourage children to offer carrots or apple pieces to the rabbit or let them watch while an adult offers food to the rabbit. Talk about how the rabbit looks, feels, moves, if it makes noise, and what it eats.

Activity 3: Animal Walk

Materials

toy animals used in Activity 1
battery-operated animal toys
carrots, apple pieces, or other appropriate foods for the animals
blocks to represent food for the animals

animal puppets
capability switch for battery-operated toys

Goals

Sensory
- to increase sensory awareness and responsiveness, especially to tactile stimulation
- to provide vestibular stimulation
- to provide proprioceptive stimulation
- to increase attention span

Gross Motor
- to improve motor planning, locomotion, balance and coordination, and weight shifting

Fine Motor
- to improve hand and finger manipulation, eye-hand coordination, and visual attention

Cognitive
- to improve understanding of cause-and-effect relationships, imitation, and concept development
- to develop generalization skills

Language
- to improve following directions; taking turns; identifying/labeling objects, actions, characteristics, and relationships; initiating; and requesting

Social
- to make choices
- to facilitate peer interaction
- to facilitate representational/pretend play

Directions

Have children imitate the animals in a variety of ways. They may move like one of the animals or allow themselves to be assisted through the movement. They can move a toy animal (help them to choose one) or "feed" a toy animal using the real food or the representative food (blocks). They can explore making the switch-activated animals move. Children who are ready may work on controlling a switch-activated animal on command. Use lots of language to describe what the children and animals are doing, how they are moving, and who is moving.

Activity 4: Baby Animal Pictures

Materials

construction paper with different animal shapes outlined on it (you may want to use only one outline per page or several smaller outlines on the same page, as appropriate for the group)

cotton balls	feathers
fake fur	glue
paintbrushes (optional)	cotton swabs (optional)
markers	table
chairs (adaptive seating as needed)	washcloths for cleanup

Goals

Sensory
- to improve sensory awareness through tactile stimulation
- to increase attention span

Fine Motor
- to improve hand/finger manipulation, eye-hand coordination, and using both hands together

Cognitive
- to improve imitation, classification, and concept development
- to develop generalization skills
- to develop recall skills

Language
- to improve following directions; taking turns; increasing vocabulary; and identifying/labeling objects, actions, characteristics, and relationships

Social
- to make choices

Directions

Position children for fine motor activity. Have children select which color paper to use and an animal shape, if appropriate. Encourage them to identify the animal shapes on their papers. Help children squeeze or spread glue onto their papers, encouraging them to stabilize paper with one hand, if possible. Vary the activity by having them spread the glue with paintbrushes or cotton swabs. Help them choose the appropriate texture for their animal shapes. Help them pat the materials into place. Use lots of language and encourage the children to describe what they are doing and the materials they are using. Remind them that the textures feel a little like the animals they were petting and playing with earlier, and that the pictures look like these animals. Let the pictures dry while completing another activity.

Snack

Materials

ice cream	ice cream scoop	bowls
vanilla wafers	spoons	napkins
small pastel candies	table	chairs (adaptive seating as needed)
juice	cups (adapted as needed)	washcloths for cleanup

Goals

Sensory
- to improve responses to sensory stimuli, especially tactile, temperature, and olfactory

Fine Motor
- to improve grasp and release, midline skills, eye-hand coordination, and hand manipulation
- to increase upper body strength
- to improve shoulder girdle strength and stability

Self-Help
- to improve self-feeding skills
- to improve oral-motor skills

Cognitive
- to improve concept development
- to develop generalization skills

Language
- to improve taking turns; identifying/labeling objects, actions, people, and characteristics; requesting; and initiating

Social
- to make choices
- to facilitate peer interaction

Directions

An adult should make ice cream bunnies, kittens, or other animals ahead of time using one scoop of ice cream for the head, two cookies for the ears, and the pastel candies for the eyes, nose, and mouth. Seat children appropriately for snack, using adaptive seating as needed. Have children help pass out napkins and spoons, if appropriate. Show children the ice cream animals and have them choose which one they want. Help them to identify their animal's eyes, nose, mouth, and ears. Talk with the children about how these animals are like the other animals they have played with and how they are different. Facilitate appropriate feeding skills as necessary for each individual. Encourage communication, including ways to request more or to indicate "all done." Offer juice as needed and provide assistance as required.

Week 2

Overall Theme: Eggs

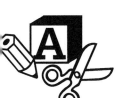

Activity 1: Obstacle Course

Materials

indoor climbing structure	toddler slide	inner tubes
indoor tunnel	ramp or other incline	carpet squares
floor pillows/beanbag chairs	benches	bolsters
steps	indoor swing	baskets

assorted plastic and/or wooden eggs (include some that open)
small treats (such as crackers or marshmallows)

Goals

Sensory
- to provide vestibular stimulation
- to provide proprioceptive stimulation
- to increase attention span

Gross Motor
- to improve balance, coordination, motor planning, locomotion, trunk rotation, and weight shifting

Fine Motor
- to improve using both hands together, reach and grasp, visual attention, midline skills, and hand/finger manipulation
- to increase upper body strength
- to improve shoulder girdle strength and stability

Self-Help
- to improve self-feeding skills
- to improve oral-motor skills

Cognitive
- to improve object permanence, imitation, problem solving, and concept development

Language
- to improve following directions; taking turns; identifying/labeling objects, actions, characteristics, and locations; requesting; and initiating

Social
- to make choices
- to facilitate peer interaction

Directions

Using the equipment available, set up an indoor obstacle course to facilitate the gross motor and vestibular goals for the individuals in the group. The materials listed above are just suggestions. Place the eggs at various points throughout the obstacle course. Have some hidden, some partially hidden, and some in plain sight. Fill the eggs that open with small treats; use some that will make noise when shaken (cereal pieces) and some that will not (marshmallows). Assist the children through the obstacle course. A "path" of carpet squares can provide a structure to follow through the course. Encourage them to use appropriate motor patterns throughout. Help them find the eggs as they go through the course. Be sure there are enough eggs for each child to find several. Give the children baskets in which to carry all the eggs they find. Assist them with opening their eggs and finding the treats inside. Encourage them to identify the treats. Assist with feeding skills as needed.

Activity 2: Hiding Eggs

Materials

box or baskets	cellophane grass (can use green or various colors)
eggs from previous activity	more treats to hide in the eggs

Goals

Sensory
- to improve responses to sensory stimuli, especially tactile
- to increase attention span

Fine Motor
- to improve using both hands together, reach and grasp, visual attention, midline skills, and hand/finger manipulation
- to improve shoulder girdle strength and stability

Self-Help
- to improve self-feeding skills
- to improve oral-motor skills

Cognitive
- to improve object permanence, imitation, problem solving, and concept development
- to develop generalization skills

Language
- to improve following directions; taking turns; identifying/labeling objects, actions, characteristics, and locations; requesting; and initiating

Social
- to make choices
- to facilitate peer interaction

Directions

As the children are watching, hide treats in the eggs again and then hide the eggs in the box or baskets of cellophane grass. Hide some eggs completely and some only partially, depending on the children's understanding of object permanence. You may want to hide additional objects in the grass as well. Help the children to explore in the grass and find the hidden treasures. Encourage them to touch and feel the grass. Describe the activity, what they are doing, and how it looks and feels. Assist the children with opening the eggs and eating the treats. Again, be aware of the tactile component to this activity. Note which children have difficulty and let them control how much they will play in the grass. Brushing and/or rubbing arms and hands with a washcloth may help make this activity more accessible for those children who show signs of tactile defensiveness.

Activity 3: Dyeing Eggs

Materials

hard-boiled eggs (1 to 2 per child)
cold-water egg dye
pitcher of cold water
vinegar (if needed for the dye)
measuring spoons
spoons or wire holders for dipping eggs into dye

cups (one for each color dye)
egg carton or other rack for drying eggs
stickers (optional)
markers (optional)
table
chairs (adaptive seating as needed)
washcloths for cleanup

Goals

Sensory
- to improve sensory awareness and responsiveness
- to increase attention span

Fine Motor
- to improve using both hands together, reach and grasp, midline skills, and visual attending and tracking
- to improve shoulder girdle strength and stability

Cognitive
- to improve object permanence, imitation, problem solving, and concept development
- to develop generalization skills

Language
- to improve following directions; taking turns; identifying/labeling objects, actions, descriptions, and locations; requesting; and initiating

Social
- to make choices
- to facilitate peer interaction

Directions

Prepare eggs ahead of time. Seat children appropriately. Let them help mix the dyes, water, and vinegar (if needed) in individual cups. Show them how to balance an egg on a spoon or holder and lower it into the cup of dye. Let each child choose which color to use and help them lower the eggs into the dye. Talk about the colors, the changes in the eggs, and the feel of the water and eggs. Help them take the eggs out and let them dry. Allow the children to decorate the colored eggs with stickers, markers, and other craft materials. This could also be done as an alternative to dyeing the eggs, if more appropriate.

Activity 4: Egg Collage

Materials

small pieces of various colored textured items (such as cloth, sponge, styrofoam, pipe cleaner, feathers, ribbon, cellophane grass, wrapping paper, tissue paper, yarn, rice, and macaroni)

stickers	markers or crayons	table
paintbrushes (optional)	cotton swabs (optional)	chairs (adaptive
construction paper	glue	seating if needed)
washcloths for cleanup	scissors	

Goals

Sensory
- to improve sensory awareness through tactile stimulation
- to increase attention span

Fine Motor
- to improve hand manipulation, eye-hand coordination, and using both hands together

Cognitive
- to improve imitation and concept development

Language
- to improve following directions; taking turns; increasing vocabulary; and identifying/labeling objects, actions, characteristics, and relationships

Social
- to make choices
- to facilitate peer interaction

Directions

Cut construction paper into egg shapes ahead of time. Alternatively, you can use one large egg-shaped piece of paper and have all the children work together on a group collage. Position children for fine motor activity. Have children select which color paper to use. Help children squeeze or spread glue onto their papers, encouraging them to stabilize the paper with one hand, if possible. Help each child choose the materials to use in the collage. Help children put the materials they have chosen onto the glue and pat the materials into place. Use lots of language and encourage the children also to describe what they are doing, the materials they are using, and how the materials feel. Let the pictures dry while completing another activity.

Snack

Materials

hard-boiled eggs	mixing bowl	plastic knives
mayonnaise or salad	cups (adapted if needed)	forks
dressing	paper plates and/	chairs (adaptive
bread	or napkins	seating as needed)
juice	table	washcloths for cleanup

Goals

Sensory
- to improve responses to sensory stimulation, especially tactile and olfactory
- to increase attention span

Fine Motor
- to improve using both hands together, midline skills, and hand/finger manipulation
- to increase upper body strength

Self-Help
- to improve self-feeding skills
- to improve oral-motor skills

Cognitive
- to improve understanding of spatial relationships, functional use of objects, imitation, and sequencing
- to develop generalization skills

Language
- to improve following directions; taking turns; identifying/labeling objects, actions, locations, and relationships; initiating; and requesting

Social
- to make choices
- to facilitate peer interaction

Directions

Encourage children to name the objects to be used (eggs, bowl, fork). Help children crack and peel the eggs. If more appropriate, peel the eggs ahead of time. Direct the children to put the peeled eggs into the bowl. Demonstrate cutting up the eggs and mashing them with a fork. Encourage children to help with these activities by taking turns. Let children help mix mayonnaise or salad dressing into the eggs. Talk about the actions involved, the items needed, and the changes they observe in the eggs. Help children to spread the egg salad onto the bread to make sandwiches. Let them pass out plates and napkins for their sandwiches. Encourage children to initiate requests for more. Use lots of language to talk about what they are doing and encourage them to label the objects, describe their actions, and indicate that they are finished. Offer juice as needed and provide assistance with feeding and drinking skills as necessary.

Week 3

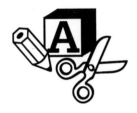

Overall Theme: Pets

Note: This would be a good time for the children to bring family pets to share with the class, if appropriate. Structure such an activity to be similar to the Pat the Bunny activity during Week 1.

Activity 1: Pet Shop

Materials

indoor climbing structure	toddler slide	inner tubes
ball pool	indoor tunnel	ramp or other incline
carpet squares	floor pillows/beanbag chairs	benches
bolsters	steps	indoor swing

assorted toys representing a variety of pets (for example, stuffed, plastic, wooden)

Goals

Sensory
- to improve responses to tactile stimulation
- to provide vestibular stimulation
- to provide proprioceptive stimulation
- to increase attention span

Gross Motor
- to improve balance, coordination, motor planning, locomotion, trunk rotation, and weight shifting

Fine Motor
- to improve using both hands together, reach and grasp, and visual attention
- to increase upper body strength
- to improve shoulder girdle strength and stability

Cognitive
- to improve object permanence, imitation, problem solving, and concept development

Language
- to improve following directions; taking turns; identifying/labeling objects, actions, descriptions, and locations; requesting; and initiating

Social
- to make choices
- to facilitate pretend play
- to facilitate peer interaction

Directions

Using the equipment available, set up an indoor obstacle course to facilitate the gross motor and vestibular goals for the individuals in the group. The materials listed above are just suggestions. At the same time, plan the course so that the equipment can be used to represent various cages for different "pets" (the toy pets you have gathered). For example, birds could live inside the climbing gym, or a parrot could use the indoor swing. Fish could live in the ball pool. Dogs, cats, or other pets could have cages or beds made from other equipment. Place the "pets" in their appropriate cages throughout the course. Tell the children that the course is a big pet shop. Assist the children through the obstacle course. A path of carpet squares can provide a structure to follow through the course. Encourage them to use appropriate motor patterns throughout. Help them find and identify the different pets as they go through the course. Encourage the children to explore how each pet lives, how it moves, what it eats, how it plays, and what sounds it makes.

Activity 2: Pet Walk

Materials

toy "pets" from previous activity
access to outdoors, if possible
strollers or other adaptive means of locomotion for children who are nonambulatory

Goals

Sensory
- to improve responses to sensory stimulation
- to provide proprioceptive stimulation
- to increase attention span
- to improve auditory and visual attending skills

Gross Motor
- to improve walking, weight shifting, balance, coordination, and motor planning

Fine Motor
- to improve eye-hand coordination, grading movements, and grasp and release
- to increase upper body strength
- to improve shoulder girdle strength and stability

Cognitive
- to improve classification, imitation, and concept development
- to develop generalization skills

Language
- to improve taking turns; following directions; increasing vocalizations/vocabulary; identifying/labeling objects, actions, characteristics, and body parts; initiating; requesting; and questioning

Social
- to make choices
- to facilitate pretend play
- to facilitate peer interaction

Directions

Have the children select "pets," if they have not already done so. Have them take their pets for a walk. Some may need leashes or cages. Have children walk along a path outdoors, if possible. Let the children who are walking help push the strollers for the children who are using them, thus helping the children who are walking improve their upper body strength. Talk with the children about their experiences on the walk. Vary this activity by having the children pretend to be the pets they have selected.

Activity 3: Pet Show

Materials

pets from the previous activities (toys or live animals)
illustrations or photos of different pets
small amounts of pet food
pet grooming materials (such as brushes or combs)

Goals

Sensory
- to increase sensory awareness and responsiveness
- to improve responses to tactile stimulation
- to increase attention span

Gross Motor
- to improve motor planning, locomotion, balance and coordination, and weight shifting

Fine Motor
- to improve eye-hand coordination, visual attention, reach and grasp, grading movement, hand/finger manipulation, and grasp and release

Cognitive
- to improve imitation, classification, object-picture association, and concept development
- to develop generalization skills

Language
- to improve following directions; taking turns; identifying/labeling objects, actions, characteristics, and relationships; initiating; and requesting

Social
- to make choices
- to facilitate peer interaction
- to facilitate pretend play

Directions

Have children prepare their pets for a pet show. Use toy or live pets as appropriate. Help children brush their pets' fur and prepare for the show. For the show, group the pets in categories; for example: dogs, cats, and birds. Talk about which pet is the biggest, smallest, quietest, and softest. Match the pictures to the pets.

Activity 4: Picture-a-Pet

Materials

construction paper with pet shapes outlined on it (you may want to use only one outline per page or several smaller outlines on the same page, as appropriate for the group)

feathers	fake fur	cotton balls
glue	paintbrushes (optional)	cotton swabs (optional)
markers	table	
washcloths for cleanup	chairs (adaptive seating as needed)	

Goals

Sensory
- to improve sensory awareness through tactile stimulation
- to increase attention span

Fine Motor
- to improve hand manipulation, eye-hand coordination, and using both hands together

Cognitive
- to improve imitation, classification, and concept formation
- to develop generalization skills
- to develop recall skills

Language
- to improve following directions; taking turns; increasing vocabulary; and identifying/labeling objects, actions, characteristics, and relationships

Social
- to make choices

Directions

Position children for fine motor activity. Have children select the color paper and animal shape they want to use. Encourage them to identify the animal shapes. Help children squeeze or spread glue onto their papers, encouraging them to stabilize the paper with one hand, if possible. Vary the activities by having them spread the glue with paintbrushes or cotton swabs. Help the children choose the appropriate textures for their animal shapes. Help them pat the materials into place. Use lots of language and encourage the children to describe what they are doing and the materials they are using. Remind them that the pictures they are making feel a little like the pets they were patting and playing with earlier and that the pictures look like the pets. Let the pictures dry while completing another activity.

Snack

Materials

cookies baked in the shapes of cats, dogs, and other pets

juice or milk	cups (adapted as needed)
napkins	table
chairs (adaptive seating as needed)	washcloths for cleanup

Goals

Sensory
- to improve responses to sensory stimuli, especially tactile and olfactory
- to increase attention span

Fine Motor
- to improve reach and grasp, grasp and release, hand/finger manipulation, and eye-hand coordination

Self-Help
- to improve self-feeding skills
- to improve oral-motor skills

Cognitive
- to improve imitation, concept development
- to develop generalization skills
- to develop recall skills

Language
- to improve following directions; taking turns; identifying/labeling objects, actions, people, and characteristics; requesting; and initiating

Social
- to make choices
- to facilitate peer interaction

Directions

Seat children appropriately for snack, using adaptive seating as needed. Have children help pass out napkins, if appropriate. Show children the cookies and have them each choose one. Explain that the cookies look like some of the pets. Ask the children to imitate their sounds. Facilitate appropriate feeding skills as necessary for each individual. Encourage communication, including ways to request more or indicate "all done." Offer juice and provide assistance as needed.

Week 4

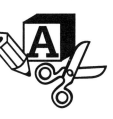

Overall Theme: Flowers

Activity 1: Planting Flowers

Materials

1 plastic flower pot for each child (yogurt cartons, cottage cheese containers, or empty margarine tubs may be substituted)

potting soil	spoons for digging
small watering can with water	1 flowering plant already in bloom for
table	each child (for example, marigolds,
chairs (adapted seating as needed)	impatiens, pansies)
washcloths for cleanup	

Goals

Sensory
- to improve sensory awareness and responsiveness

Fine Motor
- to improve reach and grasp, eye-hand coordination, and hand manipulation skills
- to increase upper body strength
- to improve shoulder girdle strength and stability

Cognitive
- to improve tool use, understanding of spatial relationships, object permanence, sequencing, imitation, and concept formation

Language
- to improve following directions; taking turns; identifying/labeling objects, actions, people, places, characteristics, and relationships; requesting; and initiating

Social
- to make choices

Directions

Assemble all of the materials, except the watering can, on a small table. Invite children to explore the flowers by looking and smelling. Have children choose the flower pots they wish to use and the flowers they wish to plant. Help children fill their pots about half full with potting soil, using the spoons to dig and fill. Position one of the flowering plants in each pot and help children fill the pots with more soil. When all the plants have been planted, help children take turns watering their plants. Throughout the activity, use lots of language to describe the plants, the soil, the sensations experienced, and what the children are doing. If the children work standing at the table, standing balance and weight-shifting goals are also incorporated into the activity.

Activity 2: Flower Walk

Materials

access to outdoors, if possible
a variety of flowers, either natural or artificial, for the children to gather
strollers or other adaptive means of locomotion for children who are
    nonambulatory
baskets for carrying the flowers (optional)

Goals

Sensory
- to increase sensory awareness and responsiveness
- to increase attention span
- to improve auditory and visual attending skills

Gross Motor
- to improve walking, stooping/squatting, weight shifting, balance, coordination, and motor planning

Fine Motor
- to improve eye-hand coordination, reach and grasp, hand manipulation, and finger isolation (pointing)
- to increase upper body strength

Cognitive
- to improve classification, imitation, and concept development
- to develop generalization skills

Language
- to improve following directions; taking turns; increasing vocalization/ vocabulary; identifying/labeling objects, actions, characteristics, relationships, and locations; initiating; requesting; and questioning

Social
- to facilitate peer interaction

Directions

Have children hike along a path outdoors, if possible. Otherwise, set up a "path" indoors with flowers placed along the way. Encouraging the children to march or hike with big, heavy steps will provide proprioceptive input and help them develop a variety of gross motor skills. Having them contrast this action with small, gentle steps will then help develop the concepts of opposite or different, as well as increasing their awareness of these sensations. Let the children who are walking push the strollers for the children who are using them, thus helping the walking children to improve their upper body strength. Talk with the children about what they see, hear, and smell. Help them pick some of the flowers. Encourage them to carry the flowers in their hands but use the baskets if needed. Ask questions about what they are doing and what they have found.

Activity 3: Potato Print Flowers

Materials

potatoes	tempera paint
paper plates, pie tins, or saucers	construction paper
smocks	table
chairs (adaptive seating as needed)	washcloths for cleanup

Goals

Sensory
- to improve sensory awareness and responsiveness

Fine Motor
- to improve reach and grasp, eye-hand coordination, hand manipulation, and using both hands together
- to increase upper body strength
- to improve shoulder girdle strength and stability

Cognitive
- to improve sequencing, imitation, and concept development
- to develop generalization skills

Language
- to improve following directions; taking turns; identifying/labeling objects, actions, people, places, characteristics, and relationships; requesting; initiating; and increasing vocabulary

Social
- to make choices

Directions

Prepare potatoes ahead of time by cutting each one in half and carving a flower-like design into each cut edge. Set up the activity on a small table. Seat children or let them work in standing, according to the needs of the group. Have children choose the color paper, the potato, and the color paint to use. Demonstrate dipping the potato in the paint and pressing it onto the paper to make a print. Assist the children as needed in making their own prints. Talk about the feel of the paint and the potato, the colors being used, and the actions involved.

Activity 4: Flower Cookies

Materials

sugar cookie dough	cutting board	flour
spatula	rolling pins	flower-shaped cookie cutters
cookie sheets	candy sprinkles	oven
potholders	table	plate for cooling cookies
	chairs (adaptive seating as needed)	washcloths for cleanup

Note: see Appendix C for a sugar cookie recipe

Goals

Sensory
- to improve sensory awareness and responsiveness, especially tactile and olfactory
- to increase attention span

Fine Motor
- to improve using both hands together, midline skills, hand/finger manipulation, eye-hand coordination, and visual attending
- to increase upper body strength

Cognitive
- to improve tool use, understanding of spatial relationships, functional use of objects, imitation, sequencing, and concept development

Language
- to improve following directions; taking turns; identifying/labeling objects, actions, characteristics, locations, and relationships; initiating; requesting; and vocabulary development

Social
- to make choices
- to facilitate peer interaction

Directions

Seat children appropriately at the table. Tell them they will be helping to make cookies. Place the cookie dough on a floured cutting board and demonstrate rolling out the dough with a rolling pin. Use small, child-sized rolling pins, if possible, to facilitate midline goals. Give each child a ball of dough and help the children to roll it out. Children may also use their hands to pat the dough flat, if preferred. Show children how to press the cookie cutters into the dough to make shapes. Let each child choose a cookie cutter to use. Help them to press the cutters into their dough and place the cookies onto cookie sheets. Let children choose which sprinkles to use to decorate their cookies. Help them shake the sprinkles onto the cookies. If possible, let the children watch you put the cookies in the oven and take them out. Throughout the activity, use lots of language to talk about how the dough feels and smells, what the children are doing, the color and texture of the sprinkles, and the shape of the cookies.

Snack

Materials

flower cookies made in previous activity
cups (adapted if necessary)
chairs (adaptive seating as needed)
washcloths for cleanup

milk or juice
paper napkins
table

Goals

Sensory
- to improve responses to sensory stimuli, especially tactile and olfactory
- to increase attention span

Fine Motor
- to improve reach and grasp, grasp and release, hand/finger manipulation, and eye-hand coordination

Self-Help
- to improve self-feeding skills
- to improve oral-motor skills

Cognitive
- to improve imitation and concept development
- to develop generalization skills
- to develop recall skills

Language
- to improve following directions; taking turns; identifying/labeling objects, actions, people, and characteristics; requesting; and initiating

Social
-
  to make choices
- to facilitate peer interaction

Directions

Seat children appropriately for snack, using adaptive seating as needed. Have children help pass out napkins, if appropriate. Show children the cookies and have them choose one. Talk about making the cookies, how the dough looked, smelled, and felt. Talk about how the cookies look, smell, and feel now. What is the same? What is different? Talk about how the cookies are shaped like flowers. How are they like the flowers found and planted in previous activities? Encourage communication, including ways to request more or indicate "all done." Assist with self-feeding skills as needed. Offer milk or juice and provide assistance as needed.

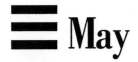

May

Week 1

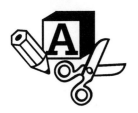

Overall Theme: Fire Trucks

Activity 1: Big Fire Truck

Materials

a visiting fire truck from the local fire station, if possible. An alternative is to make a pretend fire truck out of a climbing structure so that the children can climb up on it. A false front on a climbing gym might work. Include a hose and steering wheel.

Goals

Sensory
- to improve responses to sensory stimulation
- to improve visual attention
- to improve auditory attention
- to increase attention span

Gross Motor
- to improve motor planning, balance and coordination, trunk rotation, weight shifting, and using alternating movement patterns

Fine Motor
- to improve reach and grasp, grasp and release, and eye-hand coordination
- to increase upper body strength
- to improve shoulder girdle strength and stability

Cognitive
- to improve understanding of spatial relationships, functional object use, imitation, and concept development
- to develop generalization skills
- to develop recall skills

Language
- to improve following directions; taking turns; identifying/labeling objects, people, actions, and concepts; initiating; and requesting

Social
- to facilitate pretend play
- to facilitate peer interaction

Directions

If possible, arrange for a fire truck to visit from the local fire station. In this way the activities will proceed from the most concrete to the most abstract. If such a visit is not possible, try to create as realistic a fire truck as possible with the materials available. Be sure it is large enough that the children can climb onto it and include a steering wheel, hoses, and ladders. If possible, include a siren. Encourage the children to explore the fire truck; climb onto it (or place them on it if climbing is not possible); observe the flashing lights; hear the horn and the siren if possible, examine the wheels, hoses, and tires; and turn the steering wheel. If possible, let children examine the firefighters' boots, hats, and other gear. Sometimes fire stations have plastic firefighter's hats to give to the children if you ask ahead of time.

Activity 2: Indoor Fire Truck

Materials

large boxes
hoses (vacuum cleaner hoses work well)
rain slickers and boots (optional)

toddler or preschool climbing gym
toy firefighter hats

Goals

Sensory
- to improve responses to sensory stimulation
- to increase attention span

Gross Motor
- to improve motor planning, balance and coordination, trunk rotation, weight bearing, weight shifting

Fine Motor
- to improve eye-hand coordination, reach and grasp, and hand manipulation
- to increase upper body strength

Self-Help
- to improve dressing/undressing skills

Cognitive
- to improve understanding of spatial relationships, functional object use, imitation, classification, sequencing, and concept development
- to develop generalization skills
- to develop recall skills

Language
- to improve following directions; increasing vocalizations; taking turns; identifying/labeling objects, people, actions, and concepts; initiating; and requesting

Social
- to make choices
- to facilitate pretend play
- to facilitate peer interaction

Directions

Bring children back indoors if they have been outside exploring a real fire truck. Have the materials ready for them to make pretend fire trucks and pretend to be firefighters. Give them as much or as little facilitation as they need to initiate the play. Direct or support the children's play as needed. Encourage gross motor play as appropriate; for example, climbing into boxes or on equipment or pushing boxes to make the truck go. Remind children of what they observed and experienced with the real fire truck. Discuss how the materials they are using are like the real ones. Discuss how they are different.

Activity 3: Toy Fire Trucks

Materials

a variety of toy fire trucks
toy firefighters
capability switches
connections for capability
  switches and battery toys

equipment to fit some of the fire trucks (optional)
toy fire station (optional)
battery-operated fire truck or firefighter

Goals

Sensory
- to increase attention span

Gross Motor
- to improve motor planning, balance and coordination, trunk rotation, and weight shifting

Fine Motor
- to improve hand/finger manipulation, eye-hand coordination, and visual attention

Cognitive
- to improve imitation, concept development, and understanding of cause-and-effect and spatial relationships
- to develop generalization skills

Language
- to improve following directions; taking turns; increasing vocalizations; identifying/labeling objects, actions, characteristics, and relationships; initiating; and requesting

Social
- to make choices
- to facilitate peer interaction
- to facilitate pretend play

Directions

Set up "stations" for sets of the various toys. An adult can then assist at each station, expanding and/or guiding the play as appropriate. Activities with capability switches can also be designed to facilitate the development of pre-computer skills. Encourage children to imitate the fire sirens and honking horns. Continue to develop the concept of location (prepositions) by describing where the fire trucks are or where the people are and by directing the children to drive the trucks to specific locations. Positioning toys to a child's side or behind a child may facilitate trunk rotation and weight shifting and help develop sitting balance.

To address higher-level problem solving, mix up some of the toy sets so that the people are too big to fit in the trucks or the trucks are too big to fit in the fire station. Encourage the children to work together to match the correct pieces.

Activity 4: Fire Truck Pictures

Materials

pre-cut construction paper pieces:

rectangular "truck"	round wheels	ladders

construction paper	washcloths for cleanup	glue
yarn for "hoses"	chairs (adaptive seating as needed)	scissors
table		

Goals

Sensory
- to improve responses to sensory stimulation
- to increase attention span

Fine Motor
- to improve hand manipulation, eye-hand coordination, and using both hands together

Cognitive
- to improve understanding of spatial relationships, functional object use, imitation, and concept development
- to develop generalization skills
- to develop recall skills

Language
- to improve following directions; taking turns; increasing vocabulary; and identifying/labeling objects, actions, characteristics, and relationships

Social
- to make choices

Directions

Cut shapes for trucks and yarn "hoses" ahead of time. Position children for fine motor activity. Show the children how the fire trucks go together and how they will look when they are finished. Have children select which color paper to use for the background. Then have them choose the pieces they need for their fire trucks. Let children select pieces of yarn to use as the hoses for their trucks. Help children squeeze or spread glue onto their papers, encouraging them to stabilize the paper with one hand, if possible. Help them put their shapes onto the glue. Help them pat the materials into place. Use lots of language and encourage the children to describe what they are doing and the materials they are using. Talk about how the pictures look like fire trucks and how they look different from the fire trucks. Let the pictures dry while completing another activity.

Snack

Materials

chili	juice or milk
cooked spaghetti	spoons or forks (as appropriate)
grated cheese (optional)	napkins
plates	table
cups (adapted as needed)	chairs (adaptive seating as needed)
washcloths for cleanup	

Goals

Sensory
- to improve responses to sensory stimuli, especially tactile and olfactory
- to increase attention span

Fine Motor
- to improve grasp and release, hand manipulation, and eye-hand coordination

Self-Help
- to improve self-feeding skills
- to improve oral-motor skills

Cognitive
- to improve imitation, sequencing, and concept development

Language
- to improve following directions; taking turns; identifying/labeling objects, actions, people, and characteristics; initiating; and requesting

Social
- to make choices
- to facilitate peer interaction

Directions

Seat children appropriately for snack, using adaptive seating as needed. Have children help pass out plates, silverware, and napkins, if appropriate. Tell the children that the snack they are going to have is called "firehouse chili." Give children choices of chili with or without spaghetti, cheese, or other condiments. Encourage communication, including ways to request more or indicate "all done." Assist with self-feeding skills as needed. Offer juice and provide assistance as needed.

Week 2

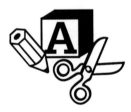

Overall Theme: Ice Cream Social

Activity 1: Human Ice Cream Cones

Materials

tunnel, inner tube, or barrel
therapy balls

Goals

Sensory
- to improve responses to proprioceptive and vestibular stimulation
- to increase body awareness

Gross Motor
- to increase use of flexion
- to improve motor planning, trunk rotation, balance and coordination, and weight shifting

Fine Motor
- to improve using both hands together, eye-hand coordination, and reach and grasp
- to increase upper body strength

Cognitive
- to improve understanding of spatial relationships, imitation, and concept development

Language
- to improve following directions; taking turns; identifying/labeling objects, people, actions, locations, and relationships; initiating; and requesting

Social
- to facilitate peer interaction
- to develop representational play

Directions

Arrange inner tube, tunnel, or similar equipment on end so that it represents a cone for the "ice cream." Use the therapy balls to represent the ice cream. Begin by having the children help scoop the therapy ball ice cream scoops into the cones. If appropriate, encourage the children to roll up in balls and pretend to be ice cream. Place them in the cones.

Activity 2: Ice Cream Cone Match

Materials

cardboard ice cream cones and cardboard scoops of ice cream, enough so that half the group has cones and the other half has ice cream scoops

record or tape player
records or tapes of children's music

Goals

Sensory
- to improve auditory attending
- to increase attention span

Gross Motor
- to improve balance, coordination, motor planning, and locomotion

Fine Motor
- to improve using both hands together, reach and grasp, and visual attention
- to improve shoulder girdle strength and stability

Cognitive
- to improve problem solving, understanding of spatial relationships, imitation, classification, and concept development
- to develop generalization skills

Language
- to improve following directions; taking turns; identifying/labeling objects, actions, locations, and relationships; initiating; and requesting

Social
- to make choices
- to facilitate peer interaction

Directions

Let children choose a cardboard ice cream cone piece. Help each child find a partner to make a complete ice cream cone. These people will be partners for the "social." When everyone has a partner, put on some music and encourage the children to dance or act out the song lyrics. Have the children take turns being the leader and the follower.

Activity 3: Big Ice Cream Cones

Materials

small pieces of various colored textured items (such as cloth, sponge, styrofoam, pipe cleaner, feathers, ribbon, cellophane grass, wrapping paper, tissue paper, yarn, rice, and macaroni)

stickers	markers or crayons
glue	paintbrushes (optional)
cotton swabs (optional)	tape
scissors	large pieces of butcher paper or newsprint
easels (optional)	washcloths for cleanup

Goals

Sensory
- to improve sensory awareness through tactile stimulation
- to increase attention span

Gross Motor
- to improve weight bearing, weight shifting, and balance

Fine Motor
- to improve hand manipulation, eye-hand coordination, using both hands together, reach and grasp, and hand/finger manipulation
- to increase upper body strength

Cognitive
- to improve imitation and concept development
- to develop generalization skills
- to develop recall skills

Language
- to improve following directions; taking turns; increasing vocabulary; identifying/labeling objects, actions, characteristics, and relationships; requesting; and initiating

Social
- to make choices
- to facilitate peer interaction

Directions

Using butcher paper or newsprint, cut out large ice cream cone shapes ahead of time and fasten them to the easels or to the wall. This activity can also be done with children seated, if that is more appropriate. In that case, use smaller paper cutouts. Have children color the cones with markers or crayons and add "toppings" with the textured materials. Encourage them to reach up to decorate the cones. Use lots of language to talk about what they are doing. Include talk involving representation and pretend; for example, "You colored your ice cream brown. Do you like chocolate?"

Activity 4: Three-Dimensional Cones

Materials

brown construction paper	tissue paper
scissors	glue
tape	table
chairs (adaptive seating as needed)	washcloths for cleanup

Goals

Sensory
- to improve responses to sensory stimulation
- to increase attention span

Fine Motor
- to improve hand/finger manipulation, eye-hand coordination, using both hands together, and grasp and release

Cognitive
- to improve understanding of spatial relationships, functional object use, imitation, and concept development
- to develop generalization skills
- to develop recall skills

Language
- to improve following directions; taking turns; increasing vocabulary; and identifying/labeling objects, actions, characteristics, and relationships

Social
- to make choices

Directions

Cut triangles ahead of time out of brown construction paper to roll into cones. Position children for fine motor activity. Show the children how the triangles roll up into cones. Give each child a triangle and help them roll their triangles into cones. Secure with tape. Have children select which color tissue paper to use for their ice cream. Show them how to crumple the tissue paper into balls to look like scoops of ice cream. Provide assistance as needed. Help children squeeze or spread glue onto the insides of their cones. Help them put their tissue paper ice cream onto their cones, gluing into place. Use lots of language and encourage the children to describe what they are doing and the materials they are using. Let the cones dry while completing another activity.

Snack

Materials

ice cream	bowls
toppings for ice cream, such as crumbled cookies and sprinkles	cups (adapted as needed) table
juice	napkins
ice cream scoop	chairs (adaptive seating as needed)
spoons	washcloths for cleanup

Goals

Sensory
- to improve responses to sensory stimuli, especially tactile, temperature, and olfactory
- to increase attention span

Gross Motor
- to improve motor planning, weight shifting, and balance and coordination

Fine Motor
- to improve using both hands together, midline skills, hand/finger manipulation, eye-hand coordination, reach and grasp, and grasp and release

Self-Help
- to improve self-feeding skills
- to improve oral-motor skills

Cognitive
- to improve functional object use, understanding of spatial relationships, object permanence, imitation, sequencing, and concept development
- to develop generalization skills
- to develop recall skills

Language
- to improve following directions; taking turns; identifying/labeling objects, actions, people, and characteristics; initiating; and requesting

Social
- to make choices
- to facilitate peer interaction

Directions

Assemble all the ingredients for making ice cream cones. If appropriate, let children stand by the table to select their combinations and help make their cones. If this is not appropriate for the group, seat children first, using adaptive seating as needed. Then let them select their combinations and help make their cones. Use lots of language to describe the cones, the combinations, and how they are put together. Describe how the cones look, taste, feel, and smell. Encourage communication, including ways to request more or indicate "all done." Offer juice and provide assistance as needed.

Week 3   Overall Theme: Grocery Store

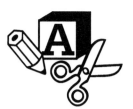

Activity 1: Going to the Store

Materials

large cardboard boxes or other containers for "cars" (as an alternative, push toys or riding toys may serve as "cars")

play purses   play keys   play sunglasses

Goals

Sensory
• to improve responses to vestibular stimulation
• to provide proprioceptive stimulation

Gross Motor
• to improve motor planning, sitting balance and coordination, and trunk rotation

Fine Motor
• to increase upper body strength
• to improve shoulder girdle strength and stability

Cognitive
• to improve understanding of spatial relationships, functional object use, sequencing, imitation, and concept development
• to develop recall skills

Language
• to improve following directions; taking turns; identifying/labeling objects, people, actions, and concepts; initiating; and requesting

Social
• to facilitate representational/pretend play
• to facilitate peer interaction

Directions

Tell children they are going on a car ride to the grocery store. Encourage them to get the items they will need for the trip; for example, play purses, sunglasses, and keys. Facilitate language as much as possible during this part of the activity. Help them into the cardboard "cars" (or alternative "vehicles"). Push the cars to the store area, which has been set up in another part of the room or in another room. Provide additional upper body strengthening by encouraging those children who are able to push cars for others. Upon arrival at the store area, help children park the cars and climb out.

Activity 2: Grocery Shopping

Materials

selection of grocery items, real and pretend, including a real jar of peanut butter, a real jar of jelly, a real loaf of bread, and a real carton of milk or juice (for safety, use nonbreakable containers)

| toy grocery carts | toy cash register | play purses |
| grocery bags | "cars" from previous activity | |

Goals

Sensory
- to improve responses to sensory stimulation
- to provide proprioceptive stimulation

Gross Motor
- to improve motor planning, balance and coordination, trunk rotation, weight bearing, weight shifting, and walking

Fine Motor
- to improve reach and grasp, eye-hand coordination, hand manipulation, and grasp and release
- to increase upper body strength
- to improve shoulder girdle strength and stability

Cognitive
- to improve understanding of spatial relationships, functional object use, classification, imitation, sequencing, and concept development
- to develop generalization skills
- to develop recall skills

Language
- to improve following directions; taking turns; identifying/labeling objects, people, actions, and concepts; initiating; and requesting

Social
- to make choices
- to facilitate representational/pretend play
- to facilitate peer interaction

Directions

Set up the "grocery store" ahead of time so that the items are easy for the children to see and reach. Use a combination of real and pretend food items, as appropriate for the group. You may want to ask families to bring in empty boxes ahead of time. Include canned goods of various sizes. Lifting and carrying the cans strengthens the shoulder girdle. Talk about the items, what the children would like to purchase, and why. Help children put their purchases in their shopping carts and pay for them at the cash register. Help them load their groceries into bags, get back in their cars, and drive home.

Activity 3: Put It Away

Materials

shelves
photos or pictures corresponding to the foods available
  from the grocery store in the preceding activity
tape

Goals

Sensory
- to provide proprioceptive stimulation
- to increase attention span

Gross Motor
- to improve balance, coordination, motor planning, weight bearing, weight shifting, trunk rotation, and locomotion

Fine Motor
- to improve using both hands together, reach and grasp, visual attention and tracking, eye-hand coordination, hand/finger manipulation, and understanding of spatial relationships
- to increase upper body strength
- to improve shoulder girdle strength and stability

Cognitive
- to improve object permanence, problem solving, picture-object association, understanding of spatial relationships, imitation, classification, and concept development
- to develop generalization skills
- to develop recall skills

Language
- to improve following directions; taking turns; identifying/labeling objects, actions, locations, and relationships; initiating; and requesting

Social
- to make choices
- to facilitate peer interaction

Directions

Set up an area, preferably in the housekeeping corner, if there is one, where the children can put away the groceries they have just purchased in the previous activity. Tape pictures that correspond to the items from the grocery store to the shelves. Help the children match the items to the pictures. Use lots of language to talk about the items and where they are going; for example, "The peanut butter is next to the jelly," or "The orange juice is in the refrigerator." Talk about what foods go together; for instance, apples and bananas go together because they are both fruits; apples and tomatoes go together because they are both red; juice and ice cream are both cold.

Snack

Materials

from the previous grocery store activity:

bread	peanut butter	jelly
table knives	plates	napkins
milk or juice	cups (adapted, if necessary)	table
chairs (adaptive seating as needed)		

Goals

Sensory
- to improve responses to sensory stimuli, especially tactile and olfactory
- to increase attention span

Fine Motor
- to improve using both hands together, grasp and release, and hand manipulation
- to improve shoulder girdle strength and stability

Self-Help
- to improve self-feeding skills
- to improve oral-motor skills

Cognitive
- to improve imitation and concept development
- to develop generalization skills
- to develop recall skills

Language
- to improve following directions; imitation; identifying/labeling objects, actions, people, and characteristics; taking turns; initiating; and requesting

Social
- to make choices
- to facilitate peer interaction

Directions

Seat children appropriately for snack, using adaptive seating as needed. Tell them they are going to make sandwiches with some of the things they bought at the store in the previous activity. As the children watch, spread the bread with peanut butter and jelly. Give each child a table knife and a slice of bread. Help them spread the peanut butter and jelly on the bread. Top with a second slice of bread. Describe what they are doing, what the snack is made of, and what it looks like. Remind the group of the previous shopping activities during which they bought the ingredients for their snack and put them away. Encourage communication, including ways to request more or indicate "all done." Offer milk or juice as needed. Assist with self-feeding and drinking skills as needed.

Week 4

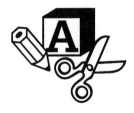

Overall Theme: Water Carnival

Activity 1: Water Painting

Materials

clean paintbrushes of various sizes	clean buckets
sunscreen (optional)	towels

Goals

Sensory
- to improve sensory awareness/body awareness and responsiveness through tactile stimulation
- to increase attention span

Gross Motor
- to improve motor planning, balance, weight bearing, and weight shifting

Fine Motor
- to improve eye-hand coordination, reach and grasp, wrist rotation, and hand manipulation skills
- to increase upper body strength
- to improve shoulder girdle strength and stability

Cognitive
- to improve understanding of spatial relationships, tool use, imitation, sequencing, and concept development

Language
- to improve following directions; taking turns; identifying/labeling objects, actions, people, places, characteristics, relationships, and body parts; requesting; and initiating

Social
- to facilitate representational/pretend play
- to facilitate peer interaction

Directions

This activity is best conducted outdoors. If it is hot and sunny, it is usually best to either leave the children's clothes on or use sunscreen. Fill several buckets with water and provide a variety of paintbrushes. Encourage children to "paint" the wall, playground equipment, and each other with the water. Use lots of language to describe what they are doing. Encourage the children to reach up high as they paint. Painting each other increases their awareness of body parts. Use lots of language to name the parts being painted and describe how it feels to paint different objects.

Activity 2: Water Slide

Materials

portable sliding board, preferably plastic   hose
small wading pool (optional)   swimsuits
sunscreen   towels

Goals

Sensory
- to improve sensory awareness/body awareness and responsiveness through tactile stimulation
- to provide vestibular stimulation
- to increase attention span

Gross Motor
- to improve motor planning, balance, weight bearing, and weight shifting

Fine Motor
- to increase upper body strength
- to increase shoulder girdle strength and stability

Self-Help
- to improve dressing/undressing

Cognitive
- to improve understanding of spatial relationships, imitation, and sequencing

Language
- to improve following directions; taking turns; identifying/labeling objects, actions, people, places, characteristics, relationships, and body parts; requesting; and initiating

Social
- to facilitate peer interaction

Directions

Set up the slide near a hose and water spout. Position the hose so the water runs down the slide from the top. The slide can also be positioned so that the children land in a small wading pool filled with water, if desired. The children may change into swimsuits if they have not already done so. They could also stay in their clothes or wear just a diaper and t-shirt. In any case, be sure tender skin is protected from the sun. Help children up the ladder and down the slide. They will go faster than usual because of the water. Use lots of language to describe what is happening; for example, "Judy is going up the slide. Whee! She came down fast!"

Activity 3: Water Balloons

Materials

balloons   hula hoops or other targets
buckets or other containers   towels

Goals

Sensory
- to provide proprioceptive stimulation
- to increase attention span

Gross Motor
- to improve balance, coordination, weight shifting, and throwing

Fine Motor
- to improve eye-hand coordination, reach and grasp, and grasp and release
- to increase upper body strength
- to improve shoulder girdle strength and stability

Cognitive
- to improve understanding of spatial and cause-and-effect relationships, imitation, conservation, sequencing, and concept development

Language
- to improve following directions; taking turns; identifying/labeling objects, actions, locations, and relationships; initiating; and requesting

Social
- to make choices
- to facilitate peer interaction

Directions

Set up the hula hoops or other targets so the children can throw the balloons through the middle. Fill the balloons with water, tie the ends closed, and place them in buckets or other containers. You will probably need to fill a lot more balloons than you think you need. Vary the amount of water in the balloons so that some are lighter and some heavier. Children can then take balloons from the bucket and toss them at the target. Adults may need to demonstrate or assist. Talk about the actions and who is throwing the balloons. Older children may enjoy trying to catch the balloons. Try this only if the children won't be too upset about getting splashed.

Activity 4: Squirt Bottles

Materials

clean spray bottles and/or squirt bottles (like those that dishwashing soap comes in)
towels

empty quart-sized milk cartons
low table

Goals

Sensory
- to improve responses to tactile stimulation
- to provide proprioceptive stimulation
- to increase attention span

Gross Motor
- to improve balance, motor planning, weight shifting, and coordination

Fine Motor
- to improve visual attending and tracking, eye-hand coordination, reach and grasp, grasp and release, and hand/finger manipulation
- to increase upper body strength

Cognitive
- to improve understanding of cause and effect, object permanence, spatial relationships; imitation; and concept development

Language
- to improve following directions; taking turns; identifying/labeling objects, actions, locations, and relationships; initiating; and requesting

Social
- to make choices
- to facilitate peer interaction

Directions

Set up several empty milk cartons or other targets on a low table. Give the children squirt bottles or spray bottles with the nozzles set to produce streams of water. Help children to aim sprays of water at the milk cartons and knock them down. Use lots of language to describe what is happening, who is taking a turn, and where the milk cartons go.

Snack

Materials

watermelon
plates
knives
table

juice
chairs (adaptive seating as needed)
washcloths for cleanup

napkins
cups (adapted as needed)

Goals

Sensory
- to improve responses to sensory stimulation, especially tactile and olfactory
- to increase attention span

Fine Motor
- to improve using both hands together, midline skills, hand/finger manipulation, eye-hand coordination, reach and grasp, and grasp and release

Self-Help
- to improve self-feeding skills
- to improve oral-motor skills

Cognitive
- to improve understanding of spatial relationships, imitation, functional use of objects, sequencing, and concept development

Language
- to improve following directions; taking turns; identifying/labeling objects, actions, locations, and relationships; initiating; and requesting

Social
- to make choices
- to facilitate peer interaction

Directions

Seat children appropriately for snack. Have children help pass out napkins, if appropriate. Children can watch as adults cut the watermelon. Talk about how it looks, feels, and tastes before and after it has been cut. Encourage children to choose a piece of watermelon. Watch out for the seeds! Provide assistance with feeding and oral-motor skills as needed. Offer juice and provide assistance as needed.

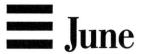 June

Week 1

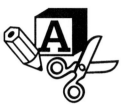

Overall Theme: Summer Clothes

Activity 1: Going Shopping

Materials

large cardboard boxes or other containers to use as pretend cars (alternative: push toys or riding toys)
play purses
play keys
play sunglasses

Goals

Sensory
- to improve responses to vestibular stimulation
- to provide proprioceptive stimulation

Gross Motor
- to improve motor planning, sitting balance, coordination, and trunk rotation

Cognitive
- to improve understanding of spatial relationships, functional object use, sequencing, imitation, and concept development
- to develop generalization skills
- to develop recall skills

Language
- to improve following directions; taking turns; identifying/labeling objects, people, actions, and concepts; initiating; and requesting

Social
- to facilitate representational/pretend play
- to facilitate peer interaction

Directions

Tell children they are going on a car ride to the store to buy new summer clothes. Encourage them to get the items they will need for the trip; for example, purses, sunglasses, and keys. Facilitate language as much as possible during this part of the activity. Help them into the cardboard "cars" (or alternative "vehicles"). Push the cars to the store area, which has been set up in another part of the room, or in another room altogether. For children who are able, encourage them to push the cars for other children. Upon arrival at the store area, help children park the cars and climb out.

Activity 2: Clothing Store

Materials

selection of summer clothing, in sizes somewhat larger than the children in the group, such as:

shorts	sun dresses	t-shirts
sun hats	bathing suits	sandals

a few items of winter clothing, for example:

coats	boots	jackets
heavy sweaters	mittens	snowsuits

rack for hanging clothes	coat hangers
mirrors	toy shopping carts
toy cash register	play purses
"vehicles" from previous activity	

Goals

Sensory
- to improve responses to sensory stimulation

Gross Motor
- to improve motor planning, balance, coordination, trunk rotation, weight bearing, weight shifting, and walking

Fine Motor
- to improve reach and grasp, eye-hand coordination, and hand/finger manipulation
- to increase upper body strength

Self-Help
- to improve dressing/undressing skills

Cognitive
- to improve understanding of spatial relationships, functional object use, classification, imitation, sequencing, and concept development
- to develop generalization skills
- to develop recall skills

Language
- to improve following directions; taking turns; identifying/labeling objects, people, actions, and concepts; initiating; and requesting

Social
- to make choices
- to facilitate pretend play
- to facilitate peer interaction

Directions

Set up the "clothing store" ahead of time so that the clothes are easy for the children to see and reach. Include as wide a variety of textures and colors in the selection as possible. Guide the children in selecting items they would use in the summer when the weather is hot. Use lots of language to discuss which clothes would be appropriate and why, to describe the items, and name who is selecting what. Incorporate dress-up activities. Provide assistance as needed. Encourage children to note the changes they see in the mirror as they try on different items. Use lots of language to describe these changes. Help children put their purchases in their shopping carts and pay for them at the cash register. If appropriate, have children get back in their vehicles and drive home.

Activity 3: Dolls

Materials

dolls in a variety of sizes
stuffed animals that can be dressed, such as teddy bears (optional)
summer clothes to fit the dolls/stuffed animals

Goals

Sensory
- to improve responses to sensory stimulation

Gross Motor
- to improve motor planning, balance, coordination, trunk rotation, weight bearing, and weight shifting

Fine Motor
- to improve reach and grasp, eye-hand coordination, and hand/finger manipulation
- to increase upper body strength

Self-Help
- to improve dressing/undressing skills

Cognitive
- to improve understanding of spatial relationships, functional object use, classification, imitation, sequencing, and concept development
- to develop generalization skills
- to develop recall skills

Language
- to improve following directions; taking turns; identifying/labeling objects, people, actions, and concepts; initiating; requesting

Social
- to make choices
- to facilitate pretend play
- to facilitate peer interaction

Directions

Display dolls and clothes so that they are easily accessible to the children. Encourage children to choose a doll or stuffed animal and select clothes for it. Show children how to dress their dolls/animals and assist them with dressing skills as needed. Use lots of language to identify the items selected, describe them, and discuss when and how they would be used. This activity can be expanded by encouraging the children to enact different summer activities with their dolls. For example, if children have selected bathing suits for their dolls, they could take the dolls to the "pool" and pretend to swim. You can modify this activity by providing more routine doll-play accessories, such as bottles and hairbrushes, if the pretend play is too abstract for your group. To emphasize gross motor skills, position children to facilitate appropriate weight bearing. To facilitate balance, weight shifting, and trunk rotation, position activities to the sides, in front of, or behind the children, or hand the children items so that they will need to reach for them.

Activity 4: Paper Dolls

Materials

large pieces of newsprint with doll shapes drawn on them
masking tape
markers or crayons

Goals

Sensory
- to increase attention span

Gross Motor
- to improve balance, coordination, weight bearing, and weight shifting

Fine Motor
- to improve hand/finger manipulation, eye-hand coordination, and midline skills
- to improve shoulder girdle strength and stability

Cognitive
- to improve imitation, tool use, and concept development
- to develop generalization skills

Language
- to improve following directions; taking turns; increasing vocabulary; and identifying/labeling objects, actions, characteristics, and relationships

Social
- to make choices
- to facilitate peer interaction

Directions

Fasten the paper dolls to the wall or other surface areas so that the children need to reach up to color them. This activity is good for working on standing balance or kneeling. Children can also be positioned in standers, if appropriate, or work from a seated position. Have the children choose which doll and which colors to use to color summer clothes on their paper dolls. Assist them as needed in reaching up to color. Use lots of language to describe what the children are doing. Emphasize the colors they are using.

Snack

Materials

gingerbread people cookies
colored frosting
juice or milk
table knives
washcloths for cleanup

napkins (optional)
cups (adapted as needed)
chairs (adapted seating as needed)
table

Goals

Sensory
* to improve responses to sensory stimuli, especially tactile and olfactory

Fine Motor
* to improve eye-hand coordination, hand/finger manipulation, reach and grasp, and grasp and release

Self-Help
* to improve self-feeding skills
* to improve oral-motor skills

Cognitive
* to improve imitation and concept development
* to develop generalization skills
* to develop recall skills

Language
* to improve following directions; taking turns; identifying/labeling objects, actions, people, and characteristics; requesting; and initiating

Social
* to make choices
* to facilitate peer interaction

Directions

Seat children appropriately for snack, using adaptive seating as needed. Have children help pass out napkins, if appropriate. Show children cookies and have them choose one. Demonstrate spreading frosting on the cookies to make "clothes." Have children choose which color frosting to use. Provide help as needed with spreading the frosting. Encourage communication, including ways to request more or indicate "all done." If possible, have children identify the kind of clothes they are putting on the cookie people—dress, bathing suit, shirt, pants. Assist with self-feeding and oral-motor skills as needed. Offer milk or juice and provide assistance as needed.

Week 2 — Overall Theme: Blue

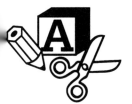

Activity 1: Obstacle Course

Materials

indoor climbing structure	toddler slide
inner tubes	indoor tunnel
ramp or other incline	carpet squares
blue contact paper	floor pillows/beanbag chairs
benches	bolsters
steps	indoor swing
blue beanbags	containers for beanbags

Goals

Sensory
- to provide vestibular stimulation
- to provide proprioceptive stimulation
- to increase attention span

Gross Motor
- to improve balance, coordination, motor planning, locomotion, trunk rotation, and weight shifting

Fine Motor
- to improve using both hands together, reach and grasp, and visual attention
- to increase upper body strength
- to improve shoulder girdle strength and stability

Cognitive
- to improve understanding of object permanence, imitation, problem solving, understanding of spatial relationships, and concept development

Language
- to improve following directions; taking turns; identifying/labeling objects, actions, descriptions, and locations; requesting; and initiating

Social
- to make choices
- to facilitate peer interaction

Directions

Using the equipment available, set up an indoor obstacle course to facilitate the gross motor and vestibular goals of the individuals in the group. The materials listed above are just suggestions. Place the blue beanbags at various points throughout the obstacle course. Have some hidden, some partially hidden, and some in plain sight. Assist the children through the obstacle course. A "path" of carpet squares, preferably blue, can provide a structure to follow through the course. Contact paper can be attached to carpet squares to enhance the color effect. Encourage the children to use appropriate motor patterns throughout. Help them find the beanbags as they go through the course. Be sure there are enough beanbags for each child to find at least two or three. Collect the beanbags in buckets or baskets, preferably blue. Depending on their abilities, children can be encouraged to carry their own buckets filled with beanbags.

Activity 2: Beanbags

Materials

several beanbags, preferably blue
basket or bin to toss them in

Goals

Sensory
- to provide proprioceptive stimulation
- to increase attention span

Gross Motor
- to improve balance, weight shifting, throwing, and coordination

Fine Motor
- to improve eye-hand coordination, grasp and release, and throwing
- to increase upper body strength
- to improve shoulder girdle strength and stability

Cognitive
- to improve understanding of spatial relationships, imitation, and concept development

Language
- to improve following directions; taking turns; identifying/labeling objects, actions, locations, and relationships; initiating; and requesting

Social
- to make choices
- to facilitate peer interaction

Directions

This activity usually works best if children are seated in a circle, with the target in the middle. Each child can take a beanbag from the basket or bin or adults can begin the activity by tossing beanbags to each child. Encourage children to throw the beanbags into the basket or bin or to each other. They may need help to accomplish this. Children who are not yet ready to throw can often begin by placing the beanbags into the container. Talk about the actions, who is throwing, and who is catching. Encourage children to name who they would like to catch the beanbag. Emphasize the blue color of the beanbags. A blue target can be painted or glued onto the side of the container as a variation of this activity.

Activity 3: Blue Toys

Materials

a variety of manipulative toys, predominately blue in color, for example:

bristle blocks	stacking blocks
pegs	beads
books	

Goals

Sensory
- to improve responses to sensory stimulation
- to increase attention span

Fine Motor
- to improve hand/finger manipulation, eye-hand coordination, reach and grasp, and grasp and release

Cognitive
- to improve understanding of spatial relationships, imitation, problem solving, picture-object association, and concept development
- to develop generalization skills

Language
- to improve following directions; taking turns; increasing vocalizations/ vocabulary; identifying/labeling objects, actions, characteristics, and locations; requesting; and initiating

Social
- to make choices
- to facilitate peer interaction

Directions

Set up "stations" for the various toys. Allow children to wander to a station and begin playing. An adult can then assist with the play, expanding and guiding as appropriate. Depending on the child's needs, gross motor goals can be incorporated into these activities by positioning the stations so that the child stands or kneels to play, for example. Encourage children to take turns with an adult or peer in stacking blocks and knocking them down. Use lots of language to describe what is happening. Emphasize the blue color of all the toys.

Activity 4: Finger Paint

Materials

blue finger paint
spoons or tongue depressors for
  scooping paint
soap for cleanup
chairs (adaptive seating as needed)

finger-paint paper
container of water
smocks
table
washcloths for cleanup

Goals

Sensory
- to improve responses to sensory stimulation
- to increase attention span

Gross Motor
- to improve balance, coordination, and control of flexion/extension patterns

Fine Motor
- to improve visual attending and tracking, hand/finger manipulation and control, and finger isolation
- to increase upper body strength
- to improve shoulder girdle strength and stability

Cognitive
- to improve imitation and concept development
- to develop generalization skills

Language
- to improve following directions; taking turns; identifying/labeling objects, actions, descriptions, relationships, and people; initiating; and requesting

Social
- to facilitate peer interaction

Directions

Give each child a piece of finger-paint paper. Sprinkle each child's paper with water and put a dab of the blue finger paint on it. Provide physical assistance to children as needed. Use lots of language to describe the motions and colors. This activity can facilitate even more peer interaction if the group works together on a single large paper.

Caution: Younger children tend to eat the paint. If you think this will happen in your group, substitute colored pudding for the paint. Although you can't hang pudding pictures on the wall, remember that it is the process that is important here, not the final product.

Snack

Materials

a variety of blue foods, such as:

blueberries	berry yogurt
berry ice cream	berry cereal
blue gelatin	blue cookies

plates	napkins
spoons (adapted as needed)	cups (adapted as needed)
blue juice	table
chairs (adapted seating as needed)	washcloths for cleanup

Goals

Sensory
- to improve responses to sensory stimulation, especially tactile and olfactory
- to increase attention span

Fine Motor
- to improve midline skills, reach and grasp, grasp and release, eye-hand coordination, and hand/finger manipulation
- to increase upper body strength
- to improve shoulder girdle strength and stability

Self-Help
- to improve self-feeding skills
- to improve oral-motor skills

Cognitive
- to improve classification, understanding of spatial relationships, imitation, functional use of objects, and concept development
- to develop generalization skills

Language
- to improve following directions; taking turns; identifying/labeling objects, actions, locations, and relationships; initiating; and requesting

Social
- to make choices
- to facilitate peer interaction

Directions

Have children help pass out plates and napkins, if appropriate. Encourage them to identify the different foods and to request the one they want to try first. Encourage each child to try each food. Describe the appearance, taste, smell, and feel of the foods with the children. Which ones do they like? Which ones do they dislike? What kinds of foods can be grouped together? (fruits, vegetables, ones you eat with a spoon, ones you eat with your fingers) Offer juice as needed.

Week 3

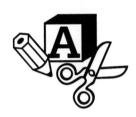

Overall Theme: Fishing

Activity 1: Fishing

Materials

rocking boat
dowels about 24" long (or appropriate size for children in group)
paper clips or washers
buckets

toddler slide or climbing structure
string
magnets
paper and/or sponge fish

Goals

Sensory
• to improve responses to sensory stimulation
• to provide vestibular stimulation

Gross Motor
• to improve balance, coordination, and motor planning

Fine Motor
• to improve midline skills, hand manipulation, grasp and release, eye-hand coordination, visual attending, and tracking
• to increase upper body strength
• to improve shoulder girdle strength and stability

Cognitive
• to improve tool use, problem solving, classification, understanding of spatial relationships, imitation, and concept development
• to develop generalization skills

Language
• to improve following directions; taking turns; identifying/labeling objects, actions, descriptions, locations, relationships, and people; initiating; and requesting

Social
• to make choices
• to facilitate representational/pretend play
• to facilitate peer interaction

Directions

Ahead of time, make fishing poles by tying string to the ends of the dowels and attaching magnets or large paper clips to the ends of the strings. Cut out paper fish and glue washers or paper clips to their mouths (if using magnets on poles) or cut sponges in the shape of fish (if using paper clips on poles). Scatter the fish on the floor near the rocking boat. Help children climb into the rocking boat. Show them how to dangle their fishing poles in the "water." Help them to catch some fish on their poles. Once they have caught a fish, help them to take it off the hook and put it in a bucket. Rock the boat gently while the activity is going on. This activity can be repeated by fishing off the "pier" or "bridge" (use toddler slide or climbing structure).

Activity 2: Edible Aquariums

Materials

blue gelatin	bowl
boiling water	measuring cup
ice cubes	chairs (adapted seating as needed)
gummy fish	clear plastic cups
spoon	table
washcloths for cleanup	

Goals

Sensory
- to improve responses to sensory stimulation
- to increase attention span

Fine Motor
- to improve visual attending and tracking, hand/finger manipulation, grasp and release, midline skills, and using two hands together

Cognitive
- to improve sequencing, functional object use, tool use, understanding of spatial relationships, problem solving, and concept development
- to develop generalization skills

Language
- to improve following directions; taking turns; identifying/labeling objects, relationships, characteristics, actions, and people; requesting; and initiating

Social
- to make choices
- to facilitate peer interaction

Directions

Position children around the table. Mix the gelatin using ½ cup boiling water and (after gelatin powder has dissolved) ½ tray of ice cubes. Use caution with the hot water. Encourage children to identify and name objects as they are used. Let them help open the gelatin package, pour it into the bowl, and take turns stirring. Encourage them to smell and taste the gelatin before and after adding the water. Remove any ice cubes that have not melted after the first few minutes. Pour the gelatin into clear plastic cups—one for each child. The gelatin should be slightly thick (if not, refrigerate briefly). Suspend gummy fish in the gelatin. Refrigerate until time for snack.

Activity 3: More Fishing

Materials

water table

nets and/or large spoons for catching fish

towels

plastic fish

buckets

Goals

Sensory
- to improve responses to sensory stimulation
- to increase attention span

Gross Motor
- to improve balance and coordination, reach and grasp, motor planning, weight bearing, and weight shifting

Fine Motor
- to improve hand manipulation, visual attending and tracking, eye-hand coordination, midline skills, and using two hands together

Cognitive
- to improve understanding of spatial relationships, tool use, functional object use, and concept development
- to develop generalization skills

Language
- to improve following directions; taking turns; identifying/labeling objects, people, actions, relationships, and characteristics; initiating; and requesting

Social
- to facilitate peer interaction

Directions

Float plastic fish in a water table. The sponge fish used in Activity 1 could also be used for this activity. Show children how they can use the nets and/or spoons to catch the fish. Have them put the fish in buckets once they have been caught. Provide physical assistance as needed. Use lots of language to describe the fish, what is happening, and who is doing what.

This kind of activity is excellent for working on standing balance and weight shifting with those children for whom these goals are indicated. Children with more physical challenges can be positioned in standers for weight bearing. This activity can also be done with children positioned in kneeling.

Activity 4: Fish Prints

Materials

sponges cut in fish shapes (from Activity 1)

trays for paint

table

washcloths for cleanup

tempera paint

construction paper

chairs (adapted seating as needed)

Goals

Sensory
- to improve responses to sensory stimulation
- to increase attention span

Fine Motor
- to improve hand/finger manipulation, eye-hand coordination, reach and grasp, grasp and release, using two hands together, and midline skills
- to improve shoulder girdle strength and stability

Cognitive
- to improve tool use, imitation, and concept development
- to develop generalization skills
- to develop recall skills

Language
- to improve following directions; taking turns; increasing vocabulary; identifying/labeling objects, actions, characteristics, and relationships; initiating; and requesting

Social
- to make choices
- to facilitate peer interaction

Directions

Position children appropriately for fine motor activity. Have each child choose which color paper to use. Demonstrate dipping the sponge fish in the paint and pressing them on the paper to make prints. Let each child choose which sponge and color paint to use. Provide help with the activity as needed. Use lots of language to describe what they are doing. Emphasize the colors of the paint and paper. Some children may want to finger-paint instead or use the sponges as if they were paintbrushes. This is fine. Remember that it is the process of exploration and learning that is important here, not the final product.

Snack

Materials

edible aquariums made in Activity 2	spoons
juice	napkins
cups (adapted as needed)	table
chairs (adapted seating as needed)	washcloths for cleanup

Goals

Sensory
- to improve responses to sensory stimulation, especially tactile and olfactory
- to increase attention span

Fine Motor
- to improve eye-hand coordination, reach and grasp, grasp and release, using both hands together, midline skills, and hand/finger manipulation
- to increase upper body strength

Self-Help
- to improve self-feeding skills
- to improve oral-motor skills

Cognitive
- to improve understanding of spatial relationships, conservation of volume, functional use of objects, imitation, sequencing, and concept development
- to develop generalization skills
- to develop recall skills

Language
- to improve following directions; taking turns; identifying/labeling objects, actions, locations, and relationships; initiating; and requesting

Social
- to make choices
- to facilitate peer interaction

Directions

Seat children appropriately for snack. Bring out the edible aquariums made earlier in the session. See if the children can identify which one is theirs. Have children help pass out napkins and spoons, if appropriate. As the children eat, talk about making the aquariums. Discuss the other events of the session as well—the different kinds of fish and what the children did. Offer juice as needed. Provide assistance with self-help and oral-motor skills as needed.

Week 4

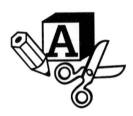

Overall Theme: Washing

Activity 1: Ball Pool Bathtub

Materials

commercial ball pool or other container filled with 3" lightweight balls
washcloths
towels

Goals

Sensory
- to improve responses to tactile and proprioceptive stimulation
- to increase body awareness

Gross Motor
- to improve motor planning, trunk rotation, sitting balance, coordination, and throwing

Fine Motor
- to improve reach and grasp, grasp and release, and eye-hand coordination
- to increase upper body strength

Cognitive
- to improve imitation, understanding of spatial relationships, functional object use, sequencing, and concept development

Language
- to improve following directions; taking turns; identifying/labeling objects, people, actions, locations, and relationships; initiating; and requesting

Social
- to facilitate pretend play
- to facilitate peer interaction

Directions

Allow children to explore the ball pool. Encourage them to climb in and out independently, assisting them to use appropriate motor patterns as necessary. Use lots of language to describe actions and who is doing what; for example, "Tiara threw the red ball." Encourage children to name objects, actions, and people. "Bury" body parts under the balls and have the children find them again; for example, "Where's Geoff's leg? There it is!" Give the children washcloths and help them scrub various body parts. Talk about the bath they are having in the big tub. When they are finished, help them out of the pool. Have them "dry off" with the towels, again telling them what parts to dry or what parts you are drying. Deep pressure, rubbing with a washcloth, and brushing may help those children with tactile defensiveness to accept this activity more comfortably.

Activity 2: Doll Bath

Materials

washable dolls	water table or plastic tubs	soap
washcloths	towels	doll-sized diapers
doll brushes and combs	lotion	powder
clothes for dolls		

Goals

Sensory
- to improve responses to sensory stimulation
- to increase attention span

Gross Motor
- to improve motor planning, trunk rotation, balance, weight bearing, and weight shifting

Fine Motor
- to improve visual attending and tracking, eye-hand coordination, grasp and release, and hand/finger manipulation

Cognitive
- to improve functional object use, object permanence, imitation, sequencing, classification, and concept development
- to develop generalization skills
- to develop recall skills

Language
- to improve following directions; taking turns; identifying/labeling objects, actions, and relationships; requesting; and initiating

Social
- to facilitate pretend play
- to facilitate peer interaction

Directions

Set up the doll bath activity. Encourage children to tell about or act out the bath sequence in order: take off the doll's clothes, put the doll in the bath, wash with soap, dry off. If children have some experience with this sort of activity, you can "forget" to put out some necessary items, such as the soap or the towels, and encourage the children to tell you what is missing. This activity can be conducted with children standing or positioned in standers at a water table or sitting around a plastic tub on the floor or table, depending on the motor needs and goals for the group. Use lots of language to talk about what the children are doing. Encourage the children to explain what they are doing and what comes next.

Activity 3: Car Wash

Materials

several riding vehicles	hose
buckets	sponges
soap	towels

Goals

Sensory
- to improve responses to sensory stimulation
- to increase attention span

Gross Motor
- to improve motor planning, trunk rotation, balance, weight bearing, and weight shifting

Fine Motor
- to improve visual attending and tracking, eye-hand coordination, grasp and release, hand manipulation, using both hands together, and midline skills
- to increase upper body strength

Cognitive
- to improve functional object use, imitation, sequencing, classification, and concept development
- to develop generalization skills

Language
- to improve following directions; taking turns; identifying/labeling objects, actions, and relationships; requesting; and initiating

Social
- to facilitate pretend play
- to facilitate peer interaction

Directions

Set up the "car wash" outside. Have available a hose with a gentle trickle of water, buckets of soapy water, and sponges of various sizes. Include a couple of really big sponges. Help the children wash the "cars" (riding toys) with the soapy sponges and rinse the soap off with the hose. Use lots of language to describe their activities. Try to get the children to tell what they are doing and what comes next. Relate this activity to the previous one. How are they the same? How are they different?

Activity 4: Washing Clothes

Materials

doll clothes   pan of soapy water
pan of fresh water   clothesline
clothespins   towels

Goals

Sensory
- to improve responses to sensory stimulation
- to increase attention span

Gross Motor
- to improve motor planning, trunk rotation, balance, coordination, weight bearing, and weight shifting

Fine Motor
- to improve visual attending and tracking, eye-hand coordination, grasp and release, hand/finger manipulation, and using both hands together

Cognitive
- to improve functional object use, imitation, sequencing, and concept development
- to develop generalization skills

Language
- to improve following directions; taking turns; identifying/labeling objects, actions, and relationships; requesting; and initiating

Social
- to facilitate pretend play
- to facilitate peer interaction

Directions

Children can be positioned in standing, sitting, or kneeling for this activity. Let the children wash the doll clothes, rinse them, and hang them up to dry. Provide help with motor skills and sequencing as needed. Encourage the children to tell what they are doing and what should come next. Relate this activity to the previous ones. How is it the same? Different?

Snack

Materials

variety of summer fruits, such as:
    strawberries   melon cubes
    grapes   bananas

straws   knives
napkins   plates
juice   cups (adapted as needed)
table   chairs (adaptive seating as needed)
washcloths for cleanup

Goals

Sensory
- to improve responses to sensory stimulation, especially tactile and olfactory
- to increase attention span

Fine Motor
- to improve midline skills, using both hands together, hand/finger manipulation, reach and grasp, grasp and release, and eye-hand coordination

Self-Help
- to improve self-feeding skills
- to improve oral-motor skills

Cognitive
- to improve understanding of spatial relationships, imitation, functional use of objects, classification, sequencing, and concept development

Language
- to improve following directions; taking turns; identifying/labeling objects, actions, locations, and relationships; initiating; and requesting

Social
- to make choices
- to facilitate peer interaction

Directions

Seat children appropriately for snack. Have children help pass out napkins, if appropriate. Fruit kabobs can be prepared ahead of time by skewering fruit pieces on straws. Encourage children to select the kabob they want and to identify the fruits. Provide assistance with feeding and oral-motor skills as needed. Offer juice and provide assistance as needed.

Week 5

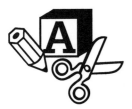

Overall Theme: Boats

Activity 1: Vestibular Boats

Materials

rocking boat   platform swing

Goals

Sensory
- to improve responses to sensory stimulation
- to provide vestibular stimulation
- to increase attention span

Gross Motor
- to improve balance, coordination, motor planning, and weight shifting

Fine Motor
- to improve grasp and release
- to increase upper body strength

Cognitive
- to improve problem solving, imitation, understanding of spatial relationships, and concept development
- to develop generalization skills

Language
- to improve following directions; taking turns; identifying/labeling objects, actions, characteristics, locations, relationships, and people; initiating; and requesting

Social
- to make choices
- to facilitate representational/pretend play
- to facilitate peer interaction

Directions

Tell children they are going for a boat ride. Let them choose whether they want to ride on the platform swing boat or the rocking boat. Let half the group use each piece of equipment, then switch. Encourage them to problem solve getting on and off the equipment, making it move, and making it stop. Use lots of language to describe these activities. Also use language to set the scene for pretend play. Describe the kind of boat they are on, where they are going, and what they are doing. Sing some boat songs in time with the movements of the boats. Impose some movements to facilitate sensorimotor goals as indicated for the group.

Activity 2: Hammock Boat

Materials

hammock swing or portable hammock

Goals

Sensory
- to improve responses to sensory stimulation
- to provide vestibular stimulation
- to increase attention span

Gross Motor
- to improve balance, coordination, motor planning, and trunk rotation

Fine Motor
- to improve grasp and release
- to increase upper body strength

Cognitive
- to improve problem solving, imitation, understanding of spatial relationships, and concept development
- to develop generalization skills

Language
- to improve following directions; taking turns; identifying/labeling objects, actions, descriptions, locations, relationships, and people; initiating; and requesting

Social
- to facilitate representational/pretend play
- to facilitate peer interaction

Directions

Set up the hammock so that several children can fit into it at the same time. Tell the children they are going for a ride in a different kind of boat. Encourage children to problem solve getting into and out of the hammock, making it move, and making it stop. Use lots of language to describe these activities. Also use language to set the scene for pretend play. Describe the kind of boat they are on, where they are going, and what they are doing. Sing some boat songs in time to the movements of the boats. Impose some movements to facilitate sensorimotor goals as indicated for the group.

Activity 3: Soap Boats

Materials

several bars of soap that will float	pencils or dowel rods
paper or fabric triangles for sails	hole puncher
water table	towels
plastic sheeting for floor (if needed)	adaptive standers (if needed)

Goals

Sensory
- to improve responses to sensory stimulation
- to increase attention span

Gross Motor
- to improve motor planning, standing balance, and weight shifting

Fine Motor
- to improve visual attending and tracking, eye-hand coordination, hand/finger manipulation, reach and grasp, and grasp and release

Cognitive
- to improve understanding of spatial relationships, functional object use, classification, imitation, and concept development
- to develop generalization skills

Language
- to improve following directions; taking turns; identifying/labeling objects, actions, people, and characteristics; requesting; and initiating

Social
- to make choices
- to facilitate pretend play
- to facilitate peer interaction

Directions

Prepare paper or cloth triangles for sails. Punch two holes in each sail. Let the children choose the bar of soap and the sail they want to use. Run the pencils or dowel rods through the holes ahead of time or let the children do this, depending on the ability level of the group. Push the pencils or dowels into the bars of soap so that the sails stand upright (adults may have to help). Help the children launch the boats into the water table.

The first part of this activity can be conducted around the water table with the table covered so that the table top is used while making the boats. The top can then be removed for the second part of the activity. Children can also be positioned in kneeling as an alternative to standing, depending on their gross motor needs and goals.

Activity 4: Boat Pictures

Materials

construction paper
glue
cotton swabs (optional)
table
washcloths for cleanup

yarn, straws, or sticks (optional)
paintbrushes (optional)
scissors
chairs (adaptive seating as needed)

Goals

Sensory
• to improve responses to sensory stimulation
• to increase attention span

Fine Motor
• to improve hand manipulation, eye-hand coordination, reach and grasp, grasp and release, and using both hands together

Cognitive
• to improve understanding of spatial relationships, functional object use, imitation, and concept development
• to develop generalization skills
• to develop recall skills

Language
• to improve following directions; taking turns; increasing vocabulary; identifying/labeling objects, actions, characteristics, and relationships; initiating; and requesting

Social
• to make choices

Directions

Cut out boat shapes from construction paper ahead of time. Use semi-circles for the boat and triangles for the sail. You can increase the tactile component by providing yarn, straws, or sticks for the masts. Position children for fine motor activity. Have children select which color paper to use. Then have them choose a boat and a sail. Help children squeeze or spread glue onto their papers, encouraging them to stabilize the paper with one hand, if possible. Help them put the boat shapes onto the glue. Help them pat the materials into place. Use lots of language and encourage the children to describe what they are doing and the materials they are using. Remind them that these pieces look like the pieces they used earlier to make their soap sailboats. Let the pictures dry while completing another activity.

Snack

Materials

bananas	napkins	ice cream scooper
ice cream	table	bowls
whipped cream	cups (adapted as needed)	juice
toppings	chairs (adaptive seating as needed)	
spoons	washcloths for cleanup	

Goals

Sensory
- to improve responses to sensory stimuli, especially tactile, temperature, and olfactory

Self-Help
- to improve self-feeding skills
- to improve oral-motor skills

Fine Motor
- to improve visual attention, eye-hand coordination, reach and grasp, grasp and release, and hand manipulation

Cognitive
- to improve understanding of spatial relationships, tool use, functional object use, and concept development
- to develop generalization skills
- to develop recall skills

Language
- to improve following directions; taking turns; identifying/labeling objects, actions, people, and characteristics; requesting; and initiating

Social
- to make choices
- to facilitate peer interaction

Directions

Seat children appropriately for snack, using adaptive seating as needed. Have children pass out napkins, if appropriate. If bowls are of different colors, let children select which color bowl to use. Tell them they are going to have banana boats for snack. Encourage them to identify each item as it is used. Peel each banana and cut in half crosswise. Then cut each piece in half lengthwise. You may want to make even smaller portions, depending on the children's appetites and abilities. Place two pieces of banana in the dish and put a scoop of ice cream on top. If you have more than one flavor, let the children choose a flavor. Add a topping, again letting children choose the flavor. Add whipped cream. Provide help with self-feeding and oral-motor skills as needed. Offer juice and give help as needed.

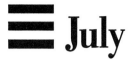

July

Week 1

Overall Theme: Parade

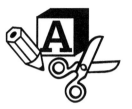

Activity 1: Rhythm Band

Materials

    selection of musical instruments; include some requiring two hands to play
      (such as cymbals, rhythm sticks, sand blocks, triangles, or tambourines);
      also include some that require the use of a stick or other tool
      (such as triangles, drums, or xylophones)

    audio player

    record or tape of marching band music (see Appendix D for resources)

Goals

Sensory
- to increase attention span
- to improve auditory awareness

Gross Motor
- to improve balance and coordination

Fine Motor
- to improve midline skills, using both hands together, grasp and release, and hand manipulation

Cognitive
- to improve understanding of cause-and-effect, tool use, imitation, and concept development

Language
- to improve following directions; taking turns; listening; identifying/labeling objects, actions, people, and concepts; initiating; and requesting

Social
- to make choices
- to facilitate peer interaction

Directions

Bring out the box of musical instruments. Encourage children to choose one to use and provide some time for them to explore the instruments. Then model the use of various instruments as all of the children play together. Put on the music and play instruments to accompany it. Allow children to exchange instruments with one another from time to time. Include music that is soft and slow as well as loud and fast. See if the children will play instruments more slowly or quietly with softer, slower music. Incorporate concepts as appropriate to the level of the group. Also, encourage singing along, even in jargon. At the close of the activity, help children put the instruments away in the box. Be aware of children who may show signs of auditory defensiveness or auditory discrimination problems during this activity. Children who are really bothered by the noise should be given a quiet space to which they can retreat, if needed.

Activity 2: Decorating Floats

Materials

riding toys and/or push toys (such as wagons, carts, and strollers)

crepe paper, stickers, balloons, paper or plastic flags, and other items to decorate the carts and riding toys

tape

scissors

Goals

Sensory
- to improve sensory awareness through visual and tactile stimulation (can incorporate auditory as well)
- to increase attention span

Gross Motor
- to improve motor planning, balance, coordination, and trunk rotation

Fine Motor
- to improve grasp and release, hand manipulation, finger isolation, and eye-hand coordination
- to increase upper body strength

Cognitive
- to develop understanding of spatial relationships, counting, imitation, and concept development

Language
- to improve following directions; taking turns; listening; identifying/labeling objects, actions, and colors; initiating; and requesting

Social
- to make choices

Directions

Bring out the riding toys and push toys to be decorated. Demonstrate and then help each child tape on streamers, tie on balloons, and stick on stickers, depending on their motor skills and interests. Those who are ready can help snip tape or streamers with child-safe scissors. For children who need assistance, tape on their selected streamers according to their preferences.

Activity 3: Parade

Materials

decorated riding and/or push toys (from Activity 2)
audio player
record or tape of marching band music (see Appendix D for resources)
rhythm instruments (optional)

Goals

Sensory
- to improve responses to sensory stimulation
- to provide proprioceptive stimulation

Gross Motor
- to improve walking, marching, pushing with feet or upper body, balance, coordination, and weight shifting

Fine Motor
- to improve reach and grasp
- to increase upper body strength
- to improve shoulder girdle strength and stability

Cognitive
- to improve understanding of spatial relationships, imitation, sequencing, and concept development

Language
- to improve following directions; listening; identifying/labeling objects, actions, people, and places; initiating; requesting; and taking turns

Social
- to facilitate representational/pretend play
- to facilitate peer interaction

Directions

Have children form a line either pushing carts, riding in carts, or riding on self-propelled riding toys. Play marching music and ask the children to march in time to the music. They may also play instruments in time to the music. If possible, have them march outdoors for at least part of the parade. Emphasize motor skills such as weight shifting over as narrow a base of support as possible, proprioceptive input into the feet through marching, and proprioceptive input into the shoulder girdle through pushing weighted carts. Children who are not yet walking may ride in carts while developing and improving skills such as sitting balance and appropriate responses to vestibular movement.

Activity 4: Playground

Materials

playground and equipment including swings, slides, and climbing structures (outdoors, if possible)

Goals

Sensory
- to improve responses to vestibular stimulation (swinging, sliding)
- to provide proprioceptive stimulation

Gross Motor
- to improve balance, coordination, motor planning, trunk rotation, and reciprocal limb movements

Fine Motor
- to improve shoulder girdle strength and stability

Cognitive
- to improve understanding of spatial relationships and imitation

Language
- to improve following directions; identifying/labeling objects, actions, people, and places; taking turns; initiating; and requesting

Social
- to make choices
- to facilitate peer interaction

Directions

Have the parade (Activity 3) end at the playground, if possible. Allow children plenty of time to explore the playground equipment. Incorporate lots of language to describe what they are doing. Encourage children to try different pieces of equipment. Assist children who may not be able to explore on their own by providing choices (for example, "Do you want to swing or slide?") and then going on the equipment with them.

Activity 5: Streamers and Bubbles

Note: This activity was devised as an alternative to fireworks, which are unsafe and possibly frightening to very young children.

Materials

cloth or paper streamers
foxtails (optional)
smaller bubble hoops (optional)

pinwheels (optional)
giant bubble hoop, bubble soap, and container for soap

Goals

Sensory
- to improve responses to sensory stimulation
- to increase attention span

Gross Motor
- to improve balance, coordination, motor planning, and trunk rotation

Fine Motor
- to improve eye-hand coordination, visual tracking, reach and grasp, and grasp and release
- to increase upper body strength
- to improve shoulder girdle strength and stability

Self-Help
- to improve oral-motor skills

Cognitive
- to improve understanding of spatial relationships, tool use, and concept development

Language
- to improve following directions; taking turns; identifying/labeling objects, actions, locations, and relationships; initiating; and requesting

Social
- to make choices
- to facilitate peer interaction

Directions

When children begin to tire of the playground activities, an adult should initiate activities with the streamers, pinwheels, or foxtails. Use one activity at a time and encourage children to reach up high to twirl the streamers or pinwheels or to throw the foxtails. Children will tend to gravitate to the activity naturally. As they tire of streamers, foxtails, or pinwheels, introduce the bubbles. Encourage children to pop them with their arms or stomp them with their feet. Those who are able can try to blow bubbles with the large bubble wand. Smaller wands may be more appropriate for younger or smaller children or children who are physically challenged. Use lots of language, showing and telling them where the bubbles, streamers, or foxtails are going and who is doing what action.

Snack

Materials

gelatin jigglers, prepared ahead of time
juice
paper plates
spoons (optional)
chairs (adaptive seating as needed)

cups (adapted as needed)
napkins
table
washcloths for cleanup

Note: see Appendix C for a gelatin jigglers recipe

Goals

Sensory
- to improve responses to sensory stimuli, especially tactile and olfactory
- to increase attention span

Fine Motor
- to improve grasp and release, hand/finger manipulation, and eye-hand coordination

Self-Help
- to improve self-feeding skills
- to improve oral-motor skills

Cognitive
- to improve imitation, sequencing, and concept development

Language
- to improve following directions; taking turns; identifying/labeling objects, actions, people, and characteristics; requesting; and initiating

Social
- to make choices
- to facilitate peer interaction

Directions

Seat children at the table. Have children help pass out plates, if appropriate. Show children the jigglers. Encourage the children to touch and describe the jigglers. Have children choose which color they would like to eat. Facilitate appropriate feeding skills as necessary for each individual. Encourage communication, including ways to request more or indicate "all done." Offer juice and provide assistance as needed. Children may be offered spoons to use with the jigglers if appropriate and if spoon feeding is a goal.

Week 2

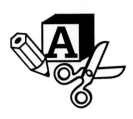

Overall Theme: Beach

Activity 1: Trip to the Beach

Materials

large cardboard boxes or other containers to use as "cars" (alternative: push toys or riding toys to serve as cars)

tote bags packed with swimsuits, towels, goggles, sunglasses, sunscreen, beach toys, swim rings, and beach sandals (tote bag contents are optional)

Goals

Sensory
- to improve responses to vestibular stimulation
- to provide proprioceptive stimulation

Gross Motor
- to improve motor planning, sitting balance, coordination, and trunk rotation

Fine Motor
- to improve reach and grasp and hand manipulation
- to increase upper body strength
- to improve shoulder girdle strength and stability

Cognitive
- to improve understanding of spatial relationships, sequencing, imitation, and concept development
- to develop generalization skills

Language
- to improve following directions; taking turns; identifying/labeling objects, actions, people, and concepts; initiating; and requesting

Social
- to facilitate representational/pretend play
- to facilitate peer interaction

Directions

Tell children they are going on a car ride to the beach. Help them into the cardboard "cars" (or alternative "vehicles"). If appropriate, have them help load the tote bags into the cars as well. Push the cars to the beach area, which has been set up in another part of the room or in another room. Encourage children who are able to help push some of the cars. Weather permitting, it is a good idea to set up the beach outside. Upon arrival at the beach area, help children climb out of the cars and unload tote bags, if these were loaded earlier.

Activity 2: At the Beach

Materials

wading pool partially filled with lukewarm water (adjust temperature to the needs of the group)

seashells (optional)

small sandbox

swimsuits for children (optional)

beach gear from previous activity

towels for drying children after activity

sand toys (such as pails, shovels, cups for scooping, windmill-type sand toy, and small objects to hide in the sand)

water toys (swim rings, beach balls of various sizes, floating objects, sponge toys, fishing toys, large spoons or nets for catching floating objects, boats, sieves for straining water)

Goals

Sensory
- to improve sensory awareness/body awareness through tactile stimulation
- to increase attention span

Gross Motor
- to improve motor planning, balance, transitional movement patterns, and trunk rotation

Fine Motor
- to improve eye-hand coordination, wrist rotation, finger isolation (poking in sand), hand manipulation, visual tracking, reach and grasp, and grasp and release
- to increase upper body strength
- to improve shoulder girdle strength and stability

Self-Help
- to improve dressing/undressing skills

Cognitive
- to improve understanding of spatial relationships, object permanence, tool use, cause-and-effect, imitation, concept development, and sequencing
- to develop generalization skills

Language
- to improve taking turns; identifying/labeling objects, actions, people, places, characteristics, relationships, and body parts; requesting; initiating; and following directions

Social
- to facilitate representational/pretend play
- to facilitate peer interaction

Directions

When children arrive at the beach area, help them unpack tote bags, remove outer garments, and change into swimsuits, if using them, and apply sunscreen. Plain oil may be substituted if children should not use sunscreen, but it will not provide the same olfactory effect. Help them find towels, sunglasses, and beach sandals and explore these items. Some children may want to play first in the sand, while others may go straight for the water. Be sure there are enough adults available to supervise both parts of this activity simultaneously.

With sand play, encourage scooping and digging with hands and tools, finding items partially or completely buried in the sand, filling containers, pouring from one container to another, lifting containers filled with sand, and watching and filling the windmill toy. If possible, let children sit in the sandbox. Bury their hands, feet, or legs in the sand, if they will allow you to do so. If you have seashells, these may be placed or hidden in the sand.

With water play, encourage scooping and dumping, filling and pouring, catching floating items with hands and tools, observing items that sink and float, throwing and catching the beach balls, passing the beach balls around the pool to others, and observing the different sizes and colors of items. Seashells can also be placed in the pool for the children to discover.

Encourage children to explore both sand and water activities. Toward the end of the activity, allow them to mix the sand and water, if possible, since the combination produces a very different kind of tactile sensation and provides opportunities for molding and building with the sand and drawing in the wet sand with fingers or a tool.

When they have tired of both activities, help them to dry off and get dressed again. If they are willing, help them back into the cars for the trip home.

Activity 3: Sand Painting

Materials

sand
glue
cotton swabs (optional)
chairs (adaptive seating as needed)

construction paper
paintbrushes (optional)
table
washcloths for cleanup

Goals

Sensory
- to improve sensory awareness through tactile stimulation
- to increase attention span

Fine Motor
- to improve hand manipulation, eye-hand coordination, using both hands together, midline skills, and grasp and release

Cognitive
- to improve imitation and concept development
- to develop generalization skills

Language
- to improve following directions; taking turns; increasing vocabulary; initiating; requesting; and identifying/labeling objects, actions, people, and characteristics

Social
- to make choices

Directions

Position children for fine motor activity. Have children select which color paper to use. A darker colored paper provides more visual contrast for this activity. Help children squeeze or spread glue onto their papers, encouraging them to stabilize the paper with one hand, if possible. Vary the activity by having them spread the glue with paintbrushes or cotton swabs. Help them sprinkle or pour sand onto the glue. Let the pictures dry while completing another activity.

Snack

Materials

frozen juice bars
"sandy beach" cookies (any simple cookie rolled in sugar for a "sandy" effect)
napkins
table
chairs (adaptive seating as needed)
washcloths for cleanup

Goals

Sensory
• to improve responses to sensory stimuli, especially tactile and olfactory

Fine Motor
• to improve reach and grasp, grasp and release, hand manipulation, and eye-hand coordination

Self-Help
• to improve self-feeding skills
• to improve oral-motor skills

Cognitive
• to improve imitation and concept development
• to develop generalization skills
• to develop recall skills

Language
• to improve following directions; taking turns; identifying/labeling objects, actions, people, and characteristics; requesting; and initiating

Social
• to make choices
• to facilitate peer interaction

Directions

Seat children appropriately for snack, using adaptive seating as needed. Show children the frozen fruit bars and have them choose one. Use the bars to facilitate oral-motor skills as appropriate. Offer "sandy beach" cookies and talk about how they are like the beach. Encourage communication, including ways to request more or indicate "all done." Assist with self-feeding and oral-motor skills as needed.

Week 3

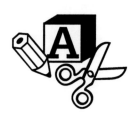

Overall Theme: At the Farm

Activity 1: Pony Rides

Materials

bolster swing
rocking horses

bolsters on floor
stick horses

Goals

Sensory
- to improve responses to vestibular stimulation
- to increase attention span

Gross Motor
- to improve balance, weight shifting, motor planning, and coordination

Cognitive
- to improve imitation, understanding of spatial relationships, and concept development

Language
- to improve taking turns; increasing vocalizations/vocabulary; following directions; identifying/labeling actions, objects, people, and characteristics; initiating; and requesting

Social
- to make choices
- to facilitate pretend play
- to facilitate peer interaction

Directions

Help children, one at a time, onto the bolster swing. Make horse noises and sing horse songs while swinging the swing back and forth. Help children adjust to the movements. Children can "ride" the bolsters on the floor while waiting their turn for the swing. Help them practice weight shifting from side to side and balancing. One end of the bolster can rear up like a horse's head with some help from an adult. Again, encourage children to make and imitate horse noises and sing horse songs during this activity. If appropriate, the children can also use rocking horses or stick horses during this activity.

Activity 2: Wagon Rides

Materials

wagons   adaptive seating to fit inside wagons if necessary

Goals

Sensory
- to improve responses to vestibular stimulation
- to provide proprioceptive stimulation
- to increase attention span

Gross Motor
- to improve balance, weight shifting, motor planning, and coordination

Fine Motor
- to improve reach and grasp and grasp and release
- to increase upper body strength
- to improve shoulder girdle strength and stability

Cognitive
- to improve imitation and concept development

Language
- to improve taking turns; increasing vocalizations/vocabulary; following directions; identifying/labeling actions, objects, people, and characteristics; initiating; and requesting

Social
- to facilitate pretend play
- to facilitate peer interaction

Directions

Help children climb into the wagons. If appropriate, some children can pull or push the wagons while others ride in them. Then they can have a turn riding while others pull or push. If children are not able to pull or push the wagons, all of the children can ride while adults do the pulling. Use adaptive seating to provide extra support for those children whose sitting balance is still unsteady. If possible, take the wagons outside and pull the children around the block, through a park, or even around the parking lot. Varied terrain that provides opportunities to go up and down hills and over small bumps is ideal. Talk with the children about what they are seeing, hearing, feeling, and even smelling during the ride. Go up and down, fast and slow, start and stop. Name these actions and encourage the children to name them or request them.

Caution: Hay could be used to create a hay ride for this activity, if staff and children are not allergic to the hay or have tactile defensiveness. Use the hay with caution because, more often than not, at least some of the children will not be able to tolerate it.

Activity 3: Farm Animal Toys

Materials

a variety of toys with a farm animal theme, for example:

puzzles	"farmer says" talking toy
farm animal scene	play farm
books	stuffed animals
puppets	

Goals

Sensory
- to increase attention span

Fine Motor
- to improve hand/finger manipulation, eye-hand coordination, finger isolation, and grasp and release

Cognitive
- to improve imitation, understanding of cause-and-effect and means-end relationships, problem solving, understanding of spatial relationships, object permanence, classification, picture-object association and matching, and concept development
- to develop generalization skills

Language
- to improve turn taking; increasing vocalizations/vocabulary; auditory awareness and attention; requesting; initiating; following directions; and identifying/labeling objects, actions, characteristics, and locations

Social
- to make choices
- to facilitate pretend play
- to facilitate peer interaction

Directions

Set up "stations" for the various toys. Allow children to wander to a station and begin playing. An adult can then assist with the play, expanding and guiding as appropriate. Puzzle pieces can be matched to pictures on the "farmer says" talking toy, for example, if children are not ready to successfully complete the puzzles themselves. Imitate animal sounds and encourage the children to do the same. Encourage children to name the animals or touch them as an adult names them. Describe the children's actions. Ask the children questions. Have them find animals who have "hidden" in the barn, behind the barn, and in the silo.

Note: It is important to let the children explore the toys as much as possible without adult interference, as long as they are not harming the toy or themselves. This is true especially with the "higher tech" toys. Eventually, they will figure out how to activate the toy and the lesson will mean more than if an adult simply shows them how to do it.

Activity 4: Rice Table

Materials

sand table (can be filled with rice, sand, beans, or other dry textured material)
toy farm set
containers for scooping and hiding
adaptive standers to allow children access to sand table, if needed

Goals

Sensory
- to sensory awareness/body awareness through tactile stimulation

Gross Motor
- to improve motor planning, standing balance, and weight shifting

Fine Motor
- to improve eye-hand coordination, wrist rotation, finger isolation (poking in rice), and hand manipulation
- to increase upper body strength
- to improve shoulder girdle strength and stability

Cognitive
- to improve understanding of spatial relationships, object permanence, tool use, imitation, and concept development
- to develop generalization skills
- to develop recall skills

Language
- to improve taking turns; identifying/labeling objects, actions, people, places, characteristics, and relationships; requesting; initiating; and following directions

Social
- to facilitate representational/pretend play
- to facilitate peer interaction

Directions

Remove the cover from the sand table and put the farm set into the rice (or sand or beans). Encourage children to "walk" animals through the rice, play with the rice with their hands, and fill containers with rice and pour them out. Hide animals in the rice and encourage children to find them. Ask children to find specific animals, to name them before picking them up, and to imitate the sounds they make. Some children may want to hide animals for the adults to find. Ask children what they are doing. Ask them to imitate different actions that an adult does with the animals. Encourage them to trade animals frequently with other children.

Snack

Materials

animal crackers	juice or milk
cups (adapted if necessary)	napkins
table	chairs (adaptive seating as needed)
washcloths for cleanup	

Goals

Sensory
- to improve responses to sensory stimuli, especially tactile and olfactory

Fine Motor
- to improve grasp and release, reach and grasp, eye-hand coordination, and hand manipulation

Self-Help
- to improve self-feeding skills
- to improve oral-motor skills

Cognitive
- to improve imitation, sequencing, and concept development
- to develop generalization skills
- to develop recall skills

Language
- to improve taking turns; identifying/labeling objects, actions, people, and characteristics; requesting; and initiating

Social
- to make choices
- to facilitate peer interaction

Directions

Seat children appropriately for snack, using adaptive seating as needed. Have children help pass out napkins, if appropriate. Show children cookies and have them choose one. Name different animals and imitate their sounds. Encourage communication, including ways to request more or to indicate "all done." Assist with self-feeding skills as needed. Offer juice as needed and provide assistance as required.

Week 4

Overall Theme: Camping

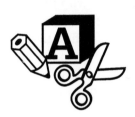

Activity 1: Trip to the Woods

Materials

large cardboard boxes or other containers to be used for "cars" (alternative: push toys or riding toys)

suitcases, duffel bags, or backpacks packed with camping gear (cook stove, canteens, binoculars, magnifying glasses, bug catchers, mess kits, flashlights, hiking boots, tarp, and insect repellent)

sleeping bags

Goals

Sensory
- to improve responses to vestibular stimulation
- to provide proprioceptive stimulation
- to increase attention span

Gross Motor
- to improve motor planning, sitting balance, coordination, and trunk rotation

Fine Motor
- to improve hand manipulation and reach and grasp
- to increase upper body strength
- to improve shoulder girdle strength and stability

Cognitive
- to improve understanding of spatial relationships, sequencing, imitation, and concept development

Language
- to improve following directions; taking turns; identifying/labeling objects, people, actions, and concepts; initiating; and requesting

Social
- to facilitate pretend play
- to facilitate peer interaction

Directions

Tell children they are going on a car ride to the woods. Help them into the cardboard "cars" (or alternative "vehicles"). If appropriate, have them help load the suitcases, duffel bags, or backpacks into the cars as well. Push cars to the woods area, which has been set up in another part of the room or in another room. Encourage the children who are able to help push the cars. Weather permitting, the woods may be located outside in a naturally wooded area, if available. Upon arrival at the woods area, help children climb out of cars and unload the camping gear, if it was loaded earlier.

Activity 2: Camping

Materials

tent
suitcases, duffel bags, or backpacks packed with camping gear
   (from previous activity)
sleeping bags
stuffed animals (optional)

Goals

Sensory
- to increase sensory awareness
- to provide proprioceptive stimulation
- to increase body awareness
- to increase attention span

Gross Motor
- to improve motor planning, balance, and coordination

Fine Motor
- to improve eye-hand coordination, visual attending and tracking, hand manipulation, reach and grasp, and grasp and release

Cognitive
- to improve understanding of spatial, means-end, and cause-and-effect relationships; tool use; imitation; object permanence; concept development; and sequencing

Language
- to improve taking turns; identifying/labeling objects, actions, characteristics, relationships, and body parts; following directions; initiating; and requesting

Social
- to facilitate representational/pretend play
- to facilitate peer interaction

Directions

Set up a tent in the classroom. Give children time to explore and describe their actions. Let children help unpack camping gear, naming items and indicating their use. Encourage children to use items appropriately and to talk about what they are doing. Rolling children in sleeping bags can provide proprioceptive input and help improve responses to sensory stimuli. Rubbing different body parts with insect repellent can increase awareness of body parts and stimulate the olfactory senses.

Other substances can be substituted for insect repellent if children are allergic to it or if there are objections to using strong chemicals unnecessarily. Inside the tent, children can turn on flashlights. Adults can direct them to shine the light in particular places or to follow an adult's light beam with their own. They can try on hiking boots and talk about big shoes and little shoes. Looking through binoculars can provide other opportunities for visual tracking as well as discussions of big and little and near and far. Children can also be encouraged to incorporate the stuffed animals into their activities; for example, preparing food for them or putting them in sleeping bags.

Activity 3: Hike

Materials

access to outdoors, if possible
a variety of natural objects (for example, stones, sticks, seeds, leaves, flowers, and feathers)
bags or baskets
strollers or other adaptive means of locomotion for children who are nonambulatory

Goals

Sensory
- to improve sensory awareness
- to provide proprioceptive stimulation
- to increase attention span
- to improve auditory and visual attending skills

Gross Motor
- to improve walking, stooping/squatting, weight shifting, balance, coordination, and motor planning

Fine Motor
- to improve eye-hand coordination, reach and grasp, grasp and release, hand/finger manipulation, and finger isolation (pointing)
- to increase upper body strength
- to improve shoulder girdle strength and stability

Cognitive
- to improve classification, imitation, and concept development
- to develop generalization skills

Language
- to improve following directions; taking turns; increasing vocalization/vocabulary; identifying/labeling objects, actions, characteristics, relationships, and locations; initiating; requesting; and questioning

Social
- to make choices
- to facilitate peer interaction

Directions

Have children hike along a path outdoors, if possible. Otherwise, set up a "path" indoors with natural objects placed along the way. Encouraging children to march or hike with big, heavy steps will provide proprioceptive input and help them develop a variety of gross motor skills. Let the children who are walking push the strollers for the children who are using them, thus helping the walking children to improve their upper body strength. Talk with the children about what they see, hear, and smell. Help them collect natural objects in their bags or baskets. Ask questions about what they are doing and about the objects they have found.

Activity 4: Collage

Materials

natural objects collected during the hike	construction paper
glue	table
chairs (adaptive seating as needed)	washcloths for cleanup

Goals

Sensory
- to improve sensory awareness through tactile stimulation
- to increase attention span

Fine Motor
- to improve hand/finger manipulation, eye-hand coordination, using both hands together, reach and grasp, and grasp and release

Cognitive
- to improve imitation, classification, and concept development
- to develop generalization skills
- to develop recall skills

Language
- to improve following directions; taking turns; increasing vocabulary; identifying/labeling objects, actions, characteristics, and relationships; initiating; and requesting

Social
- to make choices

Directions

Position children for fine motor activity. Have children select which color paper to use. Help children squeeze or spread glue onto their papers, encouraging them to stabilize the paper with one hand, if possible. Help them put the natural objects they have collected onto the glue. Encourage the children to name or describe the objects they are using and to tell about where they found each object. Let the pictures dry while completing another activity.

Snack

Materials

baked beans	plates
buns	spoons or forks (as appropriate)
hot dogs	cups (adapted as needed)
ketchup and mustard	table
juice or milk	chairs (adaptive seating as needed)
napkins	washcloths for cleanup

Note: You can use mess kits and canteens instead of plates and cups, if appropriate.

Goals

Sensory
- to improve responses to sensory stimuli, especially tactile and olfactory

Fine Motor
- to improve reach and grasp, grasp and release, hand/finger manipulation, and eye-hand coordination

Self-Help
- to improve self-feeding skills
- to improve oral-motor skills

Cognitive
- to improve imitation, sequencing, and concept development
- to develop generalization skills
- to develop recall skills

Language
- to improve following directions; taking turns; identifying/labeling objects, actions, people, and characteristics; sequencing; initiating; and requesting

Social
- to make choices
- to facilitate peer interaction

Directions

Seat children appropriately for snack, using adaptive seating as needed. Have children select a mess kit or help pass out plates, silverware, and napkins, if appropriate. Prepare the hot dogs on a grill or camp stove outdoors near the tent, if possible. Let the children watch. Give children choices of ketchup or mustard, with bun or without bun, with beans and without beans. Encourage communication, including ways to request more or indicate "all done." Discuss the activities that took place on the "camping trip." Assist with self-feeding skills as needed. Offer juice and provide assistance as needed.

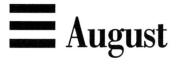

August

Week 1

Overall Theme: Sunshine

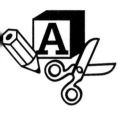

Activity 1: Parachute Sun

Materials

parachute (if a parachute is not available, you may use a sheet or blanket)

Goals

Sensory
- to increase attention span

Gross Motor
- to improve balance, coordination, and motor planning

Fine Motor
- to improve eye-hand coordination and reach and grasp
- to increase upper body strength
- to improve shoulder girdle strength and stability

Cognitive
- to improve concept development and understanding of object permanence and spatial relationships
- to develop generalization skills

Language
- to improve following directions; taking turns; identifying/labeling objects, actions, and descriptions; requesting; and initiating

Social
- to develop representational/pretend play
- to facilitate peer interaction

Directions

Spread the parachute flat on the floor. Seat the children around the edge of the parachute. Show and tell them how the parachute is shaped like the sun. Help them to grasp the edges of the parachute and wave it up and down. Have the children (one at a time or several together) go under or on the parachute. Emphasize the "up" and "down" as the parachute moves. You can also have the group try to stand up and hold the parachute open on its side at a right angle to the ground so that it looks like the sun. If the group walks with it, it will move across the "sky" like the sun. Provide children with whatever adaptive seating or physical assistance they may need.

Activity 2: Sun and Shadow

Materials

sunshine or bright light
shade

Goals

Sensory
- to increase attention span

Gross Motor
- to improve motor planning, balance, coordination, weight bearing, weight shifting, walking, and marching

Fine Motor
- to improve visual attending and tracking

Cognitive
- to improve understanding of spatial relationships, classification skills, and concept development
- to develop generalization skills

Language
- to improve following directions; taking turns; identifying/labeling objects, actions, and descriptions; requesting; and initiating

Social
- to facilitate peer interactions

Directions

This activity is best conducted outdoors during the day when the sun is bright. Some of these same ideas could be developed indoors by using a brightly lit area in contrast with a dimly lit area, but the effect will not be quite the same. Take the children outside. Explore a sunny area. Discover the children's shadows. Make shadow figures or have a shadow dance. Move fast. See if the shadows are still able to follow. Then explore a shaded area. Where are the shadows now? How does it feel to be in the shade? What is the same? What is different? Go back out into the sun. Ask the same questions again.

Activity 3: Sun Screens

Materials

sunglasses   sun visors
sunscreen   parasol

Goals

Sensory
- to improve responses to sensory stimulation
- to increase body awareness
- to increase attention span

Gross Motor
- to improve balance, coordination, and weight shifting

Fine Motor
- to improve reach and grasp, grasp and release, visual attending, eye-hand coordination, and hand manipulation
- to increase upper body strength

Self-Help
- to improve dressing/undressing skills

Cognitive
- to improve understanding of spatial relationships, functional object use, classification, imitation, and concept development
- to develop generalization skills
- to develop recall skills

Language
- to improve following directions; taking turns; identifying/labeling objects, people, actions, and concepts; initiating; and requesting

Social
- to make choices
- to facilitate pretend play
- to facilitate peer interaction

Directions

Bring out the equipment for this activity. Encourage children to spontaneously identify items and demonstrate how they are used. Contrast how things look with and without wearing sunglasses and sun visors. Help children put on or take off the items as needed. Using the sunscreen will also heighten awareness of body parts and address tactile issues. If the group decides to use sunscreen, make sure that no one is allergic to it.

Activity 4: Paper-Plate Suns

Materials

paper plates
chubby brushes (if paint is used)
yellow, orange, and red construction
   paper cut in 2" x 4" strips
stapler
table
washcloths for cleanup

yellow, orange, and red water-based
   paint or washable markers
smocks
scissors
staples
chairs (adaptive seating as needed)

Goals

Sensory
- to increase attention span

Fine Motor
- to improve hand/finger manipulation, visual attending, eye-hand coordination, and using two hands together
- to improve shoulder girdle strength and stability

Cognitive
- to improve tool use, understanding of spatial relationships, concept development, and imitation
- to develop generalization skills

Language
- to improve following directions; taking turns; increasing vocabulary; and identifying/labeling objects, actions, characteristics, and relationships

Social
- to make choices
- to facilitate peer interaction

Directions

Position children appropriately for fine motor activity. Each child will paint or color the bottoms of two paper plates. Give them the plates one at a time. Demonstrate coloring the plates and help them choose which colors to use. Describe their actions and the colors. When they each have colored two plates, have them select some construction paper strips for making sun rays. Staple the two plates together, inserting the "rays" between the edges at each staple before stapling.

Snack

Materials

rice cakes	plates
cheese slices or cream cheese with yellow food coloring added	napkins
	cups (adapted as needed)
table knives for spreading	table
toaster oven (optional)	chairs (adaptive seating as needed)
juice	washcloths for cleanup

Goals

Sensory
- to improve responses to sensory stimuli, especially tactile and olfactory
- to increase attention span

Fine Motor
- to improve using both hands together, reach and grasp, grasp and release, hand/finger manipulation, and eye-hand coordination

Self-Help
- to improve self-feeding skills
- to improve oral-motor skills

Cognitive
- to improve imitation, concept development, and sequencing
- to develop generalization skills
- to develop recall skills

Language
- to improve following directions; imitation; identifying/labeling objects, actions, people, and characteristics; taking turns; requesting; and initiating

Social
- to make choices
- to facilitate peer interaction

Directions

Seat children appropriately for snack, using adaptive seating as needed. Tell them they are going to make "sunshine snacks." Give each child a rice cake. Help each child put a cheese slice on a rice cake (if using melted cheese method) or give each child a table knife and help them spread the yellow cream cheese on the rice cake. Describe what they are doing, what the snack is made of, and what it looks like. Talk about how it looks like the sun. Heat rice cakes with cheese slices in the toaster oven just until the cheese melts. If possible, watch the cheese melt and talk about the changes the children observe. Encourage communication, including ways to request more or indicate "all done." Offer juice as needed. Assist with self-feeding and drinking skills as needed.

Week 2

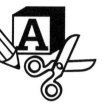

Overall Theme: Music

Activity 1: Music Walk

Materials

audio player
record or tape

Goals

Sensory
- to provide proprioceptive stimulation
- to provide vestibular stimulation
- to improve responses to auditory stimulation

Gross Motor
- to improve motor planning, balance, coordination, weight bearing, weight shifting, walking, and marching

Fine Motor
- to increase upper body strength

Cognitive
- to improve understanding of spatial relationships, imitation, and concept development

Language
- to improve following directions; listening; identifying/labeling objects, actions, people, and places; initiating; requesting; and taking turns

Social
- to facilitate representational/pretend play
- to facilitate peer interaction

Directions

Have children move in time to the music. Begin by moving in place and then expand to walking, marching, and dancing. Stop the music and have them stop their movements when the music stops. Repeat this several times. Children who are not walking can ride in strollers or carts if they wish. Children who are walking can then push the strollers. With the walkers, emphasize motor skills, such as weight shifting over as narrow a base of support as possible, proprioceptive input into the feet through marching, and proprioceptive input into the shoulder girdle through pushing strollers. Children who are riding in strollers are developing and improving sitting balance and appropriate responses to vestibular movement.

Activity 2: Music Hide and Seek

Materials

music boxes or tape players
hiding places

Goals

Sensory
- to improve responses to sensory stimulation
- to improve auditory attention
- to increase attention span

Gross Motor
- to improve balance, coordination, motor planning, locomotion, trunk rotation, and weight shifting

Fine Motor
- to improve reach and grasp, visual attention, and hand manipulation
- to increase upper body strength
- to improve shoulder girdle strength and stability

Cognitive
- to improve imitation, problem solving, understanding of spatial relationships, object permanence, and concept development

Language
- to improve sound vocalization; following directions; taking turns; identifying/ labeling objects, actions, descriptions, and locations; requesting; and initiating

Social
- to make choices
- to facilitate peer interaction

Directions

Hide a music box or tape player and have children find it by listening to the sounds it is making. Repeat until everyone has had a turn. Be sure to hide the music box at different heights to encourage a variety of motor responses and transitional movements, such as crawling, stooping, squatting, reaching above the head, and standing.

Activity 3: Explore an Instrument

Materials

musical instrument, such as a guitar, Autoharp, or piano

Goals

Sensory
- to improve responses to sensory stimulation
- to improve visual attending
- to improve auditory attending
- to increase attention span

Gross Motor
- to improve balance, coordination, trunk rotation, and weight shifting

Fine Motor
- to improve reach and grasp, hand manipulation, and finger isolation

Cognitive
- to improve imitation, understanding of cause-and-effect, and concept development
- to develop generalization skills

Language
- to improve following directions; taking turns; identifying/labeling objects, actions, descriptions, and locations; requesting; and initiating

Social
- to facilitate peer interaction

Directions

Gather children around the instrument. If possible, put it on the floor where they can see and reach it easily. Demonstrate how it is used, then let them explore as independently as possible. Use lots of language to describe the sounds, the way the instrument feels, and the way it looks. Make sure each child has a turn.

Activity 4: Rhythm Instruments

Materials

oatmeal boxes
paper plates or bowls
shoe boxes
rubber bands
jingle bells
scissors
contact paper
chairs (adaptive seating
  as needed)

aluminum pie pans
small cans with plastic lids (peanut
  cans or infant formula cans, for example)
dried beans
yarn
hole punch
table

Goals

Sensory
- to improve sensory awareness through tactile stimulation
- to increase attention span
- to improve auditory attending

Fine Motor
- to improve hand/finger manipulation, eye-hand coordination, using both hands together, reach and grasp, grasp and release, and midline skills

Cognitive
- to improve object permanence, understanding of cause-and-effect and spatial relationships, imitation, concept development, and sequencing
- to develop generalization skills
- to develop recall skills

Language
- to improve following directions; taking turns; increasing vocabulary; identifying/labeling objects, actions, characteristics, and relationships; initiating; and requesting

Social
- to make choices
- to facilitate representational play
- to facilitate peer interaction

Directions

Children may make one or more of the following rhythm instruments:

1. Tambourine—Punch holes in the edges of two paper plates or bowls. Lace them together with yarn. Tie on some bells.
2. Guitar—Stretch several rubber bands around a small shoe box. Make music by strumming or plucking the "strings."
3. Shakers—Put some dried beans in a small tin can with a plastic lid. Seal with contact paper.
4. Drum—Cover empty oatmeal boxes with contact paper.
5. Shakers II—Punch holes in the edges of two aluminum pie pans. Put some dried beans inside. Lace them together with yarn.

When the instruments are finished, have a concert. Give everyone a chance to perform solo and with the group. Talk about the experiences as the children are making the instruments. Discuss how they sound and what it feels like to play the instruments; for example, is there a vibration or a tickle?

Activity 5: Sound Match

Materials

a variety of musical instruments with which the children are familiar; such as rhythm sticks, tambourines, and drums

Goals

Sensory
- to improve responses to sensory stimulation
- to improve auditory attending
- to increase attention span

Fine Motor
- to improve reach and grasp, eye-hand coordination, visual attending and scanning, and hand manipulation

Cognitive
- to improve imitation, problem solving, tool use, object permanence, classification, and concept development
- to develop generalization skills

Language
- to improve sound vocalization; auditory discrimination; following directions; taking turns; identifying/labeling objects, actions, descriptions, and locations; requesting; and initiating

Social
- to make choices
- to facilitate peer interaction

Directions

Make sure to provide at least two sets of each instrument for this activity. Limit the number of choices based on the group's abilities. Place one set of instruments where all the children can see them. Have an adult hide nearby and play an instrument. Have the group guess which instrument it is. The one who guesses correctly may pick up the instrument and play it in response. Continue until everyone has had a turn.

Snack

Materials

bean salad (composed of the same kinds of beans used to make the musical instruments in Activity 4)
napkins
chairs (adaptive seating as needed)

plates
cups (adapted as needed)
forks (optional)
juice
washcloths for cleanup

Goals

Sensory
- to improve responses to sensory stimuli, especially tactile and olfactory
- to increase attention span

Fine Motor
- to improve reach and grasp, grasp and release, hand/finger manipulation, and eye-hand coordination

Self-Help
- to improve self-feeding skills
- to improve oral-motor skills

Cognitive
- to improve understanding of spatial relationships, imitation, and concept development
- to develop generalization skills
- to develop recall skills

Language
- to improve following directions; taking turns; identifying/labeling objects, actions, people, and characteristics; initiating; and requesting

Social
- to make choices
- to facilitate peer interaction

Directions

Seat children appropriately for snack, using adaptive seating as needed. Have children pass out plates, forks, and napkins, if appropriate. Give each child some of the bean salad. Encourage the children to identify the kinds of beans that they used in their shakers. How are they the same? How are they different? What do they taste like? Look like? Smell like? Encourage communication, including ways to request more or indicate "all done." Offer juice as needed. Assist with self-feeding and drinking skills as needed.

Week 3

Overall Theme: Bugs

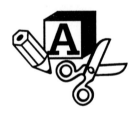

Activity 1: Bug in a Rug

Materials

sleeping bag, heavy blanket, or folding mat

Goals

Sensory
- to improve responses to sensory stimulation
- to provide proprioceptive stimulation
- to increase body awareness

Gross Motor
- to improve motor planning, crawling, rolling, and reciprocal movement patterns

Fine Motor
- to improve shoulder girdle strength and stability

Cognitive
- to improve problem solving, object permanence, classification, imitation, understanding of spatial relationships, and concept development
- to develop generalization skills

Language
- to improve following directions; taking turns; identifying/labeling objects, actions, relationships, descriptions, and people; initiating; and requesting

Social
- to facilitate pretend play
- to facilitate peer interaction

Directions

Spread the sleeping bag, blanket, or folding mat on the floor. Have the children one at a time crawl or scoot inside and roll across the floor. Adults can roll the children who cannot roll themselves. For many children, simply pressing down gently on their bodies while they are inside the "rug" will provide much-needed proprioceptive stimulation. Use lots of language to facilitate the pretend aspects of the activity for the children. Talk about the expression "snug as a bug in a rug." How does it feel?

Activity 2: Bug Hunt

Materials

access to outdoors, if possible
containers for carrying bugs and
   other objects
magnifying glass

a variety of natural objects that might
   be associated with bugs (stones,
   sticks, seeds, leaves, and flowers)
strollers or other adaptive means of
   locomotion for children who are
   nonambulatory

Goals

Sensory
- to improve sensory awareness
- to increase attention span
- to improve auditory and visual attending skills

Gross Motor
- to improve walking, stooping/squatting, weight shifting, balance, coordination, and motor planning

Fine Motor
- to improve eye-hand coordination, reach and grasp, grasp and release, hand/finger manipulation, and finger isolation (pointing)
- to increase upper body strength

Cognitive
- to improve understanding of spatial relationships, classification, imitation, concept development
- to develop generalization skills

Language
- to improve following directions; taking turns; increasing vocalizations/vocabulary; identifying and labeling objects, actions, characteristics, relationships, and locations; initiating; requesting; questioning

Social
- to make choices
- to facilitate peer interaction

Directions

Have children hike along a path outdoors, if possible. Otherwise, set up a "path" indoors with the natural objects placed along the way. Encourage them to march or hike softly and quietly so as not to frighten away the bugs. Let the children who are walking push the strollers for the children who are using them, thus helping the walking children to improve their upper body strength. Talk with the children about what they see, hear, and smell. Help them look along the path for bugs—under rocks, on sticks, and in flowers. Collect some of the bugs they find, along with related natural objects. Use the magnifying glass to examine the bugs and objects. Ask questions about what they are doing and about the items they have found.

Activity 3: Move Like a Bug/Talk Like a Bug

Materials

pictures of various bugs
bugs that were collected during the previous activity
bug puppets
costume wings and antennae (optional)

Goals

Sensory
- to increase sensory awareness and responsiveness, especially to tactile stimulation
- to provide vestibular stimulation
- to provide proprioceptive stimulation
- to increase attention span

Gross Motor
- to improve motor planning, locomotion, balance, coordination, and weight shifting

Fine Motor
- to improve hand/finger manipulation, eye-hand coordination, and visual attending and tracking

Cognitive
- to improve imitation, picture-object association, classification, and concept development
- to develop generalization skills

Language
- to improve following directions; taking turns; increasing vocalizations; identifying/labeling objects, actions, characteristics, and relationships; initiating; and requesting

Social
- to make choices
- to facilitate peer interaction
- to facilitate pretend play

Directions

Have children imitate bugs in a variety of ways. They may move like a bug or allow themselves to be assisted through the bug's motions. They can make one of the puppets move like a bug. Help them choose which bug to be by looking at and talking about the pictures and the bugs they have collected. Which bugs walk, fly, hop? Use lots of language to describe what the children are doing—how they are moving and who is moving. Encourage the children to "talk" like the bugs as well as move like them; for example, bees buzz and crickets chirp.

Note: Costume wings and antennae may help some children imagine more easily, while for others these props may be frightening.

Activity 4: Spots on a Ladybug

Materials

red construction paper cut
  in the shape of a ladybug
black pipe cleaners
smocks
table

black markers or empty roll-on type
  deodorant containers filled with
  black tempera paint
washcloths for cleanup
chairs (adaptive seating as needed)

Goals

Sensory
- to increase attention span

Fine Motor
- to improve hand/finger manipulation, eye-hand coordination, midline skills, using two hands together, reach and grasp, and grasp and release

Cognitive
- to improve imitation, tool use, and concept development
- to develop generalization skills

Language
- to improve following directions; taking turns; increasing vocabulary; identifying/labeling objects, actions, characteristics, and relationships; initiating; and requesting

Social
- to make choices
- to facilitate peer interaction

Directions

Seat children appropriately for fine motor activity. Use adaptive seating as needed. Have the children choose which paper ladybug they want to use and which marker or paint roller they would like to use. Assist them as needed in putting spots on the ladybug with the markers or paint rollers. Attach pipe cleaners for antennae. Use lots of language to describe what the children are doing. Emphasize the colors they are using.

Snack

Materials

bananas	napkins
peanut butter	plates
raisins	cups (adapted as needed)
table knives	chairs (adaptive seating as needed)
juice	table

Goals

Sensory
- to improve responses to sensory stimuli, especially tactile and olfactory
- to increase attention span

Fine Motor
- to improve using both hands together, reach and grasp, grasp and release, hand/finger manipulation, and eye-hand coordination

Self-Help
- to improve self-feeding skills
- to improve oral-motor skills

Cognitive
- to improve imitation, understanding of spatial relationships, functional use of objects, concept development, and sequencing
- to develop generalization skills
- to develop recall skills

Language
- to improve following directions; taking turns; identifying/labeling objects, actions, people, and characteristics; initiating; and requesting

Social
- to make choices
- to facilitate peer interaction

Directions

Seat children appropriately for snack, using adaptive seating as needed. Tell them they are going to make "ants on a log." Give each child a section of banana. Help each child spread peanut butter on the banana and then stick some raisins in the peanut butter (these are the "ants"). Describe what they are doing, what the snack is make of, and what it looks like. Talk about how it reminds you of bugs. Encourage communication, including ways to request more or indicate "all done." Offer juice as needed. Assist with self-feeding and drinking skills as needed.

Week 4   Overall Theme: Vegetables

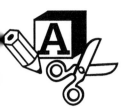

Activity 1: Obstacle Course

Materials

indoor climbing structure	indoor tunnel
inner tubes	carpet squares
ramp or other incline	benches
floor pillows/beanbag chairs	steps
bolsters	containers for vegetables (baskets would be best)
indoor swing	a variety of pretend vegetables
toddler slide	(for example, plastic, wooden, stuffed)

Goals

Sensory
- to provide proprioceptive stimulation
- to provide vestibular stimulation
- to increase visual attending
- to increase attention span

Gross Motor
- to improve balance, coordination, motor planning, locomotion, trunk rotation, and weight shifting

Fine Motor
- to improve using both hands together, reach and grasp, grasp and release, eye-hand coordination, and hand manipulation
- to increase upper body strength
- to improve shoulder girdle strength and stability

Cognitive
- to improve object permanence, imitation, problem solving, understanding of spatial relationships, classification, and concept development
- to develop generalization skills

Language
- to improve following directions; taking turns; identifying/labeling objects, actions, descriptions, and locations; requesting; and initiating

Social
- to make choices
- to facilitate pretend play
- to facilitate peer interaction

Directions

Using the equipment available, set up an indoor obstacle course to facilitate gross motor and vestibular goals for individuals in the group,. The materials listed above are just suggestions. Place the pretend vegetables at various points throughout the obstacle course. Have some hidden, some partially hidden, and some in plain sight.

Assist the children through the obstacle course. A "path" of carpet squares can provide a structure to follow through the course. Encourage the children to use appropriate motor patterns throughout. Help them find the vegetables as they go through the course. Be sure there are enough vegetables for each child to find at least two or three. Collect the vegetables in baskets or other containers. Depending on their abilities, children can be encouraged to carry their own baskets filled with vegetables.

Activity 2: Veggie Match

Materials

photos or pictures corresponding to the vegetables from the preceding activity

Goals

Sensory
- to increase attention span

Gross Motor
- to improve balance, coordination, weight shifting, and trunk rotation

Fine Motor
- to improve reach and grasp, grasp and release, visual attending and tracking, eye-hand coordination, and hand/finger manipulation

Cognitive
- to improve problem solving, picture-object association, imitation, classification, and concept development
- to develop generalization skills
- to develop recall skills

Language
- to improve following directions; taking turns; identifying/labeling objects, actions, locations, and relationships; initiating; and requesting

Social
- to make choices
- to facilitate peer interaction

Directions

Gather the children with their baskets of vegetables. Show them a picture of one of the vegetables and ask what it is. Have the children who have that vegetable in their baskets put the vegetable with the picture. Continue until all the vegetables have been "found" and identified.

Activity 3: Vegetable Soup

Materials

variety of vegetables	potholders
herbs for seasoning	spoon
water	chairs (adaptive seating as needed)
knife	table
cooking pot	washcloths for cleanup
stove	

Goals

Sensory
- to improve responses to sensory stimuli, especially tactile and olfactory
- to increase attention span

Fine Motor
- to improve using both hands together, grasp and release, hand/finger manipulation, and eye-hand coordination

Cognitive
- to improve functional object use, understanding of spatial relationships, functional use of objects, classification, sequencing, imitation, and concept development
- to develop generalization skills
- to develop recall skills

Language
- to improve following directions; imitation; identifying/labeling objects, actions, characteristics, and relationships; taking turns; initiating; and requesting

Social
- to make choices
- to facilitate peer interaction

Directions

Tell children they are going to help make vegetable soup. Show them the real vegetables and encourage the children to name the vegetables. Compare the real vegetables with the pretend vegetables from the previous activity. Have them help peel and chop the vegetables. Give each child some vegetable pieces to put into the pot. Show them the herbs. Encourage them to smell and even taste the herbs. Add water and put the pot on the stove to cook while completing the rest of the planned activities. Use lots of language to discuss the process, including the changes happening to the ingredients as they cook. How do they look, taste, feel, smell before cooking? After cooking?

Activity 4: Vegetable Prints

Materials

vegetables	knife
tempera paint	construction paper
paper plates, pie tins, or saucers	smocks
table	chairs (adaptive seating as needed)
washcloths for cleanup	

Goals

Sensory
- to improve sensory awareness and responsiveness
- to improve response to tactile stimulation

Fine Motor
- to improve reach and grasp, grasp and release, eye-hand coordination, hand manipulation skills, using both hands together, and midline skills
- to increase upper body strength
- to improve shoulder girdle strength and stability

Cognitive
- to improve sequencing, imitation, classification, and concept development
- to develop generalization skills
- to develop recall skills

Language
- to improve following directions; taking turns; identifying/labeling objects, actions, people, places, characteristics, and relationships; requesting; initiating; and increasing vocabulary

Social
- to make choices
- to facilitate peer interaction

Directions

Have children identify the vegetables as an adult cuts them in halves. Set up the activity on a small table. Seat children or let them work in standing, according to the needs of the group. Have children choose the color paper, the vegetable, and the color paint to use. Demonstrate dipping the vegetable in the paint and pressing it onto the paper to make a print. Assist the children with making their own prints. Talk about the feel of the paint and the vegetables, the colors being used, and the actions involved. Encourage children to trade vegetables and paint with each other.

Activity 5: Vegetable Garden

Materials

pictures of vegetables	scissors
brown paper	tape
glue	washcloths for cleanup

Goals

Sensory
- to improve responses to sensory stimulation
- to increase attention span

Gross Motor
- to improve weight bearing, weight shifting, trunk rotation, balance, and coordination

Fine Motor
- to improve hand/finger manipulation, eye-hand coordination, using two hands together, midline skills, reach and grasp, and grasp and release
- to increase upper body strength

Cognitive
- to improve classification, picture-object relationships, and concept development
- to develop generalization skills
- to develop recall skills

Language
- to improve following directions; taking turns; identifying/labeling objects, pictures, actions, and descriptions; initiating; and requesting

Social
- to make choices
- to facilitate peer interaction

Directions

Ahead of time, cut out a variety of pictures of vegetables. Tape a large piece of brown paper to the wall. Position it so the children can reach to the top if they extend their arms all the way. Have children select the vegetable pictures they want to use. Encourage them to identify or name the pictures and to say anything else they remember about the vegetable pictured. Help children squeeze or spread glue onto the paper. Help them pat their pictures into place. Let the pictures dry while completing another activity.

Snack

Materials

soup from Activity 3	bowls
spoons (adapted as needed)	napkins
juice	cups (adapted if necessary)
table	chairs (adaptive seating as needed)
washcloths for cleanup	

Goals

Sensory
- to improve responses to sensory stimuli, especially tactile and olfactory
- to increase attention span

Fine Motor
- to improve using both hands together, reach and grasp, grasp and release, hand/finger manipulation, and eye-hand coordination

Self-Help
- to improve self-feeding skills
- to improve oral-motor skills

Cognitive
- to improve tool use, understanding of spatial relationships, functional object use, concept development, and sequencing
- to develop generalization skills
- to develop recall skills

Language
- to improve following directions; imitation; identifying/labeling objects, actions, people, and characteristics; taking turns; initiating; and requesting

Social
- to make choices
- to facilitate peer interaction

Directions

Seat children appropriately for snack. Have them pass out napkins and spoons. Serve small quantities of the soup, possibly adding an ice cube to each bowl to cool it more quickly. Remind children about making the soup. How has it changed? How is it still the same? Provide assistance with self-feeding and oral motor skills as needed. Offer juice and provide assistance with drinking as needed.

Appendix A
Program Planning Resources

Books Related to Sample Activity Themes

Air/Wind

Baker, K. 1989. *The magic fan*. San Diego, CA: Harcourt Brace.

Ets, M. H. 1963. *Gilberto and the wind*. New York: Viking.

Hutchins, P. 1974. *The wind blew by*. New York: Macmillan.

Shaw, C. 1947. *It looked like spilt milk*. New York: Harper & Row.

Apples

Barrett, J. 1973. *An apple a day*. New York: Atheneum.

Bolliger, M. 1970. *The golden apple*. New York: Atheneum.

Brandenburg, F. 1973. *Fresh cider and apple pie*. New York: Macmillan.

Kellogg, S. 1988. *Johnny Appleseed*. New York: Morrow.

Rockwell, A. 1989. *Apples and pumpkins*. New York: Macmillan.

Autumn Leaves

Ehlert, L. 1991. *Red leaf, yellow leaf*. San Diego, CA: Harcourt Brace.

Lenski, L. 1948. *Now it's fall*. New York: H. Z. Walck.

Tresselt, A. 1948. *Johnny Maple Leaf*. New York: Lothrop.

Wheeler, C. 1982. *Marmalade's yellow leaf*. New York: Knopf.

Baby Animals

Brown, M. W. 1989. *Baby animals*. New York: Random House.

Buxton, J. 1986. *Baby bears and how they grow*. Washington, DC: National Geographic Society.

Dunbar, J. 1992. *Four fierce kittens*. New York: Scholastic.

Grunsell, A. 1983. *Baby animals*. New York: Franklin Watts.

McNaught, H. 1977. *Animal babies*. New York: Random House.

Molleson, D. 1993. *How ducklings grow*. New York: Scholastic.

Waddel, M. 1992. *Owl babies*. Cambridge, MA: Candlewick.

Beach

Brown, M. W. 1976. *The little island*. New York: Puffin.

Daniel, M. 1986. *A child's treasury of seaside verse*. New York: Dial.

De Brunhoff, L. 1969. *Babar at the seashore*. New York: Random House.

Dickens, L. 1991. *At the beach*. New York: Viking.

Florian, D. 1990. *Beach day*. New York: Greenwillow.

McClosky, R. 1952. *One morning in Maine*. New York: Viking Penguin.

McMillan, B. 1990. *One sun*. New York: Holiday House.

Zolotov, C. 1992. *The seashore book*. New York: Harper Collins.

Bird Feeders

Cox, R. K., and B. Cox. 1980. *Usborne first nature birds*. London: Usborne.

Kuchalla, S. 1982. *Now I know birds*. Mahwah, NJ: Troll Associates.

Martchenko, M. 1990. *Bird feeder banquet*. Buffalo, NY: Firefly.

Rose, G. 1987. *The bird garden*. New York: Salem House.

Blue

Hoban, T. 1978. *Is it red? Is it yellow? Is it blue?* New York: Greenwillow.

Lionni, L. 1959. *Little blue, little yellow*. New York: Obolensky.

Lobel, A. 1968. *The great blueness and other predicaments*. New York: Harper.

McClosky, R. 1989. *Blueberries for Sal*. New York: Puffin.

Wolff, R. J. 1968. *Feeling blue*. New York: Scribner's.

Boats

Allen, P. 1982. *Who sank the boat?* New York: Coward-McCann.

Flack, M. 1991. *The boats on the river*. New York: Viking.

Gramatley, H. 1939. *Little Toot*. New York: Putnam.

Spier, P. 1977. *Noah's ark*. New York: Doubleday.

Bubbles and Balls

Kellogg, S. 1978. *The mystery of the magic green ball*. New York: Dial.

Tafuri, N. 1989. *The ball bounced.* New York: Greenwillow.

Wood, A. 1985. *King Bidgood's in the bathtub.* San Diego: Harcourt Brace.

Bugs

Aylesworth, J. 1992. *Old black fly.* New York: Holt.

Cameron, P. 1961. *I can't, said the ant.* New York: Putnam.

Carle, E. 1977. *The grouchy ladybug.* New York: Crowell.

Carle, E. 1990. *The very quiet cricket.* New York: Philomel.

Conklin, G. 1962. *We like bugs.* New York: Holiday House.

Kilpatrick, C. *Usborne first nature creepy crawlies.* London: Usborne.

Wildsmith, B., and R. Wildsmith. 1993. *Look closer.* San Diego: Gulliver.

Camping

Brown, R. 1992. *The picnic.* New York: Dutton.

Mayer, M. 1977. *Just me and my dad.* New York: Western.

Romanova, N. 1985. *Once there was a tree.* New York: Dial.

Ward, L. 1958. *The biggest bear.* Boston: Houghton-Mifflin.

Corn

Asch, F. 1979. *Popcorn.* New York: Parent's Magazine Press.

Brock, E. L. 1967. *Johnny cake.* New York: Putnam's.

De Paola, T. 1978. *The popcorn book.* New York: Holiday House.

Low, A. 1993. *The popcorn shop.* New York: Scholastic.

Eggs

Eastman, P. D. 1985. *Flap your wings.* New York: Random House.

Heller, R. 1981. *Chickens aren't the only ones.* New York: Grosset and Dunlap.

Jeunesse, G., and P. de Bourgoing. *The egg: A 1st discovery book.* Broadway, NY: Scholastic.

Peppe, R. 1976. *Humpty Dumpty.* New York: Viking.

Polacco, P. 1988. *Rechenka's eggs.* New York: Philomel.

Selsam, M. 1984. *A first look at birds' nests.* New York: Walker.

Weiss, N. 1990. *An egg is an egg.* New York: Putnam.

Families

Fox, M. 1989. *Loala Lou.* San Diego: Harcourt Brace.

Guarino, D. 1989. *Is your mama a llama?* New York: Scholastic.

Hines, A. G. 1989. *Big like me.* New York: Greenwillow.

Joosse, B. 1991. *Mama, do you love me?* San Francisco: Chronicle.

Rylant, C. 1985. *The relatives came.* New York: Bradbury.

Farm

Azarian, M. 1981. *A farmer's alphabet.* Boston: D. Godine.

Hutchins, P. 1968. *Rosie's walk.* New York: Macmillan.

Lindbergh, R. 1987. *The midnight farm.* New York: Dial.

Noble, T. H. 1980. *The day Jimmy's boa ate the wash.* New York: Dial.

Parkinson, K. 1988. *The farmer in the dell.* Niles, IL: Albert Whitman.

Rae, M. M. 1988. *The farmer in the dell.* New York: Viking Kestrel.

Shone, V. 1992. *Cock-a-doodle-do: A day on the farm.* New York: Scholastic.

Feet

Aliki. 1990. *My feet.* New York: Crowell.

Dr. Seuss. 1968. *The foot book.* New York: Random House.

Hamm, D. J. 1991. *How many feet in the bed?* New York: Simon & Schuster.

Hughes, S. 1982. *Alfie's feet.* New York: Lothrop, Lee & Shepard.

Winthrop, E. 1986. *Shoes.* New York: Harper & Row.

Fire Trucks

Brown, M. W. 1938. *The little fireman.* New York: Harper-Collins.

Maass, R. 1989. *Firefighters.* New York: Scholastic.

Rey, M., and H. A. Rey. 1988. *Curious George at the fire station.* Boston: Houghton Mifflin.

Rockwell, A. 1986. *Fire engines.* New York: Dutton.

Fishing

Asch, F. 1985. *Bear shadow.* Englewood Cliffs, NJ: Prentice Hall.

Clements, A., and A. C. Yoshi. 1988. *Big Al.* Saxonville, MA: Picture Book Studio.

Keats, E. J. 1971. *Over in the meadow.* New York: Four Winds.

Langstaff, J. 1957. *Over in the meadow.* San Diego, CA: Harcourt Brace.

Pfister, M. 1992. *The rainbow fish.* New York: North-South.

Flowers

Brook, L. 1903. *Johnny Crow's garden.* New York: Warner.

Carle, E. 1991. *The tiny seed.* Natico, MA: Picture Book Studio.

Cristin, E. 1991. *In my garden.* Natico, MA: Picture Book Studio.

Ehlert, L. 1992. *Planting a rainbow.* San Diego: Harcourt Brace.

Lewis, R. 1965. *In a spring garden* (haiku). Natico, MA: Picture Book Studio.

Lobel, A. 1984. *The rose in my garden.* New York: Greenwillow.

Flying

Crews, D. 1986. *Flying*. New York: Greenwillow.

Ichikawa, S. 1991. *Nora's duck*. New York: Philomel.

McClosky, R. 1941. *Make way for ducklings*. New York: Viking.

Maris, R. 1986. *I wish I could fly*. New York: Greenwillow.

Mayer, M. 1971. *Me and my flying machine*. New York: Parent's Magazine Press.

Oppenheim, J. 1968. *Have you seen birds?* New York: Scholastic.

Rockwell, A. 1985. *Planes*. New York: Dutton.

Friends

Cohen, M. 1967. *Will I have a friend?* New York: Macmillan.

Delacre, L. 1989. *Time for school, Nathan*. New York: Scholastic.

Lionni, L. 1963. *Swimmy*. New York: Knopf Pantheon.

Wilhelm, H. 1985. *Let's be friends again*. New York: Crown.

Gingerbread House

Galdone, P. 1983. *The gingerbread boy*. Boston: Clarion.

Hunia, F. *Read it yourself Hansel and Gretel*. England: Lady Bird.

Schmidt, K. 1985. *The gingerbread man*. New York: Scholastic.

Zelinsky, P. O. 1985. *Grimm Hansel and Gretel*. New York: Putnam.

Green

Birnbaum, A. 1953. *Green eyes*. New York: Western.

Buckley, R. 1993. *The greedy python*. Natico, MA: Picture Book Studio.

Dr. Seuss. 1960. *Green eggs and ham*. New York: Random House.

Emberley, E. 1992. *Go away big green monster*. Boston: Little Brown.

Grocery Store

Grossman, B. 1989. *Tommy at the grocery store*. New York: Harper & Row.

Hutchins, P. 1976. *Don't forget the bacon*. New York: Greenwillow.

Lobel, A., and A. Lobel. 1981. *On Market Street*. New York: Greenwillow.

Rockwell, A., and H. Rockwell. 1979. *The supermarket*. New York: Macmillan.

Schotter, R. 1993. *A fruit and vegetable man*. Boston: Little Brown.

Spier, P. 1981. *Food market*. New York: Doubleday.

Hands

Brown, M. 1985. *Hand rhymes*. New York: Dutton.

Flores, A. 1987. *From the hands of a child*. Belmont, CA: David S. Lake.

Hayes, S., and T. Goffe. 1988. *Clap your hands*. New York: Lothrop, Lee & Shepard.

Okenbury, H. 1987. *Clap hands*. London: Walker.

Perkins, A. 1969. *Hand, hand, finger, thumb*. New York: Random House.

Wood, A., and D. Wood. 1991. *Piggies*. San Diego, CA: Harcourt Brace.

Ice Cream Social

Armitage, R. 1981. *Ice creams for Rosie*. New York: Elsevier-Dutton.

Rey, M., and A. Shalleck. 1989. *Curious George goes to the ice cream shop*. Boston: Houghton Mifflin.

Testa, F. 1979. *The land where ice cream grows*. New York: Doubleday.

Kites

Cooper, K. K. 1969. *The fish from Japan*. San Diego: Harcourt Brace.

Cousins, L. 1992. *Kite in the park*. Cambridge, MA: Candlewick.

Packard, M. 1990. *The kite*. Oakland, CA: Children's Press.

Peet, B. 1974. *Merle, the high flying squirrel*. Boston: Houghton Mifflin.

Wiese, K. 1948. *Fish in the air*. New York: Viking.

Lights

Asch, F. 1982. *Happy birthday moon*. Englewood Cliffs, NJ: Prentice Hall.

Brown, M. W. 1947. *Goodnight moon*. New York: Harper & Row.

Crews, D. 1981. *Light*. New York: Greenwillow.

Mittens

Brett, J. 1989. *The mitten*. New York: Putnam.

Marzollo, J. 1986. *The three little kittens*. New York: Scholastic.

Nertzel, S. 1989. *The jacket I wear in the snow*. New York: Greenwillow.

Tresselt, A. 1964. *The mitten*. New York: Lothrop, Lee & Shepard.

Multisensory Carnival

Aliki. 1962. *My five senses*. New York: Thomas Y. Crowell.

Carlstron, N. W. 1962. *Jesse bear, what will you wear?* New York: Macmillan.

Rey, M., and A. Shalleck. 1986. *Curious George goes to a costume party*. Boston: Houghton Mifflin.

Vaughn. M. K. 1985. *Wombat stew*. Morristown, NJ: Silver Burdett Press.

Music

Lionni, L. 1979. *Geraldine the music mouse*. New York: Pantheon.

McCloskey, R. 1940. *Lentil.* New York: Viking.

Sinclair, J. 1985. *The Mother Goose songbook.* New York: Derry Dale.

Webb, J. L. 1888. *The Mother Goose songbook.* New York: Cassell.

Williams, V. 1984. *Music, music for everyone.* New York: Greenwillow.

Orange
Macquire, R. 1993. *The orange book.* New York: Universe.

Miller, I. P., and K. Howard. 1979. *Do you know colors?* New York: Random House.

O'Neill, M. 1989. *Hailstones and halibut bones.* New York: Doubleday.

Rogow, Z. 1988. *Oranges.* New York: F. Watts.

Over the River and through the Woods
Child, L. M. 1974. *Over the river and through the woods.* New York: Coward, McCann and Geoghegan.

Hutchins, P. 1986. *The doorbell rang.* New York: Greenwillow.

Wood, A. 1984. *The napping house.* San Diego: Harcourt Brace.

Parade
Crews, D. 1983. *Parade.* New York: Greenwillow.

Emberley, E. 1962. *The parade book.* Boston: Little Brown.

Kroll, S. 1983. *The goat parade.* New York: Parents.

Lasky, K. 1991. *Fourth of July bear.* New York: Morrow.

Sage, J. 1991. *The little band.* New York: Margaret K. McElderry Books.

Spier, P. 1972. *Crash! bang! boom!* New York: Doubleday.

Pets
Carle, E. 1987. *Have you seen my cat?* Natico, MA: Picture Book Studio.

James, B. 1991. *He wakes me.* New York: Orchard.

Kellogg, S. 1971. *Can I keep him?* New York: Dial.

McPhail, D. 1985. *Emma's pet.* New York: Dutton.

Pumpkins
Greene, E. 1970. *The pumpkin giant.* New York: Lothrop.

Hellinsig, L. 1976. *The wonderful pumpkin.* New York: Atheneum.

Hoban, T. 1988. *Look! look! look!* New York: Greenwillow.

Kroll, S. 1984. *The biggest pumpkin ever.* New York: Holiday House.

Miller, E. 1990. *Mousekin's golden house.* New York: S & S Trade.

Red
Birdwell, N. 1988. *Clifford, the big red dog.* New York: Scholastic.

Bradbury, L. 1992. *Shapes and colors.* Auburn, ME: Ladybird.

Brown, M. W. 1989. *Big red barn.* New York: Harper & Row.

Galdone, P. 1973. *The little red hen.* New York: Seabury.

Galdone, P. 1974. *Little Red Riding Hood.* New York: McGraw-Hill.

Marshall, J. 1987. *Red Riding Hood.* New York: Dial.

Martin, B. 1967. *Brown bear, brown bear, what do you see?* New York: Holt Rinehart and Winston.

Zemach, M. 1983. *The little red hen.* New York: Farrar, Straus and Giroux.

Snow
Hader, B. H. 1948. *The big snow.* New York: Macmillan.

Keats, E. J. 1962. *The snowy day.* New York: Viking.

Keller, H. 1988. *Geraldine's big snow.* New York: Greenwillow.

Littledale, F. 1989. *Snow child.* New York: Scholastic.

Nertzel, S. 1989. *The jacket I wear in the snow.* New York: Greenwillow.

Rockwell, A., and H. Rockwell. 1962. *The first snowfall.* New York: Macmillan.

Tresselt, A. 1947. *White snow, bright snow.* New York: Lothrop, Lee & Shepard.

Summer Clothes
Carlstrom, N. W. 1986. *Jesse Bear, what will you wear?* New York: Macmillan.

Freeman, D. 1978. *A pocket for Corduroy.* New York: Viking.

Neitzel, S. 1992. *The dress I'll wear to the party.* New York: Greenwillow.

Sunshine
Asch, F. 1985. *Bear shadow.* New York: Prentice Hall.

Asch, F. 1988. *Skyfire.* New York: S & S Trade.

Belting, N. M. 1962. *The sun is a golden earring.* New York: Holt.

Dayrell, E. 1968. *Why the sun and the moon live in the sky: An African folktale.* Boston: Houghton-Mifflin.

Goudey, A. 1961. *The day we saw the sun come up.* New York: Scribner.

McDermott, G. 1974. *Arrow to the sun.* New York: Viking.

Tresselt, A. 1991. *Sun up.* New York: Lothrop, Lee & Shepard.

Toys
Crews, D. 1978. *Freight train.* New York: Greenwillow.

Kroll, S. 1983. *Toot! toot!* New York: Holiday House.

Manushkin, F. 1992. *The best toy of all.* New York: Dutton.

Williams, K. L. 1990. *Galimoto.* New York: Lothrop, Lee & Shepard.

Turkey

Balian, L. 1973. *Sometimes it's turkey, sometimes it's feathers.* Nashville: Abingdon.

Kroll, S. 1982. *One tough turkey.* New York: Holiday House.

Schatell, B. 1982. *Farmer Goff and his turkey Sam.* New York: Lippincott.

Wickstrom, S. 1990. *Turkey on the loose!* New York: Dial.

Vegetables

Ehlert, L. 1987. *Growing vegetable soup.* San Diego: Harcourt Brace.

Krauss, R. 1945. *The carrot seed.* New York: Harper & Row.

Rylant, C. 1984. *The year's garden.* Scarsdale, NY: Bradbury Press.

Sharmat, M. 1980. *Gregory the terrible eater.* New York: Scholastic.

Sobol, H. L. 1984. *A book of vegetables.* New York: Putnam.

Steele, M. 1989. *Anna's garden songs.* New York: Greenwillow.

Washing

Preston, E. M. 1969. *The temper tantrum book.* New York: Viking.

Rey, H. A. 1987. *Curious George at the laundromat.* Boston: Houghton-Mifflin.

Sutherland, H. A. 1988. *Dad's car wash.* New York: Atheneum.

Wood, A. 1985. *King Bidgood's in the bathtub.* San Diego: Harcourt Brace.

Water Carnival

Hughes, S. 1985. *Bathwater's hot.* New York: Lothrop, Lee & Shepard.

Leutscher, A. 1983. *Water.* New York: Dial.

McMillan, B. 1988. *Dry or wet?* New York: Lothrop, Lee & Shepard.

McPhail, D. 1984. *Andrew's bath.* Boston: Little Brown.

Peters, L. W. 1991. *Water's way.* New York: Arcade.

Pollock, P. 1985. *Water is wet.* New York: Putnam.

Who Am I?

Aliki. 1984. *Feelings.* New York: Greenwillow.

Carlson, N. 1988. *I like me.* New York: Viking.

Tangvald, C. H. 1985. *Me, myself, and I.* Elgin, IL: Chariot.

Waber, B. 1966. *You look ridiculous, said the rhinoceros to the hippopotamus.* Boston: Houghton Mifflin.

Winter

Burstein, F. 1989. *Anna's rain.* New York: Orchard.

Carlstrom, N. W. 1991. *Goodby geese.* New York: Philomel.

De Paola, T. 1982. *Charlie needs a cloak.* New York: Simon & Schuster.

Marzollo, J. 1993. *Happy birthday, Dr. Martin Luther King.* New York: Scholastic.

Munsch, R. 1985. *Thomas' snowsuit.* Toronto: Annick.

Yolen, J. 1988. *Owl moon.* New York: Philomel.

Ziefert, H. 1986. *A new coat for Anna.* New York: Knopf.

Books for Use throughout the Year

Ahlberg, J., and A. Ahlberg. 1979. *Each peach, pear, plum.* New York: Viking Kestrel.

Bowker, R. R. 1993. *A to zoo: Subject access to children's books* 4th ed. New Providence, NJ: Reed Reference.

First Discovery Series (excellent sources for nature information for children). New York: Scholastic. (Titles in the series include: *Airplanes & flying machines; Bears; Cats; Colors; The earth & sky; The egg; Fruit; The ladybug & other insects; The tree; Weather.*)

Lionni, L. 1992. *A busy year.* New York: Knopf.

McPhail, D. 1988. *Animals A to Z.* New York: Scholastic.

Sendak, M. 1962. *Chicken soup with rice.* HarperCollins.

Stevenson, R. L. 1946. *A child's garden of verses.* Chicago: World Book.

Tafuri, N. 1983. *All year long.* New York: Greenwillow.

Updike, J. 1965. *A child's calendar.* New York: Knopf.

Activity and Activity-Based Intervention Books

Adcock, D., and M. Segal. *Play together, grow together: A cooperative curriculum for teachers of young children.* Beltsville, MD: Gryphon House.

Atack, M. S. 1986. *Art activities for the handicapped.* Englewood Cliffs, NJ: Prentice Hall.

Barclay, K., and K. Buch. 1985. *Month by month: Language enrichment activities for early learning.* Tucson, AZ: Communication Skill Builders.

Bricker, D., and J. Cripe. 1992. *An activity-based approach to early intervention.* Baltimore: Paul H. Brookes.

Burtt, K. G., and K. Kalkstein. 1981. *Smart toys for babies from birth to two.* New York: Harper Colophon.

Cahoun, M., T. Rose, and D. Prendergast. 1991. *Charlotte Circle intervention guide for parent-child interactions.* Tucson, AZ: Communication Skill Builders.

Colgin, M. L. 1982. *One potato, two potato, three potato, four: 165 chants for children.* Beltsville, MD: Gryphon House.

Connolly, A. M., and H. Gibson. 1990. *Rainy day activities for preschoolers*. Beltsville, MD: Gryphon House.

Cromwell, L., D. Hibner, and J. Faitel. 1976. *Finger frolics: Fingerplays for young children*. Livonia, MI: Partner.

Cunningham, C., and P. Sloper. 1978. *Helping your exceptional baby*. New York: Pantheon.

Einon, D. 1985. *Play with a purpose: Learning games for children 6 weeks to 2-3 years old*. New York: St. Martin's.

Fewell, R. R., and P. F. Vasady. 1983. *Learning through play*. Hingham, MA: Teaching Resources.

Goldberg, S. 1981. *Teaching with toys*. Ann Arbor: University of Michigan Press.

Gordon, I. J. 1970. *Baby learning through baby play: A parent's guide for the first two years*. New York: St. Martin's Press.

Gordon, I. J., B. Guinagh, and J. E. Jester. 1972. *Child learning through child play: Learning activities for two and three year olds*. New York: St. Martin's Press.

Granovetter, R., and J. James. *Shift and shout: Sand play activities for children ages 1-6*. Beltsville, MD: Gryphon House.

Graves, M. 1989. *The teacher's idea book: Daily planning around the key experiences*. Ypsilanti, MI: The High/Scope Press.

Hagstrom, J., and J. Morrill. 1981. *Games babies play and more games babies play*. New York: Pocket.

Hill, D. M. 1977. *Mud, sand, and water*. Washington, DC: National Association for the Education of Young Children.

Hirsch, E., ed. 1984. *The block book*. Washington, DC: National Association for the Education of Young Children.

Honig, A. 1982. *Playtime learning games*. Syracuse, NY: Syracuse University Press.

Johnston, E. B., B. D. Weinrich, and A. R. Johnson. 1984. *A sourcebook of pragmatic activities*. Tucson, AZ: Communication Skill Builders.

Lasky, L., and R. Mukerji. 1980. *Art: Basic for young children*. Washington, DC: National Association for the Education of Young Children.

Linder, T. W. 1993. *Transdisciplinary play-based intervention: A guide for developing a meaningful curriculum for young children*. Baltimore: Paul H. Brookes.

Lynch-Fraser, D. 1982. *Danceplay: Creative movement for very young children*. New York: Walker.

Marsallo, M., and D. Vacante. 1983. *Adapted games and developmental motor activities for children*. Annandale, VA: self-published.

McCord, S. 1993. *A storybook journey: Pathways to literacy through life and play experiences*. Englewood, CO: Teacher Ideas Press.

Miller, K. 1984. *More things to do with toddlers and twos*. Beltsville, MD: Gryphon House.

Millnard, J., and P. Behrmann. 1979. *Parents as playmates: A games approach to the preschool years*. New York: Human Sciences.

Moyer, I. D. 1983. *Responding to infants*. Minneapolis, MN: T. S. Denison.

Peyton, J. L. 1986. *Puppetools*. Richmond, VA: Prescott, Durrell.

Raines, S., and R. Casady. 1991. *More story stretchers: More activities to expand children's favorite books*. Beltsville, MD: Gryphon House.

Reidlich, C. E., and M. E. Herzfeld. 1983. *Zero to three years: An early language curriculum*. Moline, IL: LinguiSystems.

Schrank, R. *Toddlers learn by doing*. Atlanta, GA: Humanics.

Schwartz, S., and J. E. H. Miller. 1988. *The language of toys: Teaching communication skills to special-needs children*. Rockville, MD: Woodbine House.

Segal, M. 1983. *Your child at play: Birth to one year*. New York: Newmarket.

Segal, M., and D. Adcock. 1985. *Your child at play: Birth to two years*. New York: Newmarket.

Shea, J. F. 1986. *No bored babies: A guide for making developmental toys for babies birth to age two*. Beltsville, MD: Gryphon House.

Sherwood, E., R. A. Williams, and R. E. Rockwell. 1990. *More mudpies to magnets: Science for young children*. Beltsville, MD: Gryphon House.

Shiller, P., and J. Rossano. 1990. *The instant curriculum: 500 developmentally appropriate learning activities for busy teachers of young children*. Beltsville, MD: Gryphon House.

Siegling, L. S., and M. Click. 1984. *At arm's length: Goals for arm and hand function*. Mesa, AZ: EdCorp.

Sobut, M., and B. Bogen. 1991. *Complete early childhood curriculum resource*. Englewood Cliffs, NJ: Center for Applied Research in Education.

Sparling, J. 1984. *Learning games for the first three years*. New York: Walker.

Sperry, V. B. 1973. *Of course I can: Sourcebook of language activities*. Palo Alto, CA: Consulting Psychologists Press.

Sullivan, M. 1982. *Feeling strong, feeling free: Movement exploration for young children*. Washington, DC: National Association for the Education of Young Children.

Weiss, D. 1990. *Goal oriented gross and fine motor lesson plans*. Palo Alto, CA: Vort.

Weissman, J. 1988. *Games to play with babies*. Beltsville, MD: Gryphon House.

_____. 1983. *Songs to sing with babies*. Beltsville, MD: Gryphon House.

Wilmes, L., and D. Wilmes. 1989. *Yearful of circle times*. Elgin, IL: Building Blocks.

Wirth, M. J. 1976. *Teacher's handbook of children's games: A guide to developing perceptual-motor skills*. West Nyack, NY: Parker.

Witt, B., and M. Klein. 1990. *PREPARE: An interdisciplinary approach to perceptual-motor readiness*. Tucson, AZ: Communication Skill Builders.

Worthley, W. J. 1978. *Sourcebook of language learning activities*. Boston, MA: Little, Brown.

Early Intervention Curricula

*Carolina Curriculum for Preschoolers
with Special Needs*
Publisher: Paul H. Brookes
P.O. Box 10624
Baltimore, MD 21285

*Carolina Curriculum for Infants and Toddlers with
Special Needs, Second Edition*
Publisher: Paul H. Brookes
P.O. Box 10624
Baltimore, MD 21285

*Developmental Programming for
Infants and Young Children*
Publisher: University of Michigan Press
839 Greene Street
Ann Arbor, MI 48109

*Early Learning Accomplishments
Profile and Activities*
Publisher: Kaplan Press
P.O. Box 5128
Winston-Salem, NC 27113

Hawaii Early Learning Profile (HELP) and Activities
Publisher: Vort Corporation
P.O. Box 60880
Palo Alto, CA 94306

Portage Guide to Early Education
Publisher: Portage Project
CESA 5, Box 564
412 East Slifer Street
Portage, WI 53901

Small Wonder
Publisher: American Guidance Service
Publisher's Building
P.O. Box 99
Circle Pines, MN 55014

Resources on Cultural Competence

Books and Journal Articles

Beginning Equal Project. 1983. *Beginning equal: A manual about non-sexist childrearing for infants and toddlers.* New York: Women's Action Alliance and Pre-School Association.

CWLA cultural competence self-assessment instrument. 1993. Washington, DC: Child Welfare League of America.

Council on Interracial Books for Children. 1980. *Guidelines for selecting bias-free textbooks and storybooks.* New York: Council on Interracial Books for Children.

Derman-Sparks, L., and the ABC Task Force. 1989. *Anti-bias curriculum: Tools for empowering young children.* Washington, DC: National Association for the Education of Young Children.

Jones, E., and L. Derman-Sparks. 1992. Meeting the challenge of diversity. *Young Children* 47(2):12-18.

Lynch, E. W., and M. J. Hanson. 1992. *Developing cross-cultural competence: A guide for working with young children and their families.* Baltimore, MD: Paul H. Brookes.

Miller, D. 1989. *First steps: Socialization in infant/toddler day care.* Washington, DC: Child Welfare League of America.

Neugebauer, B., ed. 1987. *Alike and different: Exploring our humanity with young children.* Redmond, WA: Exchange.

Saracho, O., and B. Spodek, eds. *Understanding the multicultural experience in early childhood education.* Washington, DC: National Association for the Education of Young Children.

Schniedewing, N., and E. Davidson. 1983. *Open minds to equity: A sourcebook of learning activities to promote race, sex, class and age equity.* Englewood Cliffs, NJ: Prentice Hall.

Shannon-Thornberry, M. 1982. *The alternative celebrations catalogue.* New York: Pilgrim.

Sprung, B. 1978. *Perspectives on non-sexist early childhood education.* New York: Teacher's College Press.

Materials
Multicultural materials are available from the following companies and organizations.

Afro-American Publishing Company
819 S. Wabash Avenue
Chicago, IL 60605

American Indian Resource Center
6518 Miles Avenue
Huntington Park, CA 90255

Bilingual Educational Services, Inc.
2514 S. Grand Avenue
Los Angeles, CA 90007

Children's Book Press
5925 Doyle Street, Suite U
Emeryville, CA 94608

Claudia's Caravan
P.O. Box 1582
Alameda, CA 94501

Cross Cultural Communication Centre
965 Bloor Street West
Toronto, Ontario, Canada M6H1L7

Council on Interracial Books for Children
1841 Broadway
New York, NY 10023

Educational Equity Concepts
114 E. 32nd St.
New York, NY 10016

Educational Materials, Inc.
6503 Salizar Street
San Diego, CA 92111

Faces: The Magazine About People
Cobblestone Publishing
20 Grove Street
Peterborough, NH 03458

Global Village Toys
2210 Wilshire Blvd., Suite 262
Santa Monica, CA 90403

Multicultural Project for Communication and Education
86 Lincoln Street
Boston, MA 02111

Navajo Curriculum Center Press
Rough Rock Demonstration School
P.O. Box 217
Chinle, AZ 86503

Syracuse Cultural Workers
Box 6367
Syracuse, NY 13217

United Indians of All Tribes Foundation
Community Educational Services
Discover Park
P.O. Box 99100
Seattle, WA 98199

University Bookstore
4326 University Way
Seattle, WA 89105

Resources Addressing Physical Challenges

Bly, L. 1983. *The components of normal movement during the first year of life and abnormal motor development.* Birmingham, AL: Pittenger and Associates.

Brinson, C. L. 1982. *The helping hand: A manual describing methods for handling the young child with cerebral palsy.* Charlottesville, VA: Children's Rehabilitation Center, University of Virginia.

Coling, M. C. 1991. *Developing integrated programs: A transdisciplinary approach for early intervention.* Tucson, AZ: Therapy Skill Builders.

Connor, F., G. Williamson, and J. Siepp. 1978. *Program guide for infants and toddlers with neuromotor and other developmental disabilities.* New York: Teacher's College Press.

Finnie, N. 1975. *Handling the young cerebral palsied child at home.* New York: Dutton.

Fraser, B. A., and R. N. Hensinger. 1983. *Managing physical handicaps: A practical guide for parents, care providers, and educators.* Baltimore: Paul H. Brookes.

Hanson, M. J., and S. R. Harris. 1986. *Teaching the young child with motor delays.* Austin, TX: ProEd.

Jaeger, L. 1987. *Home program instruction sheets for infants and young children.* Tucson, AZ: Therapy Skill Builders.

Levine, K. 1991. *Fine motor dysfunction: Therapeutic strategies in the classroom.* Tucson, AZ: Therapy Skill Builders.

Wright, C., and M. Nomura. 1985. *From toys to computers: Access for the physically disabled child.* San Jose, CA: Christine Wright.

Resources on Planning Environments

Coates, G. ed. 1974. *Alternative learning environments.* Stroudsburg, PA: Dowden, Hutchinson and Ross.

Greenman, J. 1988. *Caring spaces, learning places: Children's environments that work.* Beltsville, MD: Gryphon House.

Harmes, T., D. Cryer, and R. M. Clifford. 1990. *Infant/toddler environment rating scale.* New York: Teacher's College Press.

McEvoy, M. A., J. J. Fox, and M. S. Rosenberg. 1991. Organizing preschool environments: Suggestions for enhancing the development/learning of preschool children with handicaps. *Topics in Early Childhood Special Education* 11:18-20.

Shea, V., and M. Mount. 1982. *How to arrange the environment to stimulate and teach pre-language skills in the severely handicapped.* Lawrence, KS: H and H Enterprises.

Smith, J. 1980. *Play environments for movement experience.* Springfield, IL: Charles C. Thomas.

Vergeront, J. 1987. *Places and spaces for preschool and primary (indoors).* Washington, DC: National Association for the Education of Young Children.

Appendix B
Technology Resources

Sources for Switches and Battery-Operated Toys

The Able Child
325 West 11 Street
New York, NY 10014

AbleNet, Access Ability, Inc.
1081 10th Avenue South East
Minneapolis, MN 55414
(800) 322-0956

Adaptive Communication Systems, Inc.
Box 12440
Pittsburgh, PA 15231
(800) 247-3433

Don Johnston Developmental Equipment, Inc.
P.O. Box 639
1000 North Rand Road, Bldg. 115
Waconda, IL 60084
(312) 526-2682

Dunamis, Inc.
3620 Highway 317
Suwanne, GA 30174
(800) 828-2243

Linda Burkhart
8503 Rhode Island Avenue
College Park, MD 20740

Pretke Romich Company
1022 Heyl Road
Wooster, OH 44691

Steven Kanor, Ph.D., Inc.
Toys for Special Children
385 Warburton Avenue
Hastings, NY 10706
(914) 478-0960

Sunburst Communications
39 Washington Avenue
Pleasantville, NY 10570

Zygo Industries, Inc.
P.O. Box 1008
Portland, OR 97207

Sources for Software

Don Johnston Developmental Equipment, Inc.
P.O. Box 639
1000 North Rand Road, Bldg. 115
Waconda, IL 60084
(312) 526-2682

Dunamis, Inc.
3620 Highway 317
Suwanne, GA 30174
(800) 828-2243

Edmark
P.O. Box 3218
Redmond, WA 98073-3218
(206) 556-8400

Exceptional Children's Software
P.O. Box 4758
Overland Park, KS 66204

Mindscape Software
3444 Dundee Road
Northbrook, IL 60062

Sunburst Communications
39 Washington Avenue
Pleasantville, NY 10570

UCLA/LAUSD Microcomputer Software
1000 Veterans Avenue, Room 23-10
Los Angeles, CA 90024

Augmentative Communication Organizations

Activating Children Through Technology
Macomb Projects
27 Horrabin Hall
Western Illinois University
Macomb, IL 61455

Adaptive Communications Systems, Inc.
354 Hookstown Grade Road
Clinton, PA 15206

Closing the Gap
P.O. Box 68
Henderson, MN 56044

Easter Seals Communication Institute
24 Ferrand
Ontario M3C 3N2, Canada

Enabling Technologies Co.
3102 S.E. Jay Street
Stuart, FL 34997

Gallaudet University
P.O. Box 300
Washington, DC 20002

Helen Keller National Center
112 Middle Neck Road
Sands Point, NY 11050-1299

Innotek
Division of National Lekotek Center
2100 Ridge Ave.
Evanston, IL 60201

Books and Articles

Activating children through technology (ACTT). 1993. Macomb, IL: Macomb Projects, College of Education, Western Illinois University.

Beatty, J. J., and W. H. Tucker. 1987. *The computer as a paintbrush: Creative uses for the personal computer in the preschool classroom.* Columbus, OH: Merrill.

Behrmann, M. M., J. K. Jones, and M. Wilds. 1989. Technology intervention for very young children with disabilities. *Infants and Young Children* 1(4):66-77.

Blackstone, S. W. 1989. *Augmentative communication: Implementation strategies.* Bethesda, MD: American Speech-Language-Hearing Association.

Bowman, B. T. 1983. *Do microcomputers have a place in preschools?* ERIC Document Reproduction Service ED231 504.

Brady, E. H., and S. Hill. 1984. Young children and microcomputers: Research issues and directions. *Young Children* 39(3):12-22.

Brinker, R. P., and M. Lewis. 1982. Making the world work with microcomputers: A learning prosthesis for handicapped infants. *Exceptional Children* 49(2):163-70.

Budoff, M., J. Thormann, and A. Gras. 1985. *Microcomputers in special education.* Cambridge, MA: Brookline.

Burkhart, L. 1980. *Homemade battery powered toys and educational devices for severely handicapped children.* College Park, MD: self-published.

_____. 1982. *More homemade battery devices for severely handicapped children with suggested activities.* College Park, MD: self-published.

Clements, D. H. 1985. *Computers in early and primary education.* Englewood Cliffs, NJ: Prentice Hall.

Clements, D., B. Natasi, and S. Swaminathan. 1993. Young children and computers: Crossroads and directions from research. *Young Child* 48(2):56-64.

Computer use for special needs children: An instructional guide for families and professionals. 1993. Los Angeles, CA: Los Angeles Unified School District/UCLA Intervention Program.

Cuffaro, H. K. 1985. Microcomputers in education: Why is earlier better? In *The computer in education: A critical perspective,* edited by D. Sloan. New York: Teacher's College Press.

Davidson, J. 1988. Computers for preschoolers? *Pre-K Today* 2(5):28-29.

Edyburn, D., and M. Lartz. 1988. The teacher's role in the use of computers in early childhood education. *Journal of the Division for Early Childhood* 10(3):255-63.

Fallon, M. A., and J. A. S. Wann. 1994. Incorporating computer technology into activity-based thematic units for young children with disabilities. *Infants and Young Children* 6(4):64-69.

Fazlo, B. B., and H. J. Rieth. 1988. Characteristics of preschool handicapped children's microcomputer use during free-choice periods. *Journal of the Division for Early Childhood* 10(3):247-54. ERIC Document Reproduction Service No. ED 234 898.

Lewis, R. B. 1993. *Special education technology: Classroom applications.* Pacific Grove, CA: Brooks/Cole Publishing.

Meyers, L., ed. 1984. Augmenting language skills with microcomputers. *Seminars in speech and language* 5(1).

_____. 1986. *The language machine.* Boston, PA: College-Hill.

Musselwhite, C. 1986. *Adaptive play for special needs children.* Boston, PA: College-Hill.

Musselwhite, C., and K. St. Lewis. 1988. *Communication programming for persons with severe handicaps: Vocal and augmentative strategies.* Boston, PA: College-Hill.

Neiboer, R. A. 1983. *A study for the effect of computers on the preschool environment. Preschool integration through technology systems (PITTS).* 1993. Buffalo, NY: United Cerebral Palsy Association of Western New York.

Robinson, L. 1988. Designing computer intervention for very young handicapped children. *Journal for the Division for Early Childhood* 10(3):209-15.

Shane, H., and A. Bashir. 1980. Election criteria for the adoption of an augmentative communication system: Preliminary considerations. *Journal of Speech and Hearing Disorders* 45:408-14.

Silverman, F. 1980. *Communication for the speechless.* Englewood Cliffs, NJ: Prentice Hall.

Taylor, H. L. 1983. *Microcomputers in the early childhood classroom.* ERIC Educational Document Reproduction Service ED234 845.

Wright, C., and M. Nomura. 1985. *From toys to computers: Access for the physically disabled child.* San Jose, CA: Christine Wright.

Appendix C
Cooking and Snack Ideas

Books and Articles

Barrett, I. 1974. *Cooking is easy when you know how.* New York: Arco.

Burdick, A. 1972. *Look! I can cook.* New York: Crescent.

Christenberry, M. A., and B. Stevens. 1984. *Can Piaget cook?* Atlanta, GA: Humanics.

Cobb, V. 1973. *Science experiments you can eat.* Philadelphia, PA: J. B. Lippincott.

Goldberg, P. Z. 1980. *So what if you can't chew, eat hearty! Recipes and a guide for the healthy and happy eating of soft and pureed foods.* Springfield, IL: Charles C. Thomas.

Goodwin, M. T., and G. Pollen. 1974. *Creative food experiences for children.* Washington, DC: Center for Science in the Public Interest.

Johnson, B., and B. Plemons. 1978. *Cup cooking: Individual child portion picture recipes.* Lake Alfred, FL: Early Educators.

Kahan, E. H. 1974. *Cooking activities for the retarded child.* New York: Abingdon.

Lansky, V. 1974. *Feed me! I'm yours.* New York: Bantam.

Levine, L. 1968. *The kids in the kitchen.* New York: Macmillan.

Marcus, E. F., and R. F. Granovetter. 1986. *Making it easy: Crafts and cooking activities skill building for handicapped learners.* Palo Alto, CA: Vort.

Morris, S. E., and M. D. Klein. 1987. *Pre-feeding skills: A comprehensive resource for feeding development.* Tucson, AZ: Therapy Skill Builders.

Parents Nursery School. 1972. *Kids are natural cooks: Child-tested recipes for home and school using natural foods.* Boston: Houghton Mifflin.

Paul, A. 1975. *Kids cooking without a stove: A cookbook for young children.* Garden City, NY: Doubleday.

Satter, E. 1983. *Child of mine: Feeding with love and good sense.* Palo Alto, CA: Bull Publishing.

_____. 1987. *How to get your kid to eat...but not too much.* Palo Alto, CA: Bull Publishing.

Steed, F. R. 1977. *A special picture cookbook.* Lawrence, KS: H and H Enterprises.

Technical Assistance Center II. n.d. *Cooking with kids.* Harrisonburg, VA: TAC II, Early, Middle, and Special Education, James Madison University.

Wanamaker, N., K. Hearn, and S. Richarz. 1979. *More than graham crackers: Nutrition education and food preparation with young children.* Washington, DC: National Association for the Education of Young Children.

Materials

Mealtimes: A Resource for Oral-Motor, Feeding and Mealtime Programs
New Visions
Route 1, Box 175-S
Faber, VA 22938

Recipes

Corn Bread

1 cup sifted all-purpose flour	¼ cup sugar
4 tsp. baking powder	¾ tsp. salt
1 cup yellow corn meal	2 eggs
1 cup milk	¼ cup shortening

Preheat oven to 425° F. Sift dry ingredients together. Add eggs, milk, and shortening; beat just until smooth. Pour into greased 9" x 9" x 2" pan. Bake 20-25 minutes, or until done.

Homemade Play Dough

Mix in a medium saucepan:

1 cup flour	½ cup salt
2 Tbsp. cream of tartar	

Add:

1 cup water	2 Tbsp. salad oil
2 tsp. vegetable food coloring	

Cook over medium heat, stirring continuously, about 3 to 5 minutes. (Mixture will glop together in lumps just before it's finished.) Store in plastic bag or airtight container.

Gelatin Jigglers

16-oz. gelatin mix

2½ cups boiling water

Completely dissolve gelatin in boiling water. Pour into a 13" x 9" pan. Chill until firm (about 3 hours). To unmold, dip pan in hot water for 15 seconds. Cut into squares or use cookie cutters.

Peanut Butter Play Dough

½ cup peanut butter	3½ Tbsp. powdered milk
½ cup raisins	2 Tbsp. honey

Mix all ingredients together (use your hands if necessary). Adjust the amount of powdered milk to obtain the desired consistency.

Pumpkin Bread

3⅓ cups all-purpose flour	½ tsp. baking powder
2 tsp. baking soda	1½ tsp. salt
1 tsp. cinnamon	½ tsp. cloves
⅔ cup sugar	⅔ cup salad oil
4 eggs	2 cups cooked, pureed
⅔ cup water	pumpkin

Preheat oven to 350° F. Sift dry ingredients together, except sugar, and set aside. Combine sugar and oil; add eggs one at a time. Add pumpkin. Stir in flour mixture alternately with the water. Pour into two greased 9" x 5" x 3" loaf pans. Bake 1¼ hours or until done. Cool in pan.

Pumpkin Pie

1 9" unbaked pie crust	1½ cups cooked, pureed
¾ cup sugar	pumpkin
½ tsp. salt	¼ tsp. cinnamon
1 tsp. ginger	½ tsp. nutmeg
½ tsp. cloves	3 eggs
2 cups evaporated milk	

Preheat oven to 400° F. Mix pumpkin, sugar, and spices. Beat eggs and add to pumpkin mixture. Add evaporated milk. Pour into prepared, unbaked pie shell. Bake 50 minutes, or until done. Cool before serving.

Sugar Cookies

1 cup butter/margarine	1½ cups sugar
3 eggs	1 tsp. vanilla
3½ cups sifted all-purpose flour	2 tsp. cream of tartar
1 tsp. baking soda	½ tsp. salt

Cream butter and sugar. Add eggs and vanilla. Sift dry ingredients together and add to butter/sugar mixture. Chill. Preheat oven to 375° F. Roll out dough, cut shapes, and decorate, if desired. Bake on ungreased cookie sheets 6-8 minutes, or until done.

Thumbprint Cookies

½ cup sugar	½ cup butter
1 tsp. vanilla	2 eggs
2½ cups all-purpose flour, sifted	2 tsp. double-acting baking powder
½ tsp. salt	jam, jelly, or frosting

Cream butter and sugar. Add remaining ingredients, except jelly or frosting. Chill dough until manageable. Preheat oven to 375° F. Break off pieces and roll into 1" balls. Roll balls in sugar. Place on lightly greased and floured cookie sheet. Bake 5 minutes. Depress center of each cookie with your thumb. Continue baking about 8 minutes, or until done. Cool. Fill centers with jam, jelly, or frosting.

▪ Appendix D
▪ Incorporating Music in the
▪ Intervention Program*

Introducing Music into a Learning Environment

Music can play a very significant role in creating an environment in which both the child and the adult are open to learning from each other and from the activities or materials that are presented. Music supports what is being taught and learned. When combined with systematic introduction, careful observation, and responsiveness to the child's nonverbal communication signals, music can assist the process of change.

The Initial Decision to Use Music

When deciding whether music or specific musical selections are appropriate to use at home, during therapy, or in the classroom, answer the following questions:

- Does the music make a difference for the child?
- Does the music make a difference for the therapist (or teacher)?
- Does the music make a difference for the parent (or family)?
- What kinds of differences are observed when specific types or pieces of music are played?

---

* From Morris, S. E. 1991. Appendix H: Music Resources. In *Developing Integrated Programs*, by M. C. Coling. Tucson, AZ: Therapy Skill Builders. Reprinted with permission.

Selecting the Type of Music

Music can be described or categorized according to its structure (tempo, rhythm, frequencies, tonal qualities), origin (folk music, rock, opera), or its effect on the listener (dance music, superlearning music, calming music). Several specific types of music have been used successfully to support learning and change in the areas of movement, feeding, sensory organization, language, and communication.

Types of music that have been utilized in the therapy, classroom, and home environments include:

Quiet, Centering Music—To develop quieting and relaxation of the mind and emotions in order to enhance communication and learning; for example, during meals, rest periods, bedtime, and quiet times with an adult.

Superlearning Music—To enhance receptiveness to learning through a 60-beat-per-minute tempo. To provide a clear rhythmical structure similar to the rhythms of the heartbeat, sucking, and walking gait. To assist mental and physical relaxation.

Hemi-Sync Metamusic—To create a sustained focus of attention for learning. To facilitate a balanced activation of the information-processing capabilities of both the right and left hemispheres of the brain. To increase the organization and integration of sensory information. To provide physical relaxation with simultaneous mental alertness. To reduce fearfulness and negativity, which interfere with learning.

Folk Music—To provide a clear, rhythmical structure and tempo as a basis for facilitation of coordinated body movement. To provide the opportunity for exploration of vocalization, sound play patterns, gestures, and other forms of communication. To provide rhythmical opportunities for the stimulation of the face and mouth. To provide an environment of mutual enjoyment and shared rhythms for the child and adult.

It is helpful to have available two or three selections of music from each general category. A wide range of personal preferences exists in the children and adults with whom you work. It is important to find the type of music that is appropriate to use with the child and to have enough variety within that type that you don't have to consistently use the same selection.

Hemi-sync metamusic can assist children in experiencing some very profound differences in the way they physically feel and process information. Sudden changes can be frightening and can create added resistance. It may be important to introduce changes involving relaxation and focus of attention gradually. Superlearning music with a 50- to 70-beat-per-minute tempo has a similar effect for many children and is very gentle. You may wish to begin with this type of music and gradually introduce music containing the hemi-sync signals. Hemi-sync also produces a more gradual effect when played over open speakers. Listeners report a much stronger effect when they listen to hemi-sync metamusic through headphones. Thus, a continuum of experiential intensity can be created according to the type of music or sound selected and according to the way it is presented to the listener.

Observing the Effects of Music on the Individual

- Identify the child's characteristic patterns of sensorimotor, emotional, and learning behaviors that might be influenced by a musical background. These could include factors such as muscle tone, movement coordination, attending behaviors, activity level, acceptance of touch, acceptance of movement, acceptance of unfamiliar activities, and imitation abilities.

- Identify changes or directions in these specific areas that would benefit the child. What changes would you like to see happen more easily; for instance, more frequent eye contact, reduction in hypertonicity, acceptance of touch to the face, greater trust and willingness to try new activities, regular sucking rhythm?

- Identify the general type of music or characteristics of a specific piece of music that would support the changes you would like to facilitate. For example, a very rhythmical piece of music might support greater rhythm in walking or sucking; hemi-sync sounds would support greater attending and sensory organization.

- Within the category of music you have selected, choose pieces that you like and respond to positively. If you select music that is unpleasant for you or that you dislike, you automatically communicate your discomfort to the child. This can influence children's responses in a negative direction so that their reaction is more a response to you than a response to the music.

- It is helpful to listen to the selections ahead of time and become familiar with your general response to the music. This preparation can assist you in choosing the music to use with the child.

- Observe your response to the musical background as you use it with the child. Some of the changes that you may notice include: more flowing rhythms when moving with a child to folk music; enhanced intuitive knowledge of when to continue or alter an activity; stronger focus of attention in the shared activity (less mind wandering or mind chatter); easier awareness of the child's nonverbal communication; increased intuition; and increased creativity.

- Identify the child's verbal or nonverbal patterns of communication. How does the child express likes, dislikes, or preferences in other situations; for example, turning away, increasing the level of hyperactivity, reducing eye contact, arching, crying or fussing, looking toward the object, reaching, or smiling?

- Introduce the music you have selected to accompany the desired therapy or home activity.

- Observe the child's reactions for any signs that the music is aversive. If the music appears to be aversive in any way, turn it off for a period of time. Explore another selection in the same general category of music at several other sessions and observe the child's response. Decide whether the child's aversive response is to a particular piece of music or to an entire category of music.

- Observe the child's reactions for signs that the music is pleasant or enjoyed. This expression may take the form of increased relaxation, smiling, fuller participation in the activity, or looking with interest toward the tape player.

- If the music you have selected appears to be positive or helpful for at least one person in the therapy, classroom, or family setting, it may be used, providing it is not aversive to the others in the environment.

- Keep a journal describing the child's behavior and responses during sessions or time periods in which you are using the music you have selected. You may wish to select a specific area or behavior to measure during the periods in which you use the music. If you have taken the same measurements for a number of sessions before you introduce the music, you will have established a baseline for comparison. The journal and any measurements you make will allow you to decide how valuable the music background has been for the child.

- Keep a journal describing your own reactions to the background music and changes in your response to the child and the time you spend together. This procedure will enable you to decide whether the background music to your therapy, play, or learning session enhances your own learning interaction.

- The speed with which change occurs will vary with each individual. For some children and adults there is an immediate awareness of change. For others, there may be acceptance of the music and a slower or more subtle change in behavior or learning. Be aware of small changes that can occur, and resist the temptation to eliminate the music because large shifts do not occur quickly. For example, a child may engage in a familiar activity, such as working a puzzle, in the same way with or without the music. However, when the music is on, the child shares the activity with the mother and even leans against her. When the child works the puzzle without the musical background, he or she moves slightly away and prefers to play alone. If changes in working the puzzle were the sole measure of effectiveness, the more subtle interpersonal change might go unobserved.

- The frequency with which the music is used will depend upon the child's response and the desirability of using the music in different settings. Some children profit from using music throughout the day; others benefit more from brief (30- to 45-minute) periods once a day. Some music seems to create an effect primarily while it is being played, such as folk music. Hemi-sync metamusic appears to create a long-term learning or carryover effect. Because of the carryover effect, it is not necessary to use hemi-sync tapes throughout the day for them to be effective. The tapes may be used frequently during the day, however, if both the children and adults in the environment find them pleasant.

- If the music is used frequently each day, it is helpful to use breaks during which no music is played. This creates a contrast for the child and provides an opportunity to continue the behaviors facilitated by the music. Hemi-sync music is essentially training wheels for the mind that assist the brain with a new way of organizing and integrating sensorimotor experiences. Once this has been learned, the training wheels are no longer necessary.

Equipment

- Hemi-sync music is designed to be played on a stereo system. The hemi-sync effect is created by different frequencies on the two channels of the stereo. This effect will not occur if the music is played on monaural equipment.

- Equipment with a replay feature eliminates the distraction that may occur when a tape or CD reaches the end and must be re-started in the middle of an activity.

- A portable stereo with detachable speakers is helpful for creating a headphone-like effect when the speakers are placed on either side of the child's head. This may be desirable if you wish to use headphones with infants or young children who cannot tolerate anything directly touching the ears or head. If lying supine is appropriate for the child and the activity selected, the speakers can be placed within two inches of each ear. Small individual speakers can also be purchased to use with a small personal stereo. Since these players are small and often have a replay feature, this combination may offer many advantages in flexibility and price not found with larger equipment.

- Headphones may provide an advantage for specific children or environments. Headphones enable the child to listen to music at a low volume in an environment where an open-speaker system is unavailable or undesirable. Music through headphones would enable a child to listen to quiet music while in a car, in a classroom, or while taking a school examination when music is not desired for others in the same room. Since the effect of hemi-sync metamusic is more intense with headphones, listening through headphones may become important for some children.

- Commercial headphones are made for adult head sizes. They often slip and are uncomfortable for small children. Several alternatives exist in customizing headphones for infants and toddlers.

Purchase inexpensive headphones with a metal band. Most metal headbands of this type have a bump or metal hump toward the end to prevent extreme movement of the earphones as the band is adjusted for different head sizes. Use a metal file to remove this bump, giving a full range of movement of the individual earphones on the metal band. Adjust the metal band to fit the size of the child's head. Secure the band size with masking tape. Use metal cutters to remove the extra length of the band so that it doesn't poke the child. Since these headphones are relatively inexpensive, several could be constructed, either for different children or for different ranges of head size.

Another alternative is to purchase inexpensive headphones and use metal cutters to remove the earphones from the band. Alternatively, purchase the type of earphones designed to be inserted directly into the ear canal. Adapt an infant/child's cap or hat, sewing in a flap or pocket that can be closed with Velcro® or a snap. When the child wears the cap, these new pockets will be on the inside, directly at ear level. The separate earphones are inserted into the pockets on each side. The child simply wears this music hat to receive the music. This method works particularly well with infants or toddlers who generally do not adapt well to headphones. These hats should be used with caution with children who do not like wearing hats or having anything touch the head or ears.

Location

Music can be utilized during individual therapy sessions (speech and language therapy, occupational therapy, physical therapy, counseling, or psychotherapy), at home, and in the classroom to assist with relaxation and learning. Somewhat different considerations and guidelines may be followed in each setting.

Music during Individual Therapy

- It is ideal for music to be introduced initially in therapy sessions, where the child's responses to the music and to learning can be carefully observed. If the music is used in the background for therapy activities that are familiar, differences in the child's responses can be observed with greater ease.

- Therapy sessions can be utilized to identify individual areas of change that could then become generalized through using music in other environments. Therapists can work with an interested teacher to identify individual children in the classroom who might benefit from the use of music with a group.

Music in the Home

- When music is introduced into the home setting, the therapist or teacher should develop a plan with the family. This plan would include an agreement on the type of music to be used, the times or activities during which it will be used, and the frequency of use. A journal may be kept by the parents to note any changes in the child's behavior that they observe.

- It is helpful to develop a music library that consists of selections that can be loaned to the family for a period of several weeks. This library will enable them to listen to music with their child and decide which selections work well at home. When the family has identified music that they and their child like, they may purchase the music.

- Quiet music, such as centering music, superlearning music, and hemi-sync metamusic, can be used in a home or family environment at meals, bedtime, or with specific play or learning activities that would be supported by physical relaxation, mental alertness, or openness to communication.

- Music can be used during an activity or prior to it. For example, the child might spend a quiet time with soft music playing for 30 minutes before dinner; or the music might be used during the meal itself.

- Folk music tapes can be used with all of the children in the family. When siblings are involved in dancing together, singing, turn taking, and sharing with music, the child with a disability is no longer the center of attention. It is important to involve the other children in a family during activities that are fun and therapeutic for the child who needs therapy carryover activities.

Music in the Classroom

- Select quiet, organizing music to use in the background as children enter the classroom. This music creates a nonverbal message of intention to become more quiet and organized for the school day.

- Accompany specific types of activities with specific pieces of music. Children will gradually associate the music with the activity and will learn to carry over the effects experienced with the music when it is not playing. For example, one piece of music might be played during lunch while another might be used during rest time or table activities.

- To receive the benefit of the stereo presentation of hemi-sync sound, the speakers should be directed toward the children.

- If hemi-sync metamusic is to be used in the classroom with children who have neurological or emotional dysfunctions, it is particularly important to observe each child's reaction individually before presenting this music to the entire classroom. A small number of these children may show a disorganized or aversive response to the hemi-sync signal. It is helpful to identify children who appear to benefit and those who may indicate that they do not like the sounds. If there are children in the classroom who are clearly irritated by hemi-sync metamusic, this type of music should not be used while the sensitive children are in the room. This music, however, might be used with other children while the sensitive child is involved in a pull-out activity or if the speakers are directed so that they are not facing children who might be irritated by the sounds.

Selection of Music for the Development of Movement

1. Music selections should be clear and rhythmical. They should not contain a great deal of fancy elaboration and instrumentation. They should be performed as straightforwardly as possible, emphasizing a basic rhythm and melody that are strong and uncluttered. Many variations in tempo are appropriate. Syncopation and irregularity in the underlying rhythm pattern should be avoided. We are striving for a clearer rhythm pattern in the child's movement. The structure of the music should mirror the type of movement being worked on.

2. Music should have a rhythmical structure and tempo that meet the needs of the individual child. A tape with slower songs and rhythms might be developed for a child who needs a slower response time for postural reactions. Baroque music or folk dance music could be used in place of songs with lyrics. Instrumental music is less distracting for some children and is more appropriate if you wish to incorporate visual and movement imagery with the movement. It is generally easier to create custom-made tapes for a child or group of children than to find a commercial product that is totally appropriate.

3. Music should be conducive to health and growth. Despite its popularity with today's children and adolescents, rock music should be avoided during treatment sessions. Data shows that the irregular rhythm of rock music has a negative effect on growth (in plant research), that it weakens muscle responses, and that it reduces the amount of coordinated activity of the hemispheres of the brain. The precise structure of baroque music, on the other hand, has been associated with greater growth and health (in plants), and with accelerated learning. This type of music can be used as an initial background for movement awareness or to provide a background for sensory integration activities that create the foundation for movement facilitation.

4. Folk music can be extremely effective. It contains many themes of interest to children (animals, people, humor) and utilizes a simple melody structure with a great deal of rhythmical repetition of melodic and lyric phrases. Folk music that contains a sincere feeling tone and an underlying honesty and respect for children should be selected. This type of music is often identified intuitively rather than through a logical sequential analysis of the song. Most traditional folk songs have withstood time and many generations of children and adults who have loved them and played them. Many of these songs are already familiar to the adult who is working/playing with the child. Contemporary songs composed in a folk style are also appropriate. It is important to sense whether the song was written as an expression of childhood and with a knowledge and appreciation of children, or whether the underlying theme is simply to teach something with music. Many of the songs written for straight educational purposes lack the spark and feeling tone of pleasure and playfulness that is carried in the more traditional folk song. Some music written specifically for children is patronizing or overly cute. An emotional tone of respect for the child and the sheer enjoyment of the music is crucial.

5. If you wish to develop recorded materials for your program, the following suggestions and observations are helpful:

    a. Determine the kind of music that is appropriate for one or more of the children with whom you work. Assess the initial needs of your program. It is not necessary to create a full program immediately.

    b. Begin listening to different types of music that would be appropriate. Listen first at an intuitive, feeling level for what the specific piece has to offer. Move with the music and let it create images for you. Imagine yourself moving with children to the music. Listen again to the music with a more analytical ear. What does it have to offer a specific child or family in your program? What is the tempo? the rhythm? the theme of the song?

    c. Broaden your exposure to music that is available in your community. Check listings of specific compositions, records, and artists in books or articles on the therapeutic use of music (see the discography). Begin to listen to selections on records borrowed from your library or school or in your own music collection. Include music from the cultural traditions of the children and families with whom you work.

    d. Create several custom tapes for your program. These may include songs or instrumental pieces from a single record or artist or they may include a mixture of artists and recordings. Consider your purposes for creating the tape as you decide whether a given song or composition belongs on the tape. For example, you may wish to begin a tape with slow to moderately paced music that has a clear, steady rhythm. The slow tempo and steady rhythm lend themselves well to activities that build postural tone and stability. Add songs that create an appropriate background for more complex movement and coordination. These songs may be interspersed with songs that have slower tempos and that are specifically appropriate for building and steadying postural tone. As overall movement control improves throughout the first half of the tape, songs can be added that include active vocalization, play with the mouth, gestures, or use of a communication miniboard, for instance.

    e. Explore the use of the new tape with specific children. You will gain a clearer sense of which materials work for you and for the child. Look for an overall pleasurable response from the child. The child may become more playful and willing to work/play with you as the tape is playing. The child may become more alert to a specific song. There may be smiling, vocalization, increased relaxation, or increased body movement with the music. Watch for an increase in endurance and tolerance in treatment. The child may be able to focus on activities for longer periods and not tire as quickly. Touch and movement may be accepted more readily with the music. You may observe a child become more interactive and communicative when the tape or specific songs are used during the session.

    f. As you use the tape, make written notes of the types of activity that seem particularly appropriate with each song. This written listing can be typed and given to parents, teachers, or other therapists who are using a copy of your tape with the child.

Music for the Development of Learning, Communication, and Movement

Quiet, Centering Music

Purpose: To develop quieting and relaxation of the mind and emotions in order to enhance communication and learning (for example, during meals, rest periods, bedtime, or quiet times with an adult).

*Comfort Zone
Steven Halpern
Halpern Sounds

Spectrum Suite
Steven Halpern
Halpern Sounds

Ancient Echoes
Steven Halpern
Halpern Sounds

Dawn
Steven Halpern
Halpern Sounds

Eventide
Steven Halpern
Halpern Sounds

Birds of Paradise
Georgia Kelly
Heru Records

Tarashanti
Georgia Kelly
Heru Records

Seapeace
Georgia Kelly
Heru Records

Harp and Soul
Georgia Kelly
Heru Records

Silk Road
Kitaro
Canyon Records

*Fairy Ring
Mike Rowland
Music Design

*Golden Voyage: Vol. 1
Bearns and Dexter
Awakening Productions

Golden Voyage: Vol. 4
Bearns and Dexter
Awakening Productions

Gregorian Chant from Hungary: Medieval Christmas
Hungaroton Melodies

Christopher Parkening Plays J.S. Bach
Christopher Parkening
Angel

The Pachelbel Canon in D
Jean-Francois Paillard
Chamber Orchestra
RCA

Mother Earth's Lullaby
Synchestra
Synchestra

Silver Ships
Synchestra
Synchestra

December
George Winston
Wyndam Hill Productions

Autumn
George Winston
Wyndam Hill Productions

Winter into Spring
George Winston
Wyndam Hill Productions

Childhood and Memory
Will Ackerman
Wyndam Hill Productions

*Transitions
Burt Wolf and Joe Wolff
Placenta Music

Lullabies from around the World
Steven Bergman
Steven Bergman

Sweet Baby Dreams
Steven Bergman
Steven Bergman

Dream Passage
Daniel Kobialka
LiSem Enterprises

Fragrances of a Dream
Daniel Kobialka
LiSem Enterprises

*Going Home
Daniel Kobialka
LiSem Enterprises

Timeless Motion
Daniel Kobialka
LiSem Enterprises

When You Wish upon a Star
Daniel Kobialka
LiSem Enterprises

Miracles
Rob Whitesides-Woo
Serenity Music

Chistofori's Dream
David Lanz
Narada Music

Superlearning Music

Purpose: To enhance receptivity to learning through a 60-beat-per-minute tempo. To provide a clear rhythmical structure similar to the rhythms of the heartbeat, sucking, and walking gait.

*Comfort Zone
Steven Halpern
Halpern Sounds

Superlearning Music
(baroque classical music)
Superlearning Inc.

*Relax with the Classics: Vol. 1
Largos (baroque classical music)
LIND Institute

*Relax with the Classics: Vol. 2
Adagios (baroque classical music)
LIND Institute

*Relax with the Classics: Vol. 3
Pastorale (baroque classical music)
LIND Institute

*Relax with the Classics: Vol. 4
Andante (baroque classical music)
LIND Institute

Music for Mellow Minds
Janalea Hoffman
Mellow Minds

Mind-Body Tempo
Janalea Hoffman
Mellow Minds

*Alleluia
Robert Grass and On Wings of Sing
Spring Hill Music

*Om Namaha Shivaya
Robert Grass and On Wings of Sing
Spring Hill Music

Hemi-Sync Music

Purpose: To create a more sustained focus of attention for learning. To facilitate a more balanced activation of the information-processing capabilities of both the right and left hemispheres of the brain. To reduce fearfulness and negativity, which interfere with the learning of new skills.

Metamusic Back Room
Robert Monroe
Alan Phillips
The Monroe Institute

Metamusic Blue
Robert Monroe
The Monroe Institute

*Metamusic Converse
Robert Monroe
Alan Phillips
The Monroe Institute

*Metamusic Downstream
Robert Monroe
Alan Phillips
The Monroe Institute

*Metamusic Eddys
Robert Monroe
Alan Phillips
The Monroe Institute

Metamusic Green
Robert Monroe
The Monroe Institute

Metamusic Highland Ring
Robert Monroe
Alan Phillips
The Monroe Institute

Metamusic Limbic
Robert Monroe
Alan Phillips
The Monroe Institute

*Metamusic Midsummer Night
Robert Monroe
Alan Phillips
The Monroe Institute

*Metamusic Modern
Robert Monroe
Alan Phillips
The Monroe Institute

Metamusic Nostalgia
Robert Monroe
Alan Phillips
The Monroe Institute

Metamusic Outreach
Robert Monroe
Alan Phillips
The Monroe Institute

Metamusic Random Access
Robert Monroe
Alan Phillips
The Monroe Institute

Metamusic Sam and George
Robert Monroe
Alan Phillips
The Monroe Institute

Soft and Still
Robert Monroe
The Monroe Institute

Metamusic Sunset
Robert Monroe
Alan Phillips
The Monroe Institute

*Metamusic Trailing Edge
Robert Monroe
Alan Phillips
The Monroe Institute

Folk Music

Purpose: To provide a clear, rhythmical structure and tempo as a basis for facilitation of coordinated body movement. To provide the opportunity for exploration of vocalization, sound play patterns, gestures, and other forms of communication. To provide an environment of mutual enjoyment and shared rhythms for the child and adult.

*I've Got a Song
Sandy and Carolyn Paton
Folk-Legacy Records

*When the Spirit Says Sing
Sandy and Carolyn Paton
Folk-Legacy Records

*Teaching Peace
Red Grammer
Smilin' Atcha Music

Birds, Beasts, Bugs, and Little Fishes
Pete Seeger
Folkways

Birds, Beasts, Bugs, and Bigger Fishes
Pete Seeger
Folkways

Song and Playtime with Pete Seeger
Pete Seeger
Folkways

American Game and Activity Songs for Children
Pete Seeger
Folkways

American Folk Songs
Pete Seeger
Folkways

Marching across the Green Grass and Other American
  Children's Game Songs
Jean Ritchie
Folkways

14 Numbers, Letters, and Animal Songs
Alan Mills
Folkways

I'll Sing You a Story
Sam Hinton
Folkways

Woody Guthrie's Children's Songs
Logan English
Folkways

Songs to Grow On
Woody Guthrie
Folkways

Animal Folksongs for Children
Peggy Seeger
Folkways

*Lullabies and Other Children's Songs
Nancy Raven
Pacific Cascades

*People and Animal Songs
Nancy Raven
Pacific Cascades

Songs for the Holiday Season
Nancy Raven
Pacific Cascades

Singing, Prancing, and Dancing
Nancy Raven
Pacific Cascades

*Many Blessings
On Wings of Song
Spring Hill Music

Let's Sing Fingerplays
Tom Glazer
CMS Records

Rhythms of Childhood
Ella Jenkins
Scholastic

My Street Begins at My House
Ella Jenkins
Folkways

Growing Up with Ella Jenkins
Ella Jenkins
Folkways

You'll Sing a Song and I'll Sing a Song
Ella Jenkins
Folkways

Howjadoo
John McCutcheon
Rounder Records

Grandma Slid Down the Mountain
Cathy Fink and Friends
Rounder Records

Monsters in the Closet
Gerri Gribi and Tom Pease
Makin' Jam, Etc.

My Rhinoceros and Other Friends
Guy Carawan
A Gentle Wind

A Home in Tennessee
Sparky Rucker
A Gentle Wind

A Song or Two for You
Nick Seeger
A Gentle Wind

Sing a Song, Sing Along
Faith Petric
A Gentle Wind

Down in the Valley
Robin and Linda Williams
A Gentle Wind

Camels, Cats, and Rainbows
Paul Strausman
A Gentle Wind

*The Dildine Family
The Dildine Family
A Gentle Wind

Hello Everybody
Rachel Buchman
A Gentle Wind

Singable Songs for the Very Young
Raffi
A & M Records

More Singable Songs
Raffi
A & M Records

—

* Available from New Visions

Addresses of Distributing Companies

Folk Legacy Records
Sharon, CT 06069

A Gentle Wind
Box 3103
Albany, NY 12203

The Monroe Institute
Route 1, Box 175
Faber, VA 22938

Music Design
207 East Buffalo
Milwaukee, WI 53202

Music for Little People
P.O. Box 1460
Redway, CA 95560-1460

New Leaf Distributing Company
5425 Tulane Dr. S.W.
Atlanta, GA 30336

New Visions
Route 1, Box 175-S
Faber, VA 22938

Rounder Records
One Camp Street
Cambridge, MA 02140

Silo
P.O. Box 429
Waterbury, VT 05676

Superlearning, Inc.
450 Seventh Ave.
New York, NY 10123

References

Anastasiow, N. J. 1990. Implications of the neurobiological model for early intervention. In *Handbook of early childhood education*, edited by S. J. Meisels and J. P. Shonkoff, 196-216. Cambridge, England: Cambridge University Press.

Blackstone, S. W. 1989. *Augmentative communication: Implementation strategies.* Bethesda, MD: American Speech-Language-Hearing Association.

Bredekamp, S., ed. 1986. *Developmentally appropriate practice.* Washington, DC: National Association for the Education of Young Children.

Bricker, D., and J. Cripe. 1992. *An activity-based approach to early intervention.* Baltimore, MD: Paul H. Brookes.

Brinker, R. P., and M. Lewis. 1982. Making the world work with microcomputers: A learning prosthesis for handicapped infants. *Exceptional Children* 49(2):163-70.

Bronfenbrenner, U. 1979. *The ecology of human development: Experiments by nature and design.* Cambridge, MA: Harvard University Press.

Brown, F., P. Belz, L. Corsi, and B. Wenig. 1993. Choice diversity for people with severe disabilities. *Education and Training in Mental Retardation* 28(4):318-26.

Burkhart, L. 1980. *Homemade battery powered toys and educational devices for severely handicapped children.* College Park, MD: self-published.

———. 1982. *More homemade battery devices for severely handicapped children with suggested activities.* College Park, MD: self-published.

Butler, J. A., S. Rosenbaum, and J. S. Palfrey. 1987. Ensuring access to health care for children with disabilities. *New England Journal of Medicine* 317:162-65.

Corey, G. 1990. *Theory and practice of group counseling,* rev. ed. Pacific Grove, CA: Brooks/Cole.

Crnic, K. A., W. N. Friedrick, and M. T. Greenberg. 1983. Adaptation of families with mentally retarded children: A model of stress, coping and family ecology. *American Journal of Mental Deficiency* 88:125-38.

Daniels, W. R. 1986. *Group power: A manager's guide to using meetings.* San Diego, CA: University Press.

Derman-Sparks, L., and the ABC Task Force. 1989. *Anti-bias curriculum: Tools for empowering young children.* Washington, DC: National Association for the Education of Young Children.

Destefano, D., A. Howe, and E. Horn. 1991. *Best practices: Evaluating early childhood special education programs.* Tucson, AZ: Communication Skill Builders.

Dunlap, W. R. 1979. How do parents of handicapped children view their needs? *Journal of the Division of Early Childhood* 1:1-9.

Dyer, K., G. Dunlap, and V. Winterling. 1990. Effects of choice making on the serious problem behaviors of students with severe handicaps. *Journal of Applied Behavior Analysis* 23(4):515-24.

Elkind, D. 1986. Formal education and early childhood education: An essential difference. *Phi Delta Kappan* May:631-36.

Farran, D. C., J. Metzger, and J. Sparling. 1986. Immediate and continuing adaptations in parents of handicapped children: A model and an illustration. In *Families of handicapped persons*, edited by J. J. Gallagher and P. M. Vietze, 143-156. Baltimore, MD: Paul H. Brookes.

Featherstone, H. 1980. *A difference in the family: Living with a disabled child.* New York: Penguin.

Fewell, R. 1986. A handicapped child in the family. In *Families of handicapped children*, edited by R. R. Fewell and P. F. Vadasy, 3-34. Austin, TX: Pro-Ed.

Fromberg, D. 1987. Play. In *The early childhood curriculum: A review of current research*, edited by C. Seefeldt, 35-74. New York: Teacher's College Press.

Gallagher, J. J., P. Beckman, and A. H. Cross. 1983. Families of handicapped children: Sources of stress and its amelioration. *Exceptional Children* 50:10-19.

Garrett, J. N. 1993. *Parents of young children with Down syndrome: An investigation of stress and coping.* Unpublished manuscript.

Garvey, C. 1977. *Play.* Cambridge, MA: Harvard University Press.

Gossens, C., and S. Crain. 1986. *Augmentative communication: Intervention resources.* Wauconda, IL: Don Johnston Developmental Equipment.

Hoffman, E. 1988. Time management from the kitchen. *Academic Therapy* 23(3):275-77.

Johnson-Martin, N., K. G. Jens, and S. M. Attermeier. 1991. *The Carolina curriculum for infants and toddlers with special needs,* 2d ed. Baltimore: Paul H. Brookes.

Jones, H., and S. Warren. 1991. Enhancing engagement in early language teaching. *Teaching Exceptional Children* 23:48-50.

Kornblatt, E. S., and J. Heinrich. 1985. Needs and coping abilities of children with developmental disabilities. *Mental Retardation* 20:2-6.

Linder, T. 1990. *Transdisciplinary play-based assessment.* Baltimore: Paul H. Brookes.

———. 1993. *Transdisciplinary play-based intervention.* Baltimore: Paul H. Brookes.

MacKeith, R. 1973. The feelings and behavior of parents of handicapped children. *Developmental Medicine and Child Neurology* 25:524-27.

Miller, L. 1989. Classroom based language intervention. *Language Speech and Hearing Services in the Schools* 20:153-69.

Mineo, B. A., and R. A. Cavalier. 1987. An ultrasonic bladder sensor for persons with incontinence. *Proceedings of the Tenth Annual Conference on Rehabilitation Technology.* Washington, DC: RESNA.

Minuchin, P. 1985. Families and individual development: Provocations from the field of family therapy. *Child Development* 56:289-302.

Musselwhite, C. 1986. *Adaptive play for special needs children.* Boston, PA: College-Hill.

Musselwhite, C., and K. St. Lewis. 1988. *Communication programming for persons with severe handicaps: Vocal and augmentative strategies.* Boston, PA: College-Hill.

Piaget, J. 1962. *Play, dreams and imitation in childhood.* New York: W. W. Norton.

Sameroff, A. J., and M. J. Chandler. 1975. Reproductive risk and the continuum of caretaking casualty. In *Review of child development research,* edited by F. D. Horowitz, M. Hetherington, S. Scarr-Salapatek, and G. Siegel, 187-244. Chicago: University of Chicago Press.

Schulz, J. B. 1985. The parent-professional conflict. In *Parents speak out: Then and now,* edited by H. R. Turnbull III and A. P. Turnbull, 11-22. Columbus, OH: Charles E. Merrill.

Shane, H., and A. Bashir. 1980. Election criteria for the adoption of an augmentative communication system: Preliminary considerations. *Journal of Speech and Hearing Disorders* 45:408-14.

Shonkoff, J. P., and P. C. Marshall. 1990. Biological bases of developmental dysfunction. In *Handbook of early childhood education,* edited by S. J. Meisels and J. P. Shonkoff, 35-52. Cambridge, England: Cambridge University Press.

Shonkoff, J. P., and S. J. Meisels. 1990. Early childhood intervention: The evolution of a concept. In *Handbook of early childhood education,* edited by S. J. Meisels and J. P. Shonkoff, 3-32. Cambridge, England: Cambridge University Press.

Smith, D., and J. Smith. 1978. Trends. In *Systematic instruction of the moderately and severely handicapped,* edited by M. E. Snell, 478-493. Columbus, OH: Charles E. Merrill.

Swan, W. W., and J. L. Morgan. 1993. *Collaborating for comprehensive services for young children and their families: The local interagency coordinating council.* Baltimore, MD: Paul H. Brookes.

Turnbull, A. P., and H. R. Turnbull III. 1990. *Families, professionals and exceptionality: A special partnership,* rev. ed. Columbus, OH: Charles E. Merrill.

Warren, S., and A. Kaiser. 1986. Incidental language teaching: A critical review. *Journal of Speech and Hearing Disorders* 51:291-99.

Werner, E. E. 1990. Protective factors and individual resilience. In *Handbook of early childhood education,* edited by S. J. Meisels and J. P. Shonkoff, 97-116. Cambridge, England: Cambridge University Press.

Widerstrom, A. 1991. *Adapting developmentally appropriate practice for young children with special needs.* Reston, VA: Council for Exceptional Children.

Wikler, L. 1981. Chronic stresses of families of mentally retarded children. *Family Relations* 30:281-88.

Add these language products to your resource library . . .

CLAS EARLY CHILDHOOD
by Lynn Plourde, M.A., CCC-SLP

Take a whole-language approach to early childhood education. Reinforce target vocabulary by engaging your students in active learning. You'll capture your students' attention with eight engaging thematic units. **0761671773-YCS**

CLAS PRESCHOOL
by Lynn Plourde, M.A., CCC-SLP

Here's a complete 10-month program of listening and speaking activities to use in a day-care center or preschool setting. Weekly activities develop oral language skills such as auditory memory and question-asking abilities. Get parents involved too, with home activities based on classroom lesson plans. The program is organized so completely that substitute teachers can use it easily! **0761675701-YCS**

Take a look at these early intervention materials written by well-known authorities . . .

INCLUSIVE EARLY CHILDHOOD EDUCATION
A Model Classroom
by Marie R. Abraham, M.A., Lori M. Morris, M.A., and Penelope J. Wald, Ed.D.

Include all your students in this new curriculum. You'll find successful techniques on how to integrate children with mild through moderate developmental delays with other students. Create an instructional program that's based on the current theory that children learn through active exploration in an interactive environment. **0761678840-YCS**

MOTOR DEVELOPMENT KIT
Activity Sessions for Children
by M. Kay Mason, with Shelia Alkins Preddy, OTR, and Glenda Bridges, SLP

Help your students with motor delays or difficulties improve their skills using this motor development program. Working through seven activity stations, your school-age students will increase muscle tone, correct posture, and build confidence. Each station addresses basic concepts that encourage the develoment of a wide range of motor, cognitive, and language skills. Within each station, activities vary in difficulty. Materials needed for the activities are included in the kit or can easily be made from everyday items. **0761643370-YTS**

EVERY MOVE COUNTS
Sensory-Based Communication Techniques (VHS videotape)
*by Jane E. Korsten, M.A., Dixie K. Dunn, M.A., OTR, Teresa Vernon Foss, M.Ed., and
Mary Kay Francke, COTA*

Empower children and adults unable to use formal language with effective sensory-based communication strategies. Clients learn how to control their environment—the prerequisite for communication! You'll have everything you need—assessments, intervention strategies, activity guide, positioning suggestions, recordkeeping forms, and carryover materials. **076164749X-YTS**

NORMAL DEVELOPMENT COPYBOOK
by Marsha Dunn Klein, M.Ed., OTR/L, Nancy Harris Ossman, B.S., OTR, and Barbara Tracy, B.S., PT

Completely reproducible, you'll find all your favorite pictures from the *Normal Development Poster Set.* Each page features a developmental age, skill illustration, and space for you to suggest "Helpful Hints." Individualize pages by writing at-home activities for reaching goals. As a special plus, 24 "Developmental Sequence" pages illustrate skill acquisition in a glance. On one convenient page you'll have pictures and steps showing a task through completion— a great overview for parents! **0761647325-YTS**

THE TRANSITION SOURCEBOOK
A Practical Guide for Early Intervention
by Andrea M. Lazzari, Ed.D.

Structure and evaluate positive transitions for children with special-needs and their families with this practical, hands-on guide. The systematic approach outlines the steps in transition, preparing staff and families, supporting children, follow-up, and case studies. A wealth of sample forms gets you started right away! **0761677437-YCS**

SENSORY INTEGRATION THERAPY
by Toronto Sensory Integration Study Group

This 20-minute, full-color videotape allows you to explore the unique environment of sensory integration therapy. Use it to train therapists, students, teachers, or to educate parents. The program discusses the process of SI and shows characteristics and behaviors of children with SI disorders. It also outlines target areas for therapy. Plus, a balance of therapeutic activities provides the sensory motor foundation for learning. **0761647155-YTS**

COMBINING NEURO-DEVELOPMENTAL TREATMENT AND SENSORY INTEGRATION PRINCIPLES
An Approach to Pediatric Therapy
by Erna I. Blanche, M.A., M.O.T., Tina M. Botticelli, M.S., PT, and Mary K. Hallway, OTR

Use this guide to help you combine the two most prevalent methods of treatment in pediatric therapy: Neuro-Developmental Treatment (NDT) and Sensory Integration (SI). Focus on remediating sensory and movement problems that affect the daily activities of your clients, birth to 12 years. Create an individualized therapy program that is appropriate for each client, using the techniques you find most helpful. **0761643346-YTS**

MULTI-PLAY
Sensory Activities for School Readiness
by Gerri A. Duran, OTR/L, and Sharon Klenke-Ormiston, M.A., CCC-SLP

Build on your kindergarten clients' natural play experiences to increase their school readiness. Strengthen motor skills, language, and speech with play-based multisensory activities. Plus, use this collaborative model to involve teachers in classroom carryover. **0761643060-YTS**

For current prices on these practical resources, please call 1-800-228-0752.

ORDER FORM

Ship to:

Institution: _____

Name: _____

Occupation/Dept: _____

Address: _____

City: _____ State: _____ Zip: _____

Please check here if this is a permanent address change.

Telephone No. _____ ☐ work ☐ home

Payment Options:

☐ Bill me.   ☐ My check is enclosed.

☐ My purchase order is enclosed. P.O. # _____

☐ Charge to my credit card: ☐ VISA ☐ MasterCard ☐ American Express

Card No. ☐☐☐☐☐☐☐☐☐☐☐☐☐☐☐☐

Expiration Date: Month _____ Year _____

Signature _____

Qty.	Cat. #	Title	Amou

Prices are in U.S. dollars. Payment must be made in U.S. fund

- If your account is not currently listed as "tax exempt," applicable destination charges will be added to your invoice.
- Orders are shipped by United Parcel Service (UPS) unless otherwise requested. If another del service is required, please specify.
- For regular delivery service, your order will be charged 5% handling plus actual shipping cha
- We occasionally backorder items temporarily out of stock. If you do not accept backorders, please tell us on your purchase order or on this form.

Money-Back Guarantee
You'll have up to 90 days of risk-free evaluation of the products your ordered. If you're not completely satisfied with any product, we'll pick it up within the 90 days and refund the full purchase price! **No questions asked!**

For Phone Orders
Call 1-800-228-0752. Please have your credit and/or institutional purchase order informat ready. Monday-Friday 7am-7pm Central Time.
1-800-723-1318 TDD
FAX 1-800-232-1223

Send your order to:
Therapy Skill Builders
a division of The Psychological Corporation
555 Academic Court / San Antonio, Texas 78204-2498